Management of *Helicobacter pylori*–Related Diseases

Editors

AKIKO SHIOTANI
DAVID Y. GRAHAM

GASTROENTEROLOGY CLINICS OF NORTH AMERICA

www.gastro.theclinics.com

Consulting Editor
GARY W. FALK

September 2015 • Volume 44 • Number 3

ELSEVIER

1600 John F. Kennedy Boulevard • Suite 1800 • Philadelphia, Pennsylvania, 19103-2899
http://www.theclinics.com

GASTROENTEROLOGY CLINICS OF NORTH AMERICA Volume 44, Number 3
September 2015 ISSN 0889-8553, ISBN-13: 978-0-323-39565-6

Editor: Kerry Holland
Developmental Editor: Alison Swety

Gastroenterology Clinics of North America (ISSN 0889-8553) is published quarterly by Elsevier Inc., 360 Park Avenue South, New York, NY 10010-1710. Months of issue are March, June, September, and December. Business and Editorial Offices: 1600 John F. Kennedy Blvd., Suite 1800, Philadelphia, PA 19103-2899. Customer Service Office: 6277 Sea Harbor Drive, Orlando, FL 32887-4800. Periodicals postage paid at New York, NY and additional mailing offices. Subscription prices are $320.00 per year (US individuals), $160.00 per year (US students), $530.00 per year (US institutions), $350.00 per year (Canadian individuals), $651.00 per year (Canadian institutions), $445.00 per year (international individuals), $220.00 per year (international students), and $651.00 per year (international institutions). Foreign air speed delivery is included in all *Clinics* subscription prices. All prices are subject to change without notice. **POSTMASTER:** Send address changes to *Gastroenterology Clinics of North America*, Elsevier Health Sciences Division, Subscription Customer Service, 3251 Riverport Lane, Maryland Heights, MO 63043. **Telephone: 1-800-654-2452 (U.S. and Canada); 314-447-8871 (outside U.S. and Canada). Fax: 314-447-8029. E-mail: journalscustomerservice-usa@elsevier.com (for print support); journalsonlinesupport-usa@elsevier.com (for online support).**

Reprints. For copies of 100 or more, of articles in this publication, please contact the Commercial Reprints Department, Elsevier Inc., 360 Part Avenue South, New York, New York 10010-1710. Tel. 212-633-3874, Fax: 212-633-3820, E-mail: reprints@elsevier.com.

Gastroenterology Clinics of North America is also published in Italian by Il Pensiero Scientifico Editore, Rome, Italy; and in Portuguese by Interlivros Edicoes Ltda., Rua Commandante Coelho 1085, 21250 Cordovil, Rio de Janeiro, Brazil.

Gastroenterology Clinics of North America is covered in *MEDLINE/PubMed (Index Medicus), Excerpta Medica, Current Contents/Clinical Medicine, Science Citation Index, ISI/BIOMED*, and *BIOSIS*.

Contributors

CONSULTING EDITOR

GARY W. FALK, MD, MS
Professor of Medicine, Division of Gastroenterology, Hospital of the University of Pennsylvania, University of Pennsylvania Perelman School of Medicine, Philadelphia, Pennsylvania

EDITORS

AKIKO SHIOTANI, MD, PhD
Professor, Department of Internal Medicine, Kawasaki Medical School, Kurashiki, Okayama, Japan

DAVID Y. GRAHAM, MD
Professor of Medicine, Molecular Virology, and Microbiology, Department of Medicine, Michael E. DeBakey Veterans Affairs Medical Center, Baylor College of Medicine, Houston, Texas

AUTHORS

TAIJI AKAMATSU, MD, PhD
Endoscopy Center, Suzaka Prefectural Hospital, Nagano Prefectural Hospital Organization, Suzaka, Nagano, Japan; Gastroenterology, Department of Internal Medicine, Shinshu University School of Medicine, Matsumoto, Nagano, Japan

MASAHIRO ASAKA, MD, PhD
Cancer Preventive Medicine, Hokkaido University Graduate School of Medicine, Sapporo, Japan

LUCIE BÉNÉJAT, MS
Engineer, Bacteriology Laboratory, INSERM U853, University of Bordeaux, Bordeaux, France

THOMAS G. BLANCHARD, PhD
Associate Professor, Department of Pediatrics, University of Maryland School of Medicine, Baltimore, Maryland

XAVIER CALVET, MD, PhD
Professor, Digestive Diseases Unit, Corporació Sanitària Universitària Parc Taulí, Sabadell, Spain; Centro de Investigación Biomédica en Red de Enfermedades Hepáticas y Digestivas (CIBERehd), Instituto de Salud Carlos III, Madrid, Spain; Departament de Medicina, Universitat Autònoma de Barcelona, Barcelona, Spain

TSUTOMU CHIBA, MD, PhD
Department of Gastroenterology and Hepatology, Graduate School of Medicine, Kyoto University, Kyoto, Japan

STEVEN J. CZINN, MD
Department of Pediatrics, University of Maryland School of Medicine, Baltimore, Maryland

FRANCESCO DI MARIO, MD
Department of Clinical and Experimental Medicine, University of Parma, School of Medicine, Parma, Italy

MARIA P. DORE, MD
Dipartimento di Medicina Clinica e Sperimentale, University of Sassari, Sassari, Italy; Department of Medicine, Michael E. DeBakey Veterans Affairs Medical Center, Baylor College of Medicine, Houston, Texas

ELISABETTA GONI, MD
Department of Gastroenterology, Hepatology and Infectious Diseases, Otto-von-Guericke University, Magdeburg, Germany

DAVID Y. GRAHAM, MD
Professor of Medicine, Molecular Virology, and Microbiology, Department of Medicine, Michael E. DeBakey Veterans Affairs Medical Center, Baylor College of Medicine, Houston, Texas

YUGO IWAYA, MD, PhD
Gastroenterology, Department of Internal Medicine, Shinshu University School of Medicine, Matsumoto, Nagano, Japan

ERNST J. KUIPERS, MD, PhD
Professor of Medicine, Department of Gastroenterology and Hepatology, Erasmus MC University Medical Center, Rotterdam, The Netherlands

SUN-YOUNG LEE, MD, PhD
Department of Internal Medicine, Konkuk University School of Medicine, Seoul, Korea

PHILIPPE LEHOURS, Pharm, PhD
Associate Professor, Bacteriology Laboratory, INSERM U853, University of Bordeaux, Bordeaux, France

KATSUHIRO MABE, MD, PhD
Cancer Preventive Medicine, Hokkaido University Graduate School of Medicine, Sapporo, Japan

HIROYUKI MARUSAWA, MD, PhD
Department of Gastroenterology and Hepatology, Graduate School of Medicine, Kyoto University, Kyoto, Japan

TAKAYUKI MATSUMOTO, MD, PhD
Division of Gastroenterology, Department of Internal Medicine, School of Medicine, Iwate Medical University, Morioka, Japan

RUMIKO MATSUSHIMA, MD
Department of Gastroenterology, Hokkaido University Graduate School of Medicine, Sapporo, Japan

FRANCIS MÉGRAUD, MD
Professor, Bacteriology Laboratory, INSERM U853, University of Bordeaux, Bordeaux, France

JAVIER MOLINA-INFANTE, MD
Department of Gastroenterology, Hospital San Pedro de Alcantara, Caceres, Spain

SHOTARO NAKAMURA, MD, PhD
Division of Gastroenterology, Department of Internal Medicine, School of Medicine, Iwate Medical University, Morioka, Japan

TAKUMA OKAMURA, MD, PhD
Gastroenterology, Department of Internal Medicine, Shinshu University School of Medicine, Matsumoto, Nagano, Japan

ESTHER NINA ONTSIRA NGOYI, MD
Assistant Professor, Bacteriology Laboratory, INSERM U853, University of Bordeaux, Bordeaux, France

MASSIMO RUGGE, MD, FACG
Surgical Pathology and Cytopathology Unit, Department of Medicine - DIMED, University of Padova, Padova, Italy

TAKAHIRO SHIMIZU, MD, PhD
Department of Gastroenterology and Hepatology, Graduate School of Medicine, Kyoto University, Kyoto, Japan

AKIKO SHIOTANI, MD, PhD
Professor, Department of Internal Medicine, Kawasaki Medical School, Kurashiki, Okayama, Japan

TOMOAKI SUGA, MD, PhD
Gastroenterology, Department of Internal Medicine, Shinshu University School of Medicine, Matsumoto, Nagano, Japan

MOMOKO TSUDA, MD
Department of Gastroenterology, Hokkaido University Graduate School of Medicine, Sapporo, Japan

NIMISH VAKIL, MD, FACP, FACG, AGAF, FASGE
Clinical Professor of Medicine, University of Wisconsin School of Medicine and Public Health, Madison, Wisconsin; Aurora Summit Medical Center, Summit, Wisconsin

NORIHIKO WATANABE, MD, PhD
Department of Gastroenterology and Hepatology, Graduate School of Medicine, Kyoto University, Kyoto, Japan

Contents

> Proton pump inhibitors (PPI) are a major cause of false-negative *Helicobacter pylori* test results. Detecting PPI use and stopping it 2 weeks before testing is the preferred approach to improve the reliability of *H pylori* diagnostic tests. Immunoblot and molecular methods may be useful for the detection of *H pylori* infection in difficult cases. When conventional tests are negative and eradication is strongly indicated, empirical *H pylori* treatment should be considered. In this article, an updated critical review of the usefulness of the various invasive and noninvasive tests in the context of extensive PPI use is provided.

> Cure rates greater than 90% to 95% should be expected with an antimicrobial therapy for *Helicobacter pylori* infection. Standard triple therapy does not guarantee these efficacy rates in most settings worldwide anymore. The choice of eradication regimen should be dictated by factors that can predict the outcome: (1) *H pylori* susceptibility; (2) patients' history of prior antibiotic therapy; and (3) local data, either resistance patterns or clinical success. Currently, the preferred first-line choices are 14-day bismuth quadruple and 14-day non-bismuth quadruple concomitant therapy. Bismuth quadruple (if not used previously), fluoroquinolone-, furazolidone- and rifabutin-containing regimens might be effective rescue treatments.

> Bismuth triple therapy was the first effective *Helicobacter pylori* eradication therapy. The addition of a proton pump inhibitor helped overcome metronidazole resistance. Its primary indication is penicillin allergy or when clarithromycin and metronidazole resistance are both common. Resistance to the primary first-line therapy have centered on complexity and difficulties with compliance. Understanding regional differences in effectiveness remains unexplained because of the lack of studies including susceptibility testing and adherence data. We discuss regimen variations including substitutions of doxycycline, amoxicillin, and twice a day therapy

Helicobacter pylori infection plays a crucial role in gastric carcinogenesis. *H pylori* exerts oncogenic effects on gastric mucosa through complex interaction between bacterial virulence factors and host inflammatory responses. On the other hand, gastric cancer develops via stepwise accumulation of genetic and epigenetic alterations in *H pylori*-infected gastric mucosa. Recent comprehensive analyses of gastric cancer genomes indicate a multistep process of genetic alterations as well as possible molecular mechanisms of gastric carcinogenesis. Both genetic processes of gastric cancer development and molecular oncogenic pathways related to *H pylori* infection are important to completely understand the pathogenesis of *H pylori*-related gastric cancer.

Helicobacter pylori eradication therapy for chronic gastritis achieved world-first coverage by the Japanese national health insurance scheme in 2013, making a dramatic decrease of gastric cancer–related deaths more realistic. Combining *H pylori* eradication therapy with endoscopic surveillance can prevent the development of gastric cancer. Even if it develops, most patients are likely to be diagnosed at an early stage, possibly resulting in fewer gastric cancer deaths. Success with the elimination of gastric cancer in Japan could lead other countries with a high incidence to consider a similar strategy, suggesting the potential for elimination of gastric cancer around the world.

Recent trends and current knowledge on the diagnosis and treatment strategy for gastric mucosa-associated lymphoid tissue (MALT) lymphoma are reviewed. *Helicobacter pylori* infection plays the causative role in the pathogenesis, and *H pylori* eradication is the first-line treatment of this disease, which leads to complete remission in 60% to 90% of cases. A Japanese multicenter study confirmed that the long-term outcome of gastric MALT lymphoma after *H pylori* eradication is excellent. Treatment strategies for patients not responding to *H pylori* eradication including "watch and wait" strategy, radiotherapy, chemotherapy, rituximab immunotherapy, and combination of these should be tailored in consideration of the disease extent in each patient.

Conflicting data have been published on the effect of long-term proton pump inhibitor therapy on the gastric mucosa in *Helicobacter pylori*–infected subjects. In this article, the available data are reviewed and a

The purpose of this study was to elucidate the prevalence and effect of *Helicobacter pylori* infection in Japanese teenagers. The study subjects were students ages 16 to 17 from one high school studied between 2007 and 2013. Students who tested positive on this screening examination underwent esophagogastroduodenoscopy and biopsy samples to determine their *H pylori* status using culture and histology. Cure of *H pylori* infections was determined by urea breath test. The low rate of prevalence of *H pylori* infection in present Japanese teenagers makes it possible and cost effective to perform examinations and carry out treatment of this infection in nationwide health screenings of high school students.

Helicobacter pylori infection contributes to a variety of gastric diseases. *H pylori*-associated gastric cancer is diagnosed in advanced stages, and a vaccine against *H pylori* is desirable in parts of the world where gastric cancer remains a common form of cancer. Some of the strategies of vaccine development used in animals have been tested in several phase 3 clinical trials; these trials have been largely unsuccessful, although *H pylori*-specific immune responses have been induced. New insights into promoting immunity and overcoming the immunosuppressive nature of *H pylori* infection are required to improve the efficacy of an *H pylori* vaccine.

GASTROENTEROLOGY
CLINICS OF NORTH AMERICA

RELATED INTEREST

Infectious Disease Clinics of North America
March 2015 (Vol. 29, Issue 1)
Clostridium difficile Infection
Mark H. Wilcox, *Editor*

THE CLINICS ARE AVAILABLE ONLINE!
Access your subscription at:
www.theclinics.com

Foreword
Helicobacter pylori

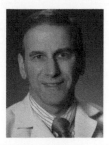

Gary W. Falk, MD, MS
Consulting Editor

Helicobacter pylori infection is no longer given as much attention as it was in its early days with the pioneering work of Warren and Marshall. However, *H pylori* remains a major worldwide problem as a cause of peptic ulcer disease and gastric neoplasia. Furthermore, there remains considerable confusion regarding modern approaches to diagnosis and treatment of this infection. Given current antibiotic resistance patterns of *H pylori*, these issues have considerable importance today. In this issue of *Gastroenterology Clinics of North America*, Drs Shiotani and Graham have addressed these and other pertinent matters of *H pylori* infection in a timely and comprehensive update for clinicians around the world, which should get everybody on the "same page" in the modern era of *H pylori*.

Gary W. Falk, MD, MS
Division of Gastroenterology
University of Pennsylvania Perelman School of Medicine
PCAM South Pavilion, 7th Floor
3400 Civic Center Boulevard
Philadelphia, PA 19104-4311, USA

E-mail address:
gary.falk@uphs.upenn.edu

Gastroenterol Clin N Am 44 (2015) xiii
http://dx.doi.org/10.1016/j.gtc.2015.07.012
0889-8553/15/$ – see front matter © 2015 Published by Elsevier Inc.

gastro.theclinics.com

Preface

Helicobacter pylori: New Thoughts and Practices

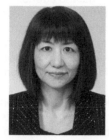 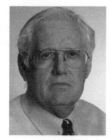

Akiko Shiotani, MD, PhD   David Y. Graham, MD
Editors

Research and thinking about *Helicobacter pylori* have recently experienced a paradigm shift. The Kyoto Consensus Conference on *H pylori* concluded that (a) *H pylori* gastritis was defined as an infectious disease even when patients have no symptoms and irrespective of complications such as peptic ulcers and gastric cancer, and (b) *H pylori*–infected individuals should be offered eradication therapy, unless there are competing considerations. *H pylori* is now recognized as the cause of the vast majority of gastric cancers, one of the major causes of cancer deaths worldwide. Recently, the World Health Organization published an IARC monograph entitled "*H pylori* eradication as a strategy for preventing gastric cancer." Japan approved global *H pylori* therapy along with a program of surveillance for those at high risk of gastric cancer, and pilot studies of mass *H pylori* eradication have been started in China, Taiwan, and Europe. The second aspect of the paradigm shift relates to *H pylori* eradication therapy. Until recently, identification of a new therapy, or study of the usefulness of a therapy in a new region, was largely done using a trial-and-error approach. It became clear that effective *H pylori* therapy, like that of other bacterial infectious diseases, must be susceptibility-based. The reasons therapy fails include the presence of resistant strains, poor choice of doses and/or duration of therapy, and poor patient adherence. There are a now a number of regimens that will reliably achieve 95% or greater cure rates with susceptible strains. As a general rule, they all contain a double dose of proton pump inhibitors (eg, 40 mg of omeprazole or an equivalent twice a day) and are for 14 days. In most regions, clarithromycin and fluoroquinolone resistance has increased sufficiently that they should no longer be used in empiric triple therapies.

This issue has several general themes. One theme is the modern approaches to the diagnosis and treatment of *H pylori* infections, which also includes an article on the current and future role of probiotics in therapy and in reducing side effects of current therapies. It remains a paradox that almost every hospital in the world offers culture and susceptibility testing for common infections and yet few extend this service to the

Gastroenterol Clin N Am 44 (2015) xv–xvi
http://dx.doi.org/10.1016/j.gtc.2015.07.001
0889-8553/15/$ – see front matter © 2015 Published by Elsevier Inc.

culture of *H pylori*. The recognition of the importance of susceptibility data in choosing effective therapy prompted an article on the molecular approaches to identification of antimicrobial resistance. The article on *H pylori* diagnosis focuses on the problems the widespread use of proton pump inhibitors causes in the interpretation of currently available tests. There is also an article regarding when it is appropriate to follow up therapy with endoscopy.

There are four articles on *H pylori* in malignancy, three regarding gastric adenocarcinomas, and one on MALT lymphoma. These include an update on the role of *H pylori* in the molecular pathogenesis of gastric cancer, stratification of patients with *H pylori* in relation to risk of gastric cancer, and a discussion of the ground-breaking current Japanese approach to *H pylori* eradication and the elimination of gastric cancer. Finally, there is an up-to-date discussion of treatment strategies for the management of MALT lymphoma.

The final grouping consists of new information about *H pylori* in children based on recent experiences in Japan, the rationale for a test-and-treat strategy in patients with GERD, and an update on vaccination to prevent and potentially treat *H pylori*. Recent success in China with a vaccine strategy shows that vaccination is an option and potentially opens the way to eradication of *H pylori* in developing countries, where the prevalence of *H pylori* is high.

Akiko Shiotani, MD, PhD
Department of Internal Medicine
Kawasaki Medical School
577 Matsushima Kurashiki City
Okayama Prefecture 701-0192, Japan

David Y. Graham, MD
Department of Medicine
Michael E. DeBakey VAMC
Baylor College of Medicine
2002 Holcombe Boulevard
Room 3A-318B (111D)
Houston, TX 77030, USA

E-mail addresses:
shiotani@med.kawasaki-m.ac.jp (A. Shiotani)
dgraham@bcm.edu (D.Y. Graham)

Diagnosis of *Helicobacter pylori* Infection in the Proton Pump Inhibitor Era

Xavier Calvet, MD, PhD[a,b,c,*]

KEYWORDS

- *Helicobacter pylori* • Proton pump inhibitors • Diagnosis • Treatment

KEY POINTS

- Proton pump inhibitors (PPI) are a major cause of false-negative *Helicobacter pylori* test results.
- Detecting PPI use and stopping it 2 weeks before testing is the preferred approach to improve the reliability of *H pylori* diagnostic tests in this setting.
- Immunoblot and molecular methods may be useful for the detection of *H pylori* infection in difficult cases.
- When conventional tests are negative and eradication is strongly indicated, empirical *H pylori* treatment should be considered.

INTRODUCTION

Helicobacter pylori is the major cause of peptic ulcer and gastric cancer. It is estimated that more than 50% of the world population is affected by this chronic gastric infection.[1] Diagnostic methods for the infection have been classically divided into invasive (those that require endoscopy) and noninvasive (those that not). The invasive methods available in clinical practice are histology, rapid urease test (RUT), and culture. In addition, molecular methods (in particular, biopsy polymerase chain reaction [PCR]) have been gaining popularity, although their use is still mainly restricted to research. Practical noninvasive methods include urea breath test (UBT), stool test, and serology.[2]

a Digestive Diseases Unit, Corporació Sanitària Universitària Parc Taulí, Parc Taulí, 1, Sabadell 08208, Spain; b Centro de Investigación Biomédica en Red de Enfermedades Hepáticas y Digestivas (CIBERehd), Instituto de Salud Carlos III, Madrid, Spain; c Departament de Medicina, Universitat Autònoma de Barcelona, Parc Taulí, 1, Sabadell 08208, Spain
* Digestive Diseases Unit, Corporació Sanitària Universitària Parc Taulí, Sabadell 08208, Spain.
E-mail address: xcalvet@tauli.cat

Gastroenterol Clin N Am 44 (2015) 507–518
http://dx.doi.org/10.1016/j.gtc.2015.05.001
0889-8553/15/$ – see front matter © 2015 Elsevier Inc. All rights reserved.

In the last decade, we have become increasingly aware of the strengths and limitations of diagnostic techniques for *H pylori* infection. In particular, (1) molecular methods have suggested that an undetermined percentage have low-density infection, that is not detected by the traditional tests; (2) the current widespread use of proton pump inhibitors (PPI) or antibiotics may markedly reduce the sensitivity of diagnostic techniques, and (3) diffuse mucosal damage associated with mucosal-associated lymphoid tissue (MALT) lymphoma or extensive intestinal metaplasia may produce false-negative results in diagnostic tests (**Table 1**). These drawbacks have led to a search for improved techniques and have highlighted the need for changes in the diagnostic approach to particular situations (**Table 2**).

In this article, an updated critical review of the usefulness of the various invasive and noninvasive tests in the context of extensive PPI use is provided.

INVASIVE TESTS
Histology

Histology has been the mainstay of the invasive diagnosis of *H pylori* infection. Its global reliability remains high in recent studies, with sensitivity and specificity rates higher than 95%.[3,4] However, although histology remains one of the most accurate diagnostic tests, its performance in clinical practice may be lower because of generalized use of PPI, inadequate biopsy sampling, and inadequate staining.

The active use of PPI or antibiotics is known to cause false-negative results in all invasive tests. The rate of false-negative results is reported to be at least 30%. Current guidelines recommend stopping PPI at least 2 weeks before testing for *H pylori* infection[2] and antibiotics at least 4 weeks beforehand. However, a recent study in Canada[5] showed that 47% of the patients who were tested by histology were actively receiving a PPI.

Regarding sampling, the recommended standards for histology are those of the updated Sydney classification system, which requires at least 1 biopsy from 5 different sites: (1) the lesser curvature of the corpus about 4 cm proximal to the angulus; (2) and (3) the lesser and greater curvature of the antrum, both within 2 to 3 cm of the pylorus; (4) the middle portion of the greater curvature of the corpus, approximately 8 cm from the cardia; and (5) the incisura angularis.[6] However, this approach is not widely

Table 1		
Factors that may reduce *H pylori* reliability		
Factor	**Potential Mechanisms**	**Effect**
Extensive atrophy	Low acid secretion, diffuse mucosal damage, overgrow of urease-positive bacteria	Decreased sensitivity Decreased specificity?
Extensive intestinal metaplasia	Low acid secretion, overgrow of urease-positive bacteria	Decreased sensitivity Decreased specificity?
MALT lymphoma	Diffuse mucosal damage	Decreased sensitivity
Use of antibiotics	Direct antibacterial effect, low density of infection	Decreased sensitivity
Use of PPI	Decreased acid secretion, low density of infection, direct antibacterial effect?	Decreased sensitivity
Use of histamine 2 receptor antagonists	Decreased acid secretion, low density of infection	Decreased sensitivity

Table 2
Approaches to potentially improve the reliability of *H pylori* diagnostic tests

Measure	Test Involved	Mechanism
Avoid antibiotics	Histology, culture, UBT, RUT, SAT	Increase gastric *H pylori* density
Avoid acid secretion, especially PPI	Histology, culture, UBT, RUT, SAT	Increase gastric *H pylori* density
Locally validate the test	SAT, serology, Immunoblot	Accurate test selection
Antrum and gastric corpus sampling	Histology, culture, RUT	May detect residual, low-density *H pylori* infection in gastric corpus glands
Use of ancillary stains/ immunohistochemistry	Histology	May detect residual, low-density *H pylori* infection in gastric corpus glands
Use of citric acid pretest meal	UBT	Increase urease activity, inhibits non–*H pylori* urease, decreases gastric overgrow

Abbreviation: SAT, stool antigen test.

followed in clinical practice, and fewer than 5% of gastric biopsies in the United States comply with these standards.[7] Additional data from the Canadian study also show that 60% of the biopsies had samples from only 1 gastric site, mainly from the antrum.[5]

Gastric antrum biopsies seem reliable enough for most patients.[8] The sensitivity of histology decreases in patients with extensive inflammation or atrophy, and the antrum-only approach is not recommended in areas in which atrophic changes are common. In this regard, sampling of the corpus greater curvature is recommended, because it increases the likelihood of a positive biopsy in patients with atrophy.[9,10]

Similarly, in their retrospective study including a large series of biopsies, Lash and Genta[7] reported that the use of at least 2 antral and 2 corpus biopsies increased the diagnostic yield of histology for *H pylori* infection. However, the increase in the number of positive biopsies was moderate, from 10% to 15%. No cost analyses have been performed to ascertain whether this modest increase in sensitivity justifies routine performance and analysis of 2 or 3 sets of biopsies, although placing several specimens on 1 slide may decrease the pathology costs.

Obtaining adequate sampling and corpus biopsies is especially important in patients receiving PPI therapy. Histologic changes induced by PPI in individuals infected by *H pylori* were first described by Graham and colleagues.[11,12] Although the changes vary,[13] patients with *Helicobacter* infection using PPI tend to have an almost normal antrum with minimal chronic inflammation, no neutrophils, and no detectable bacteria; in contrast, the corpus may show chronic active gastritis. The few remaining bacteria may occasionally be found in deeper portions of the oxyntic glands. Therefore, because infection seems to remain in the corpus, antrum-only sampling may further reduce the sensitivity of histology in PPI users.

With regard to the staining of biopsies, Giemsa is generally preferred to hematoxylin-eosin. Giemsa stain is routinely performed at most centers and is cheap and highly reliable for the diagnosis of *H pylori* infection. By contrast, it has been suggested that hematoxylin-eosin alone has a lower sensitivity for diagnosing *H pylori* infection.[14–17] However, pathologists consider the 2 stains to be equivalent.[18]

Other staining techniques including inmunohistochemical detection of the bacteria or silver staining are routinely not indicated, because they do not clearly increase the diagnostic accuracy. However, ancillary tests may be useful when the result is uncertain, particularly in PPI users, in whom other bacteria are likely to be present.[18–20] It has been suggested that immunohistochemical staining may help to identify low-density infection in oxyntic glands in patients receiving PPI, especially when minimal inflammation is present.[20] However, it remains unclear whether H pylori–negative active gastritis represents a new entity or is caused by low-density infection not detected by histology or other conventional diagnostic methods.[21–23]

PPI use reduces the sensitivity of histology for diagnosing H pylori infection. Whether corpus sampling, or the use of immunohistochemical staining, or a combination of the 2 may reduce the false-negative results associated with PPI use is an issue that needs further investigation.

Culture

The feasibility and usefulness of H pylori culture has been a matter of debate among microbiologists and clinicians since the bacterium was first isolated. Culture allows the determination of antibiotic resistances to design an optimal therapy. However, it is time and resource consuming and is routinely performed only at a few centers. Specificity of culture is high, approaching 100%, but sensitivity is lower; although some reference centers claim sensitivity rates more than 90%,[24] in most settings they range between 40% and 80%.

The Maastricht consensus[2] states that culture is important before first-line therapy, should be considered before second-line therapy (statement 5), and is mandatory (whenever possible) before third-line therapy (statement 18). However, the scientific evidence supporting the Maastricht recommendations is weak. Two recent meta-analyses[25,26] showed that treatment guided by antibiotic susceptibility was superior to empirical treatment of first-line therapy. However, a major limitation of all the studies included was that all patients were randomized after endoscopy had been performed. Because no study has randomized patients to empirical treatment versus endoscopy and culture plus culture-guided treatment, the effectiveness of susceptibility-guided treatment in clinical practice has never been evaluated. In second-line therapy there was also a nonsignificant trend favoring culture-guided treatment.[25]

No comparative studies of empirical versus susceptibility-guided treatment after 2 treatment failures have been performed. Nor do the results of the observational studies reporting culture-guided third-line therapies show especially good results.[25] Overall, then, there is little evidence in favor of routine culture and susceptibility-guided treatment in H pylori treatment.

Although it is thought that PPI use reduces culture efficacy by decreasing bacterial density, few data have been reported. In a recent study, Siavoshi and colleagues[27] evaluated the results of H pylori tests in 530 dyspeptic patients and reported that the rate of positive culture was 30% in patients receiving PPI versus 56% in those not receiving the drugs. It is unclear whether sampling an additional corpus biopsy for culture might increase culture sensitivity, as it has been shown to increase histology sensitivity.[10]

Rapid urease test

RUT is an indirect test based on the activity of the H pylori urease enzyme, which degrades urea to form ammonia. This situation increases the pH level, which can be detected by a pH indicator.[28] It requires a sample of gastric mucosa, which is introduced in the mixture of urea and the pH indicator. There are many different commercial RUT kits, including gel-based tests (CLOtest, Kimberly-Clark Ballard Medical Products, Roswell, GA, HpFast, GI supply, Camp Hill, Pennsylvania) paper-based tests (PyloriTek, Serim Laboratories, Elkhart, IN, ProntoDry HpOne, Medical

Instruments Corporation, Solothurn, Switzerland), and liquid-based tests (CPtest, Yamanouchi, Milan, Italy, EndoscHp, Cambridge Life Sciences, UK).

Commercial RUTs have a sensitivity of 80% to 95% and specificity higher than 95% to 100%.[4,29,30] These figures are slightly lower than those for histology but are still acceptable for clinical practice.[4] The number of bacteria present in the biopsy is the main cause of the reduction in sensitivity. It is estimated that densities lower than 10^4 to 10^5 organisms may result in false-negative tests.[28] This situation may often occur in bleeding patients or after treatment. In these situations, RUT is not indicated as a sole test. Extensive atrophy or intestinal metaplasia may also be associated with low density and false-negative RUT results. In addition, any treatment that reduces bacterial density, such as the use of antibiotics, bismuth compounds, or PPI, may result in false-negative tests. Reviews recommend obtaining 2 samples (1 from the antrum and 1 from normal-appearing corpus) and avoiding areas of ulceration and obvious intestinal metaplasia to obtain optimal results. Combining the 2 samples in the same tests seems to accelerate positive results.[31] Whether or not the inclusion of a corpus sample is useful for increasing the yield of RUT remains to be determined. False-positive tests are less frequent but may occur if the sample is kept beyond 24 hours.

Overall, the test is cheap and rapid and provides adequate screening. Positive results should prompt *H pylori* treatment. By contrast, after negative RUT, a second confirmatory test may be considered depending on the importance of treating the infection, the degree of suspicion, and the presence of factors that may cause false-negative results as described earlier.

Molecular tests

Both in situ hybridization and PCR are sensitive tests and can be used to detect *H pylori* in biopsies. Furthermore, these tests can determine antibiotic resistances (see the article of Francis Megraud in this issue).

There is growing evidence that, even when performed in optimal conditions, the sensitivity of conventional tests for detecting *H pylori* infection may be suboptimal. If this situation occurs, it is most probably caused by low-density occult infection, and many studies have shown that molecular methods can detect at least a part of these occult or low-density cases. Bik and colleagues[32] characterized the gastric microbiota of *H pylori*–positive and *H pylori*–negative individuals by using broad-range PCR and 16S ribosomal DNA sequence analysis in 23 healthy volunteers. *H pylori* infection was detected in 12 individuals by conventional tests and in 19 of the 23 by molecular tests. In another important article, Raderer and colleagues[33] reported 6 patients with gastric MALT lymphoma with negative results for all *H pylori* conventional tests who presented with complete resolution of the disease after *H pylori* treatment, thus suggesting that the patients had an undetectable active infection. Weiss and colleagues[34] evaluated 60 gastric biopsies from patients with dyspepsia, performing immunohistochemistry, RUT, and a multiplex PCR. PCR consistently identified *H pylori* in more patients, including those positive by the other methods. The same group claimed that multiplex PCR was able to detect the infection in patients on PPI therapy even when RUT was negative.[35]

However, even molecular tests may not be sensitive enough to detect all cases of low-density infection. Guell and colleagues[36] reported that 79% of the patients with peptic ulcer bleeding who tested negative for *H pylori* during the bleeding episode had active infection, which was detected when the tests were repeated a few weeks after the acute bleeding episode. Real-time PCR performed in the biopsy obtained during the bleeding episode detected 64% of all the infected patients.[37]

Some investigators have suggested that the molecular test should be used as a gold standard for diagnosis of infection, because of its superior sensitivity.[38] However, PCR tests are prone to false-positive results. There are many examples of positive PCR tests (eg, from saliva or oral samples) in patients with no evidence of *H pylori* using any other test, suggesting that cross-reacting DNA from as yet uncultured organisms may be a significant obstacle to the use of PCR-based tests as a gold standard.[39] Therefore, a single PCR should not be used as a gold standard. Reliable demonstration of *H pylori* infection by PCR may require the positivity of more than 1 gene.[40]

PCR has not been adopted as a routine test because of its many drawbacks. It is technically demanding and expensive compared with conventional tests; it requires special laboratory conditions, and it is prone to false-positive results as a result of contamination. In addition, these tests may be inappropriate for determining cure after treatment (it has been suggested that residual death organisms of DNA fragments might cause false-positive results) and have not been evaluated in this setting.

PCR in feces may be an attractive alternative for noninvasive evaluation of not only the presence of infection but also the bacterial resistances to clarithromycin. However, some studies have found its sensitivity to be low, mainly because of the presence of PCR inhibitors.[41]

Noninvasive Tests

Urea breath test

H pylori urease splits urea into ammonia and carbon dioxide. In the UBT, patients ingest urea labeled with either ^{13}C or ^{14}C. Although the ^{14}C test is safe, cheap, and reliable, nonradioactive ^{13}C is generally preferred.

The test mechanism involves urease, an enzyme that is not present in mammals. By contrast, *H pylori* has a strong urease activity. An individual infected with *H pylori* presents urease activity in the stomach. Hydrolysis of urea occurs, causing the production of labeled CO_2, which diffuses into the blood vessels and appears in the subject's breath within a few minutes. UBT is probably the most reliable noninvasive test, with reported sensitivity and specificity of more than 95%.[2,42]

However, the reliability of UBT is affected by many factors. As in the case of most of the tests detecting active infection, its sensitivity is markedly decreased by recent antibiotic use. In addition, PPI use reduces the sensitivity of the test by 30%[43] and histamine 2 receptor antagonist use by approximately 10%[44] unless the test used citric acid. Technical characteristics may also affect the reliability of the test; it has been shown that the use of a test meal including citric acid enhances the activity of *H pylori* urease.[44–50] This enhancing of urease activity may help to increase sensitivity in patients with low-density infection caused by PPI use.

In addition, false-positive results have been attributed to the activity of urease-producing bacteria other than *Helicobacter*, such as *Proteus mirabilis* or *Staphylococcus aureus*, which may colonize gastric lumen in situations of achlorhydria.[51] In this case, acidification of the media by citric acid might help to bring down the number of false-positive results by reducing the density of the contaminating bacteria.

However, there are many commercial tests that skip the use of the citric acid pretreatment. Many recent reports have reported an unacceptably high rate of false-positive results with these tests.[4,52] This finding is especially relevant in terms of posttreatment evaluation, in which a positive UBT must be followed by a second expensive and burdensome antibiotic treatment and then another test to confirm the cure of the infection.

Stool antigen tests

The stool test detects bacterial antigens of *H pylori* that are present in stool in infected patients. It has been shown that these antigens disappear when *H pylori* infection is cured. Because each commercial stool antigen test (SAT) detects different antigens, the results change from one test to another. Furthermore, because of the marked genetic variability of *H pylori*, the accuracy of the same test may vary according to population. For this reason, the Maastricht consensus recommends local validation before using a given SAT.[2] SAT may use polyclonal or monoclonal antibodies. Polyclonal antibodies are obtained by immunizing laboratory animals. This method produces extremely variable sets of antibodies, which differ from batch to batch. This finding may explain why the excellent results obtained in the first SAT validation studies[53] have not been reproduced in later research. Meta-analyses have shown that SAT using polyclonal antibodies are consistently inferior to those using monoclonal antibodies.[54] Regarding the test method, in the office, immunochromatographic tests have generally produced slightly worse results than laboratory enzyme-linked immunosorbent assay (ELISA) tests.[4,55–57]

A major problem with the use of SAT is that many commercial tests are available but have never been validated; in addition, in some areas, sensitivity and specificity of even the best monoclonal ELISA SAT barely reaches 90%.[56,57] Many recent tests did not even achieve these minimal rates for sensitivity or specificity.[58–61]

Although there is no consensus on the minimal values that a diagnostic test should achieve, a sensitivity of less than 90% seems inadequate for the diagnosis of the infection, and a specificity less than 90% may generate many false-positive results, thus rendering the test inadequate for posttreatment evaluation.

PPI use may also cause false-negative results with SAT.[2] In this case, little is known about possible corrective measures. SAT may be preferable in patients who have very recently initiated PPI therapy; Gisbert and colleagues[62] reported a high sensitivity of monoclonal ELISA tests in SAT performed immediately after admission for upper gastrointestinal bleeding.

SEROLOGY

Serology tests detect circulating antibodies against *H pylori* in patients' serum. Antibodies can be detected by a variety of methodologies, including immunohistochemical or latex agglutination on-site tests, laboratory ELISA, and Western blot. In this last test, the specific antigens are separated by gel electrophoresis and transferred to a filter-paper strip. This strip is reacted with the patient's serum. Immunoblot allows detection of all the immunoglobulin isotypes and can evaluate many different specific antigens in a single assay.

Serology is the most frequently used diagnostic test, because of its availability, low cost, and accuracy. Its sensitivity and specificity vary markedly depending on the method of diagnosis, the antibody detected by the test, and the setting. On-site immunohistochemical or latex agglutination tests achieve very low accuracy and should not be used.[63] Although the ELISA test is more accurate than on-site tests, its accuracy depends on the antigen used for antibody detection.[63] An additional limitation of serology is that levels of circulating antibodies remain high for years even after treatment of the infection, and so, they cannot be used to determine cure after treatment. For all these reasons, the Maastricht consensus[2] does not recommend the use of serology for routine diagnosis.

Western blot analysis is the most sensitive serologic technique. Although (as all serologic tests) they cannot be used to evaluate the efficacy of *H pylori* treatment, Western blot tests are generally able to detect the infection with sensitivity and specificity rates higher than 95% in untreated patients. In addition, Western blot determines antibodies against other *H pylori* proteins such as CagA (cytotoxin-associated gene A).

Although it has mostly been used in research, it offers high sensitivity and may be useful for detecting infection in difficult cases.[64,65]

Serology and Western blot are the only tests that are not affected at all by PPI use. In the absence of previous eradication therapy, a positive serologic test may suggest active infection and indicate the need for prompt therapy, especially when it is not possible or advisable to withdraw the PPI and the direct tests are negative.

SUMMARY: DIAGNOSIS OF *HELICOBACTER PYLORI* INFECTION IN THE PROTON PUMP INHIBITORS ERA

Choice of the best available test and its appropriate performance are especially important in the current situation of widespread use of PPI. PPI are probably the most important (although not the only) reason for a decreased sensitivity and false-negative *H pylori* test results (**Fig. 1**). Detecting PPI use and stopping it 2 weeks before testing is the preferred approach to improve the reliability of diagnostic tests in this setting.

When stopping PPI is not possible, measures than might improve test reliability include (1) adequate sampling (including a corpus biopsy) and staining (including inmunohistochemical techniques when necessary) for histology, (2) corpus sampling to increase RUT sensitivity, (3) the use of locally validated SAT, and (4) use of UBT protocols with citric acid pretreatment. All these measures may help to improve the accuracy of *H pylori* diagnosis in patients receiving ongoing PPI therapy. However, they all require further evaluation to clearly establish their usefulness in patients treated with a PPI.

We have evidence that the sensitivity of current tests for detecting *H pylori* may be suboptimal in many different settings. In patients in whom eradication might be particularly beneficial (eg, in MALT lymphoma or after peptic ulcer bleeding), the use of extensive workup including serology or Immunoblot or molecular methods is favored when conventional tests do not show infection. These methods may increase

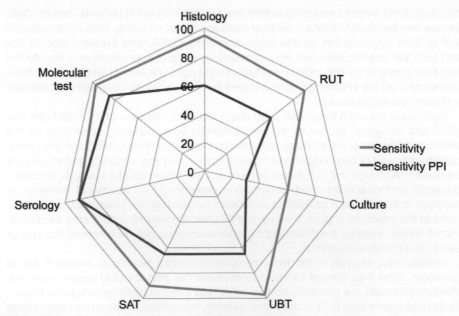

Fig. 1. Effect of PPI use in the sensitivity of the different *H pylori* tests.

detection of the infection. Furthermore, in cases in which eradication is strongly indicated, empirical *H pylori* treatment should be considered when all tests are negative or cannot be performed.

Future developments in *H pylori* diagnosis should include (1) the consensus definition of the minimum criteria to consider a given test as acceptable in clinical practice, (2) the design of easy, cheap, and commercially available PCR kits, (3) the careful local validation of serology or SAT before introducing a given test in clinical practice, and (4) the evaluation of the usefulness of corpus biopsy sampling in improving the sensitivity of histology, culture, and RUT results.

ACKNOWLEDGMENTS

I thank Michael Maudsley for his help with the English, and Prof, David Y. Graham, Sergio Lario, Albert Villoria, and Jordi Sanchez for their useful comments on the article.

REFERENCES

1. McColl KE. Clinical practice. *Helicobacter pylori* infection. N Engl J Med 2010; 362:1597–604.
2. Malfertheiner P, Megraud F, O'Morain CA, et al. Management of *Helicobacter pylori* infection–the Maastricht IV/Florence consensus report. Gut 2012;61: 646–64.
3. Lee HC, Huang TC, Lin CL, et al. Performance of routine *Helicobacter pylori* invasive tests in patients with dyspepsia. Gastroenterol Res Pract 2013;2013:184806.
4. Calvet X, Sánchez-Delgado J, Montserrat A, et al. Accuracy of diagnostic tests for *Helicobacter pylori*: a reappraisal. Clin Infect Dis 2009;48:1385–91.
5. El-Zimaity H, Serra S, Szentgyorgyi E, et al. Gastric biopsies: the gap between evidence-based medicine and daily practice In the management of gastric *Helicobacter pylori* infection. Can J Gastroenterol 2013;27:e25–30.
6. Dixon MF, Genta RM, Yardley JH, et al. Classification and grading of gastritis. The updated Sydney system. International workshop on the histopathology of gastritis, Houston 1994. Am J Surg Pathol 1996;20:1161–81.
7. Lash JG, Genta RM. Adherence to the Sydney system guidelines increases the detection of *Helicobacter* gastritis and intestinal metaplasia in 400738 sets of gastric biopsies. Aliment Pharmacol Ther 2013;38:424–31.
8. Genta RM, Graham DY. Comparison of biopsy sites for the histopathologic diagnosis of *Helicobacter pylori*: a topographic study of *H. pylori* density and distribution. Gastrointest Endosc 1994;40:342–5.
9. Lan HC, Chen TS, Li AF, et al. Additional corpus biopsy enhances the detection of *Helicobacter pylori* infection in a background of gastritis with atrophy. BMC Gastroenterol 2012;12:182.
10. Lee JH, Park YS, Choi KS, et al. Optimal biopsy site for *Helicobacter pylori* detection during endoscopic mucosectomy in patients with extensive gastric atrophy. Helicobacter 2012;17:405–10.
11. Graham DY, Genta R, Evans DG, et al. *Helicobacter pylori* does not migrate from the antrum to the corpus in response to omeprazole. Am J Gastroenterol 1996;91: 2120–4.
12. Graham DY, Genta RM. Long-term proton pump inhibitor use and gastrointestinal cancer. Curr Gastroenterol Rep 2008;10:543–7.
13. Kumar KR, Iqbal R, Coss E, et al. *Helicobacter* gastritis induces changes in the oxyntic mucosa indistinguishable from the effects of proton pump inhibitors. Hum Pathol 2013;44:2706–10.

14. Laine L, Lewin DN, Naritoku W, et al. Prospective comparison of the H&E, Giemsa and Genta stains for the diagnosis of *Helicobacter pylori*. Gastrointest Endosc 1997;45:463–7.
15. Rotimi O, Cairns A, Gray S, et al. Histological identification of *Helicobacter pylori*: comparison of staining methods. J Clin Pathol 2000;53:756–9.
16. Garza-González E, Perez-Perez GI, Maldonado-Garza HJ, et al. A review of *Helicobacter pylori* diagnosis, treatment, and methods to detect eradication. World J Gastroenterol 2014;20:1438–49.
17. Fallone CA, Loo VG, Lough J, et al. Hematoxylin and eosin staining of gastric tissue for the detection of *Helicobacter pylori*. Helicobacter 1997;1:32–5.
18. Batts KP, Ketover S, Kakar S, et al. Appropriate use of special stains for identifying *Helicobacter pylori*: recommendations from the Rodger C. Haggitt Gastrointestinal Pathology Society. Am J Surg Pathol 2013;37:e12–22.
19. Chitkara Y. Upfront special staining for *Helicobacter pylori* in gastric biopsy specimens is not indicated. Am J Clin Pathol 2015;143:84–8.
20. Panarelli NC, Ross DS, Bernheim OE, et al. Utility of ancillary stains for *Helicobacter pylori* in near-normal gastric biopsies. Hum Pathol 2015;46(3): 397–403.
21. Genta RM, Lash RH. *Helicobacter pylori*-negative gastritis: seek, yet ye shall not always find. Am J Surg Pathol 2010;34:e25–34.
22. Genta RM, Sonnenberg A. *Helicobacter*-negative gastritis: a distinct entity unrelated to *Helicobacter pylori* infection. Aliment Pharmacol Ther 2015;41: 218–26.
23. Kilincalp S, Ustun Y, Akinci H, et al. Letter: effect of proton pump inhibitor use on invasive detection of *Helicobacter pylori* gastritis. Aliment Pharmacol Ther 2015; 41:599.
24. Hirschl AM, Makristathis A. Methods to detect *Helicobacter pylori*: from culture to molecular biology. Helicobacter 2007;12(Suppl 2):6–11.
25. Góngora SL, Puig I, Calvet X, et al. Systematic review and meta-analysis: susceptibility-guided versus empirical antibiotic treatment for *Helicobacter pylori* infection. J Antimicrob Chemot 2015, in press.
26. Wenzhen Y, Yumin L, Quanlin G, et al. Is antimicrobial susceptibility testing necessary before first-line treatment for *Helicobacter pylori* infection? Meta-analysis of randomized controlled trials. Intern Med 2010;49:1103–9.
27. Siavoshi F, Saniee P, Khalili-Samani S, et al. Evaluation of methods for *H. pylori* detection in PPI consumption using culture, rapid urease test and smear examination. Ann Transl Med 2015;3:11.
28. Ricci C, Holton J, Vaira D. Diagnosis of *Helicobacter pylori*: invasive and non-invasive tests. Best Pract Res Clin Gastroenterol 2007;21:299–313.
29. Redéen S, Petersson F, Törnkrantz E, et al. Reliability of diagnostic tests for *Helicobacter pylori* infection. Gastroenterol Res Pract 2011;2011:940650.
30. Vaira D, Perna F. How useful is the rapid urease test for evaluating the success of *Helicobacter pylori* eradication therapy? Nat Clin Pract Gastroenterol Hepatol 2007;4:600–1.
31. Uotani T, Graham DY. Diagnosis of *Helicobacter pylori* using the rapid urease test. Ann Transl Med 2015;3:9.
32. Bik EM, Eckburg PB, Gill SR, et al. Molecular analysis of the bacterial microbiota in the human stomach. Proc Natl Acad Sci U S A 2006;103:732–7.
33. Raderer M, Streubel B, Wohrer S, et al. Successful antibiotic treatment of *Helicobacter pylori* negative gastric mucosa associated lymphoid tissue lymphomas. Gut 2006;55:616–8.

34. Weiss J, Tsang TK, Meng X, et al. Detection of *Helicobacter pylori* gastritis by PCR. Correlation with inflammation scores and immunohistochemical and CLO test findings. Am J Clin Pathol 2008;129:89–96.
35. Chen T, Meng X, Zhang H, et al. Comparing multiplex PCR and rapid urease test in the detection of *H. pylori* in patients on proton pump inhibitors. Gastroenterol Res Pract 2012;2012:898276.
36. Guell M, Artigau E, Esteve V, et al. Usefulness of a delayed test for the diagnosis of *Helicobacter pylori* infection in bleeding peptic ulcer. Aliment Pharmacol Ther 2006;23:53–9.
37. Ramirez-Lazaro MJ, Lario S, Casalots A, et al. Real-time PCR improves *Helicobacter pylori* detection in patients with peptic ulcer bleeding. PLoS One 2011; 6:e20009.
38. Patel SK, Pratap CB, Jain AK, et al. Diagnosis of *Helicobacter pylori*: what should be the gold standard? World J Gastroenterol 2014;20:12847–59.
39. Sugimoto M, Wu JY, Abudayyeh S, et al. Caution regarding PCR detection of *Helicobacter pylori* in clinical or environmental samples. J Clin Microbiol 2009; 47:738–42.
40. Ramírez-Lázaro MJ, Lario S, Calvet X, et al. Occult *H. pylori* infection partially explains "false positive" results of C13-urea breath test. United European Gastroenterol J 2015, in press.
41. Scaletsky IC, Aranda KR, Garcia GT, et al. Application of real-time PCR stool assay for *Helicobacter pylori* detection and clarithromycin susceptibility testing in Brazilian children. Helicobacter 2011;16:311–5.
42. Gisbert JP, Pajares JM. Review article: 13C-urea breath test in the diagnosis of *Helicobacter pylori* infection: a critical review. Aliment Pharmacol Ther 2004;20: 1001–17.
43. Laine L, Estrada R, Trujillo M, et al. Effect of proton-pump inhibitor therapy on diagnostic testing for *Helicobacter pylori*. Ann Intern Med 1998;129: 547–50.
44. Graham DY, Opekun AR, Jogi M, et al. False negative urea breath tests with H2-receptor antagonists: interactions between *Helicobacter pylori* density and pH. Helicobacter 2004;9:17–27.
45. Pantoflickova D, Scott DR, Sachs G, et al. 13C urea breath test (UBT) in the diagnosis of *Helicobacter pylori*: why does it work better with acid test meals? Gut 2003;52:933–7.
46. Agha A, Opekun AR, Abudayyeh S, et al. Effect of different organic acids (citric, malic and ascorbic) on intragastric urease activity. Aliment Pharmacol Ther 2005; 21:1145–8.
47. Graham DY, Opekun AR, Hammoud F, et al. Studies regarding the mechanism of false negative urea breath tests with proton pump inhibitors. Am J Gastroenterol 2003;98:1005–9.
48. Shiotani A, Saeed A, Yamaoka Y, et al. Citric acid-enhanced *Helicobacter pylori* urease activity in vivo is unrelated to gastric emptying. Aliment Pharmacol Ther 2001;15:1763–7.
49. Graham DY, Malaty HM, Cole RA, et al. Simplified 13C-urea breath test for detection of *Helicobacter pylori* infection. Am J Gastroenterol 2001;96:1741–5.
50. Graham DY, Runke D, Anderson SY, et al. Citric acid as the test meal for the 13C-urea breath test. Am J Gastroenterol 1999;94:1214–7.
51. Osaki T, Mabe K, Hanawa T, et al. Urease-positive bacteria in the stomach induce a false-positive reaction in a urea breath test for diagnosis of *Helicobacter pylori* infection. J Med Microbiol 2008;57:814–9.

52. Kwon YH, Kim N, Lee JY, et al. The diagnostic validity of citric acid-free, high dose ^{13}C-urea breath test after Helicobacter pylori eradication in Korea. Helicobacter 2015;20:159–68.
53. Vaira D, Malfertheiner P, Mégraud F, et al. Diagnosis of Helicobacter pylori infection with a new non-invasive antigen-based assay. HpSA European study group. Lancet 1999;354:30–3.
54. Gisbert JP, de la Morena F, Abraira V. Accuracy of monoclonal stool antigen test for the diagnosis of H. pylori infection: a systematic review and meta-analysis. Am J Gastroenterol 2006;101:1921–30.
55. Calvet X, Lehours P, Lario S, et al. Diagnosis of Helicobacter pylori infection. Helicobacter 2010;15(Suppl 1):7–13.
56. Calvet X, Lario S, Ramírez-Lázaro MJ, et al. Comparative accuracy of 3 monoclonal stool tests for diagnosis of Helicobacter pylori infection among patients with dyspepsia. Clin Infect Dis 2010;50:323–8.
57. Calvet X, Lario S, Ramírez-Lázaro MJ, et al. Accuracy of monoclonal stool tests for determining cure of Helicobacter pylori infection after treatment. Helicobacter 2010;15:201–5.
58. Korkmaz H, Findik D, Ugurluoglu C, et al. Reliability of stool antigen tests: investigation of the diagnostic value of a new immunochromatographic Helicobacter pylori approach in dyspeptic patients. Asian Pac J Cancer Prev 2015;16:657–60.
59. Lee YC, Tseng PH, Liou JM, et al. Performance of a one-step fecal sample-based test for diagnosis of Helicobacter pylori infection in primary care and mass screening settings. J Formos Med Assoc 2014;113:899–907.
60. Okuda M, Osaki T, Kikuchi S, et al. Evaluation of a stool antigen test using a mAb for native catalase for diagnosis of Helicobacter pylori infection in children and adults. J Med Microbiol 2014;63:1621–5.
61. Osman HA, Hasan H, Suppian R, et al. Evaluation of the Atlas Helicobacter pylori stool antigen test for diagnosis of infection in adult patients. Asian Pac J Cancer Prev 2014;15:5245–7.
62. Gisbert JP, Trapero M, Calvet X, et al. Evaluation of three different tests for the detection of stool antigens to diagnose Helicobacter pylori infection in patients with upper gastrointestinal bleeding. Aliment Pharmacol Ther 2004;19:923–9.
63. Burucoa C, Delchier JC, Courillon-Mallet A, et al. Comparative evaluation of 29 commercial Helicobacter pylori serological kits. Helicobacter 2013;18:169–79.
64. Veijola L, Oksanen A, Sipponen P, et al. Evaluation of a commercial immunoblot, Helicoblot 2.1, for diagnosis of Helicobacter pylori infection. Clin Vaccine Immunol 2008;15:1705–10.
65. González CA, Megraud F, Buissonniere A, et al. Helicobacter pylori infection assessed by ELISA and by immunoblot and noncardia gastric cancer risk in a prospective study: the Eurgast-EPIC project. Ann Oncol 2012;23:1320–4.

Practical Aspects in Choosing a *Helicobacter pylori* Therapy

Javier Molina-Infante, MD[a],*, Akiko Shiotani, MD, PhD[b]

KEYWORDS

- *Helicobacter pylori* • Therapy • Eradication • Triple • Quadruple • Concomitant
- Bismuth • Resistance

KEY POINTS

- Antibiotic resistance is the critical factor responsible for eradication treatment failure. Because of increasing clarithromycin resistance, first-line triple therapy for *Helicobacter pylori* (*H pylori*) infection is currently ineffective in most settings worldwide.
- Treatment results for infectious diseases are best (>90%–95%) when regimens are reliably used to treat patients with organisms susceptible to the antimicrobials chosen. Most eradication therapies, however, are prescribed empirically.
- The choice of therapy may depend on patient previous antibiotic treatment, local patterns of antibiotic resistance, and drug availability. Currently, the most effective first-line eradication regimens are 14-day bismuth and nonbismuth concomitant quadruple therapies.
- Fluoroquinolone-, furazolidone-, and rifabutin-containing regimens might be effective rescue treatments, as well as bismuth quadruple therapy if not used previously.
- Optimization of all eradication regimens (increased duration, adequate proton pump inhibitor, and antibiotic doses and dosing intervals) is key to maximize their efficacy.
- Besides antibiotic resistance, compliance is a major concern with increasing complex eradication therapies. Probiotics show promise as an adjuvant treatment to reduce side effects and improve adherence to therapy. Whether probiotics can also increase eradication rates should be further elucidated.
- On large variations in *H pylori* resistance patterns, the golden rule for choice of treatment is only to use what works locally (>90%–95% success) and to closely monitor its effectiveness over time.

Disclosure Statement: The authors have no conflict of interest to declare.
[a] Department of Gastroenterology, Hospital San Pedro de Alcantara, C/Pablo Naranjo s/n, Caceres 10003, Spain; [b] Department of Internal Medicine, Kawasaki Medical School, 577 Matsushima, Kurashiki, Okayama Prefecture 701-0114, Japan
* Corresponding author.
E-mail address: xavi_molina@hotmail.com

INTRODUCTION

Thirty years after the transcendental discovery of the originally termed *Campylobacter pyloridis* as a causative agent for gastritis and peptic ulceration in 1984,[1] *Helicobacter pylori (H pylori)* remains the most common bacterial infection in humans. It is estimated that approximately 50% of the world's population is infected; this infection is currently the main cause of gastritis, gastroduodenal ulcer disease, and gastric cancer. Eradication of *H pylori* infection has dramatically changed the natural history of peptic ulcer disease.[2] Furthermore, the World Health Organization classified *H pylori* as a definite carcinogen in 1994 for its established role in the pathogenesis of gastric cancer and gastric mucosa–associated lymphoid tissue lymphoma.[3] Emphasis has been lately made on the importance of primary and secondary gastric cancer prevention, starting with *H pylori* eradication.[4] In fact, Japan has recently embarked on population-wide *H pylori* eradication coupled with surveillance targeted to those with significant remaining risk.

Standard triple therapy, consisting of a proton pump inhibitor (PPI) plus amoxicillin and either clarithromycin or metronidazole, has been (and unfortunately still remains in many settings) the gold standard eradication therapy for *H pylori* infection over the last 2 decades. However, the efficacy of triple therapy at the present time is seriously challenged in many parts of the world, where eradication rates have declined to unacceptably low levels, largely related to the development of resistance to clarithromycin.[5] Moreover, *H pylori* resistance to metronidazole is prevalent as well in certain geographic areas (ie, South America, Turkey, Iran, China) and fluoroquinolone resistance is rapidly growing worldwide due to widespread use of levofloxacin for ear, nose and throat, bronchial and urinary tract infections. Failure of *H pylori* treatment, in addition, selects antibiotic-multiresistant strains, which will be even more difficult to treat. Complicating this scenario, rescue drugs may be unavailable (eg, bismuth, tetracycline, furazolidone) or may lead to severe adverse effects (eg, rifabutin).

This article aims to revisit all practical aspects that should be taken into consideration when choosing an *H pylori* eradication regimen. Increasing antibiotic resistance coupled with a lack of new therapeutic alternatives can seriously hamper the fight against *H pylori* infection. Now more than ever, a clear understanding of the interplay between the bacteria, the individual patient, its geographic area, and the drugs selected becomes pivotal to select and optimize the best therapeutic strategy for each patient, maximizing the efficacy of eradication regimens and minimizing treatment failures, selection of resistant strains, and need for step-up antibiotic therapy.

Why Is Helicobacter pylori Difficult to Treat?

The *H pylori* infection should be treated by means of a combination of acid-suppressive agents and several antibiotics, yet it has proven challenging to cure. Several factors may account for difficulties associated with cure of the infection, including bacteria-, environmental-, host-, and drug-associated variables. All of these factor influencing eradication rates and potential solutions to overcome these obstacles are summarized in **Table 1**. By far, the most important factor is the development of *H pylori* resistance to many antimicrobial agents, especially clarithromycin, metronidazole, and fluoroquinolones. In *H pylori* infection, resistance usually develops because of the outgrowth of a small existing population of resistant organisms. Clarithromycin must bind to ribosomes in order to kill *H pylori*. Acquired resistance is associated with failure to bind to ribosomes, such that resistance cannot be overcome by increasing the dose or duration. Likewise, resistance to fluoroquinolones (eg, levofloxacin, moxifloxacin) is not responsive to changes in dose or duration. Metronidazole

Table 1
Theoretic causes explaining why *H pylori* is difficult to cure and potential solutions to circumvent these difficulties

Causes	Mechanisms	Potential Solutions
Microorganism itself	Phenotypical antibiotic resistance (persistence of nonreplicating microorganisms)	Increasing amoxicillin/metronidazole duration and doses or shortening dosing interval
	High bacterial load	Increasing PPI doses and/or shortening interval dosing
		Increasing the dose and duration of antibiotic therapy
		Combining several antibiotics *(one of which will probably kill the resistant organisms)*
		Pretreatment with PPI and bismuth, reducing the bacterial load *(which would make survival of the minor populations less likely)*
Gastric environment	Acid gastric pH (*H pylori* becomes phenotypically resistant with a pH range between 3 and 6, usually in the mucus. Increasing the pH in this layer to 6 or 7 allows the bacteria to enter the replicative state, where they become susceptible to amoxicillin and clarithromycin.)	Increasing PPI doses and/or shortening interval dosing
Antibiotics	Clarithromycin and fluoroquinolone resistance	Not responsive to increasing doses or duration
	Metronidazole resistance	Increasing the dose and duration can partially overcome bacterial resistance.
	Amoxicillin and clarithromycin require microbial replication to kill microorganisms.	Increasing duration of therapy Increasing PPI doses and/or shortening interval dosing

resistance can be partially overcome by increasing the dose and duration. In contrast, bismuth resistance does not occur and acquired resistance to either amoxicillin or tetracycline is rare in most regions.

However, treatment may also fail while the organism remains susceptible to the antibiotic.[5] This treatment failure is most commonly seen with amoxicillin, for which acquired resistance is rare. This form of reversible resistance is termed *phenotypical antibiotic resistance*, and it is often caused by the presence of nonreplicating population of organisms. Bacteria usually oscillate between a nonreplicating (phenotypically resistant) and replicating state (phenotypically susceptible), during which they cannot and can be eradicated, respectively.[5] As shown in **Table 1**, short duration or shortage of antibiotic drugs may limit the presence of antibiotic drugs during susceptibility periods. Furthermore, insufficient acid suppression, keeping acid gastric pH between 3 and 6, may predispose microorganisms to a nonreplicative state; this is a phenotypically resistant state. Additionally, amoxicillin and clarithromycin are effective antibiotics against *H pylori* provided microbial replication is present.

Another *H pylori* intrinsic obstacles for eradication regimens might be the high bacterial load of *H pylori* organisms in the stomach, resulting in an inoculum effect, and the wide variety of niches where the microorganism can reside (intracellularly, mucus layer).[5] Therefore, drug regimens, including PPI and antibiotics doses and dosing intervals, should be specifically designed to target all of these problems (see **Table 1**).

CHOICE OF THERAPY

The strongest predictor of *H pylori* treatment failure using a regimen proven to be effective elsewhere is antimicrobial resistance. From a microbiological standpoint, treatment results are best when regimens are used to treat patients with organisms susceptible to the antimicrobials chosen. Pretreatment susceptibility testing, either by direct culture of the organism from gastric biopsies or indirectly by molecular testing in gastric biopsies/stools, can be used for this purpose. Nonetheless, this strategy is hampered by the wide unavailability of these techniques, besides the need for an invasive procedure (endoscopy), cost, or time consumption. Another choice would be using bismuth quadruple therapy because resistance to tetracycline is negligible and metronidazole resistance can be partially overcome by increasing doses and duration. Nonetheless, this approach is limited to regions where bismuth salts and tetracycline are both available.[6] The launch of Pylera (the 3-in-1 capsule containing bismuth, tetracycline, and metronidazole, therefore, decreasing pill burden and theoretically improving compliance) might be a good therapeutic option where available.[7]

Therefore, one often must choose antibiotic therapy empirically; the best approach is using regimens that have proven to be reliably excellent locally. Considering *H pylori* is an infectious disease and 100% success might be obtainable, the efficacy of an antimicrobial therapy should be scored as excellent (>95% success), good (>90% success), borderline acceptable (85%–89% success), poor (80%–84% success), or unacceptably low (<80%).[8] The choice should take advantage of knowledge of local resistance patterns, clinical experience, and patient history. The history of patients' prior antibiotic use and any prior therapies will help identify which antibiotics are likely to be successful and those where resistance is probable.[6] In fact, treatment outcome in a population or a patient can be calculated based on the effectiveness of a regimen for infections with susceptible and with resistant strains coupled with knowledge of the prevalence of resistance (ie, based on formal measurement, clinical experience, or both). The formula and calculations for predicting the outcome of any antimicrobial therapy have been recently reported.[6] The therapeutic expectations for an individual patient with clarithromycin-based therapies (triple, sequential, concomitant) and bismuth quadruple therapy, depending on the rate of clarithromycin and metronidazole resistance, are shown in **Table 2**.

In this current era of increasing antibiotic resistance, all therapies should be optimized. High-dose PPI therapy (eg, 40 mg of omeprazole or equivalent twice a day) is recommended in order to guarantee effective and prolonged gastric acid suppression. All PPI molecules are metabolized by cytochrome P450 (*CYP*) *2C19*. Four different genotypes have been described: ultrarapid, rapid/extensive, intermediate, and poor metabolizers. The prevalence of CYP2C19 rapid metabolizer genotype has been shown to be highest in Europe and in North America (56%–81%), whereas the proportion is lower (27%–38%) in the Asian population. Plasma PPI levels and intragastric pH levels during PPI treatment are inversely related to the CYP2C19 genotype. Accordingly, several meta-analyses have shown eradication rates are inversely related to the ability to metabolize the PPIs (eg, the ultrarapid and rapid metabolizer groups have lower eradication rate compared with other groups).[9,10] Therefore, it is

Table 2
Example of efficacy of clarithromycin-containing regimens for an individual patient, based on predicted resistance to clarithromycin and metronidazole

Antimicrobial Prediction	7-d Triple Therapy	14-d Triple Therapy	10-d Sequential Therapy	14-d Sequential Therapy	10-d Concomitant Therapy	14-d Concomitant Therapy	14-d Bismuth Quadruple Therapy
Clarithromycin and metronidazole susceptible (%)	94	97	95	98	94	97	99
Clarithromycin resistant-metronidazole susceptible (%)	<20	50	80	88	94	97	99
Clarithromycin susceptible-metronidazole resistant (%)	94	97	75	75	94	97	95
Clarithromycin and metronidazole resistant (%)	<20	50	<20	<20	<25	<50	95

Data from Graham DY, Lee YC, Wu MS. Rational *Helicobacter pylori* therapy: evidence based medicine rather than medicine based evidence. Clin Gastroenterol Hepatol 2014;12:177–86.

conceivable that all patients, especially in Europe and North America, should receive high-dose PPI therapy with a proper dosing interval (twice or more than a day) in order to circumvent the selection of nonreplicative *H pylori* strains, increase the effectiveness of amoxicillin and clarithromycin, and achieve similar efficacy rates in either rapid and poor *CYP2C19* metabolizers[5,6] (see **Table 1**). Moreover, a 14-day duration is recommended, given the fact it has proven a therapeutic benefit for triple, bismuth quadruple, and nonbismuth quadruple sequential and concomitant therapy.[6,11–13]

FIRST-LINE REGIMENS

Available first-line regimens, with preferred drug doses and dosing intervals, along with caveats for each treatment, are summarized in **Table 3**. The preferred empirical choices are currently 14-day bismuth quadruple therapy or 14-day nonbismuth quadruple concomitant or hybrid (sequential-concomitant) therapy, depending on local resistance pattern, clinical experience, and patient history of antibiotic use.

Table 3
Current first-line therapeutic recommendations in the era of increasing clarithromycin and metronidazole resistance

Eradication Regimens	Preferred Dosages and Dosing Intervals	Caveat
14-d Bismuth-containing classic quadruple therapy	Bismuth salts qid PPI (double doses) bid Tetracycline 500 mg qid Nitroimidazole 500 mg tid	Availability Complexity Side effects Compliance
14-d Bismuth-containing quadruple therapy using Pylera	PPI (double doses) bid Pylera 3 pills qid	Availability Cost Relatively low tetracycline doses
14-d Nonbismuth quadruple concomitant therapy	PPI (double doses) bid Amoxicillin 1 g bid Clarithromycin 500 mg bid Nitroimidazole 500 mg bid	Cure rates ≤90% if dual resistance rate ≥15%

14-d Nonbismuth quadruple hybrid therapy	7 d
	  PPI (double doses) bid
	  Amoxicillin 1 g bid
	7 d
	  PPI (double doses) bid
	  Amoxicillin 1 g bid
	  Clarithromycin 500 mg bid
	  Nitroimidazole 500 mg bid
		Cure rates <90% if dual resistance rate >9%

14-d Nonbismuth quadruple sequential therapy	7 d
	  PPI (double doses) bid
	  Amoxicillin 1 g bid
	7 d
	  PPI (double doses) bid
	  Clarithromycin 500 mg bid
	  Nitroimidazole 500 mg bid
		Cure rates <90% if dual resistance rate >5%
		Not recommended as an empirical therapy

14-d Triple therapy	PPI (double doses) bid Amoxicillin 1 g bid Clarithromycin 500 mg bid	Cure rates <90% if clarithromycin resistance >15% Not recommended as an empirical therapy

Dual resistant *H pylori*: microorganism resistant to both clarithromycin and metronidazole.

The Achilles heel of standard triple therapy is clarithromycin resistance. Because of the increasing worldwide clarithromycin resistance, triple therapy should no longer be prescribed on an empirical basis and its use should be strictly restricted to a minority of settings where clarithromycin resistance is known to be low (ie, Northern Europe[14] or Thailand[15]) or where cure rates greater than 90% to 95% have been documented in clinical practice.[16] When used, it should be given for 14 days with double-dose PPI twice a day, because this strategy can increase eradication rates by 10%.[11]

The Achilles heel of clarithromycin-containing nonbismuth quadruple therapies (sequential, hybrid, and concomitant) is dual *H pylori* resistance to clarithromycin and metronidazole. Sequential, hybrid, and concomitant therapies have been shown to fail when the rate of dual resistant strains is greater than 5%, greater than 9%, or greater than 15%, respectively.[6] Therefore, any empirical nonbismuth quadruple therapy would likely be a poor choice in settings with documented high clarithromycin and metronidazole resistance (eg, Turkey,[17,18] Korea[19,20]; see later discussion) or in some specific high-risk patients for acquired antibiotic resistance (eg, patients who previously used clarithromycin- and/or metronidazole-containing eradication regimens, women who used metronidazole for trichomonas infections, immigrants from developing countries).[6] A decision-making algorithm taking all these considerations into account for first-line eradication regimens is displayed in **Fig. 1**.

Nonbismuth Quadruple Therapies

Sequential therapy
Sequential therapy was developed in Italy in 2000 as a replacement for triple therapy in order to overcome the problem of clarithromycin resistance. It initially consisted of

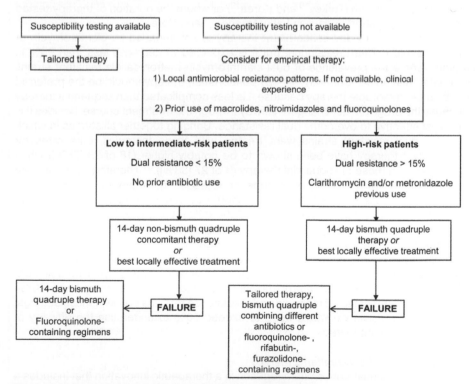

Fig. 1. Recommended approach for *Helicobacter pylori* therapy.

5 days of PPI plus amoxicillin, followed by a further 5 days of PPI with 2 other antibiotics, usually clarithromycin and a nitroimidazole.[21,22] Several meta-analyses and pooled data analyses, mostly from Italy, confirmed between 2007 and 2009 the advantage of 10-day sequential over 7- or 10-day triple therapy, with mean cure rates greater than 90%.[23–26] In 2012 and 2013, 2 updated meta-analyses[27,28] and 2 systematic reviews,[29,30] including studies from Asia, Europe, and Latin America, exhibited mean eradication rates notably lower (79%–84%) than those reported in early Italian trials. These poor results were confirmed in a global meta-analyses in 2013 with overall cure rates of 84% (95% confidence interval 82.1%–86.4%), besides confirming the lack of advantage over 14-day triple therapy.[31] Further analyses have shown that metronidazole resistance and dual clarithromycin-metronidazole resistance undermined the efficacy of sequential therapy.[6,32]

Concomitant therapy

The concept of a nonbismuth quadruple regimen or concomitant regimen consists of converting standard triple therapy to a quadruple therapy by the addition of 500 mg of metronidazole or tinidazole twice daily. This therapeutic regimen resurfaced in 2010 as an alternative therapy to triple and sequential therapy. Recent meta-analyses have consistently shown its advantage over triple therapy.[33,34] In addition, several recent studies over the last 4 years[18,19,35–50] evaluating the efficacy of concomitant therapy have been conducted in Latin America,[35] Asia (Thailand,[36] Japan,[37] Taiwan,[38,39] China,[40] and Korea[19,41,42]), and Europe (Spain,[43–45] Greece,[46,47] Italy,[48,49] and Turkey[18,50]). Regardless of the duration of therapy, all studies showed intention-to-treat cure rates ranging between 85% and 94%, with the exceptions of regions where dual resistance is high (Turkey[18] and Korea[19]) or where the duration of therapy tested was possibly too short (5 days in Latin America[35] and Korea[37]).

The efficacy of 14-day concomitant therapy is not impaired by clarithromycin or metronidazole isolated resistance, but it is expected to decrease less than 90% in regions where the prevalence of dual clarithromycin-metronidazole resistant strains is greater than 15%.[6] Currently, 14-day concomitant therapy should be the preferred nonbismuth quadruple therapy because it is less complicated than sequential therapy because the drugs are not changed halfway through the treatment course, besides it is the most effective to overcome dual resistance. Bringing together all studies in which H pylori dual resistant strains were treated with these therapies, cure rates for concomitant therapy have been shown to be notably higher (18 of 23 [78%]) when compared with those of sequential therapy (9 of 27 [33%]).[51] Therefore, concomitant therapy would always be equal or superior to sequential therapy.[6] However, it is important to stress that neither therapy should be recommended in settings with high rates of metronidazole resistance (>50%–60%) along with high clarithromycin resistance (eg, Latin America, Turkey, Korea) or in populations at high risk of dual resistance (eg, following clarithromycin or metronidazole treatment failures).[6] These recommendations are in agreement as well with good to excellent results in some Asian countries[36–40] and Southern Europe,[43–49] where clarithromycin ranges from low (9%) to high (40%); but metronidazole resistance remains relatively low (<30%–40%). As a matter of fact, if metronidazole resistance remains stable in these settings, clarithromycin resistance would need to exceed 50% to undermine the efficacy of 14-day concomitant therapy.

Hybrid (sequential-concomitant) therapy

The hybrid sequential-concomitant regimen is a therapeutic innovation that includes a PPI plus amoxicillin for 14 days, adding clarithromycin and a nitroimidazole for the final

7 days.[52] In other words, it is a 7-day first dual-phase (PPI + amoxicillin) followed by a 7-day quadruple phase (PPI + amoxicillin + clarithromycin + nitroimidazole). Several recent studies conducted between 2011 and 2014 have consistently shown cure rates of 86% or greater in Taiwan,[52,53] Iran,[54] and Spain/Italy[44]; but poor results have been reported in other studies conducted in Italy[48,49] and Korea.[20] It could be considered in the same populations where concomitant therapy is recommended; however, 14-day hybrid therapy is expected to decrease less than 90% when clarithromycin-metronidazole resistance exceeds 9%.[6] Hybrid therapy provides the advantage of improved safety, convenience, and better compliance. A recent first meta-analyses on hybrid therapy has not shown relevant differences in terms of efficacy with the sequential and concomitant therapy.[55] Further studies, however, are required to validate this therapy in settings with different patterns of resistance.

Bismuth Quadruple Therapy

This therapy is the oldest effective therapy, mostly underappreciated, and a resurfacing one on account of increasing failure of clarithromycin-containing therapies. Doses and duration are critical to the outcome, especially in the presence of metronidazole resistance. Using this regimen at full doses and for 14 days, one can expect 95% or greater treatment success, irrespective of the level of metronidazole resistance.[6,56] The main disadvantages are its complexity and frequent side effects, both of which may hamper compliance with therapy. In addition, bismuth salts or tetracycline are not widely available now. Doxycycline cannot successfully substitute for tetracycline and should not be used.[6] This regimen is the regimen most in need of clinical trials to simplify and to improve compliance. Recent studies conducted in Italy and China have shown similar success rates using twice-a-day bismuth and full 4-times-a-day antibiotic doses.[57,58] In this context, bismuth-based quadruple therapy in its most recent galenic formulation, bismuth subcitrate potassium, metronidazole, and tetracycline (bismuth, metronidazole and tetracycline [BMT], sold under license as Pylera), may be an attractive therapeutic option.[7] However, its use is currently limited by its high cost, the fact that only a 10-day regimen is available in a prepackaged form, and the dose of tetracycline is only 1500 mg. Moreover, it remains unknown if these more convenient formulations produce improved compliance, especially when considering that side effects are often the reason for poor compliance with bismuth therapy. Head-to-head comparisons with standard bismuth triple therapy and with twice-a-day dosing for bismuth are needed, especially in populations with high rates of metronidazole resistance.

RESCUE THERAPY

Even with the current most effective treatment regimens, a variable proportion of patients will fail to eradicate *H pylori* infection at the first attempt.[6,12] Despite the number of studies, the optimal retreatment regimen has not yet been defined. Our therapeutic target, similar to first-line regimens, should be at least 90% cure rates. The empirical choice of a rescue treatment primarily depends on which treatment was used initially (eg, bismuth or nonbismuth quadruple therapy), the local rate of fluoroquinolone resistance, and availability of either bismuth salts/tetracycline. After failure of a clarithromycin- or metronidazole-containing treatment, clinicians should assume that *H pylori* are likely resistant to the antibiotic used, so it is not appropriate to repeat the same antibiotics. An exception to this rule is amoxicillin, which rarely induces resistance. Most will be cured by using bismuth quadruple therapy after failure of clarithromycin-containing regimens.[58,59] In the absence of pretreatment antibiotic resistance testing, the most commonly used strategies for a second-line therapy in regions where bismuth quadruple therapy is unavailable is a fluoroquinolone-containing therapy. This therapy should only be considered if no fluoroquinolone, including ciprofloxacin, was used before.[6] Rescue therapy is defined as therapy after 2 treatment failures with 2 different regimens.[6,60] At this stage, recent European guidelines recommend that treatment should be guided by antimicrobial susceptibility testing, whenever possible.[11] The available regimens for rescue therapy, with preferred duration, doses, and interval dosing, besides potential caveats, are summarized in **Table 4**. Furazolidone quadruple therapy (where available) and rifabutin triple therapy are typically reserved as salvage therapies of last resort. A recommended therapeutic algorithm for *H pylori* rescue therapy is displayed in **Fig. 1**.

Fluoroquinolone-Containing Therapy

Levofloxacin is a fluoroquinolone with a broad spectrum of activity against *H pylori*. Fluoroquinolone-based therapy has been proposed in several international guidelines as a rescue therapy. However, prevalence of fluoroquinolone resistance has increased rapidly in recent years, mostly because of widespread use of levofloxacin for respiratory tract, urinary, and ear, nose, and throat infections. Recent studies have reported high levofloxacin resistance rates, ranging from 63% in China to 14% in Europe.[6,14] A recent review revealed a weighted efficacy of 76% for levofloxacin-containing rescue regimens.[60] Indeed, 7-day triple therapy, including PPI, amoxicillin, and levofloxacin, provides cure rates of typically less than 80%; extending the duration to 10 days improves outcomes, but the treatment success has remained typically less than 90%.[60–63] Treatment success would decrease to less than 90% with 14-day

Table 4
Current rescue therapeutic recommendations, in the era of increasing fluoroquinolone resistance, in patients with high risk of acquired clarithromycin and/or metronidazole resistance after failure of first eradication regimen

Eradication Regimens	Preferred Dosages	Caveat
14-d Fluoroquinolone triple therapy	PPI (double doses) bid Amoxicillin 1000 mg bid Levofloxacin 500 mg	Cure rates ≤90% if levofloxacin resistance ≥12%
14-d Bismuth-containing fluoroquinolone quadruple therapy	Bismuth salts 240 mg bid PPI (double doses) bid Amoxicillin 1000 mg bid Levofloxacin 250 mg bid	Cure rates ≤90% if levofloxacin resistance ≥25%
14-d Bismuth quadruple concomitant therapy	PPI (double doses) bid Bismuth salts 240 mg bid *Plus a combination of 2 antibiotics among the following:* Amoxicillin 1 g tid/bid Nitroimidazole 500 mg tid Tetracycline 500 mg qid Furazolidone 100 mg tid	Availability Side effects Complexity Compliance Potential genotoxic and carcinogenetic effects of furazolidone
14-d Rifabutin-containing therapy	PPI (double doses) bid, tid Amoxicillin 1000 mg tid Rifabutin 150 mg bid	Cost Potential severe side effects *(myelotoxicity and hepatotoxicity)* Risk of development of resistance in *M tuberculosis*

fluoroquinolone triple therapy when fluoroquinolone resistance rates exceed approximately 12%,[64] whereas 14-day bismuth-containing fluoroquinolone quadruple therapy will not reach 90% cure rates in areas with a fluoroquinolone resistance of up to approximately 25%.[65] Therefore, awareness of local resistance rates or close monitoring of cure rates are mandatory in order to promptly detect inefficacy of these therapies. The role of newer fluoroquinolones, such as sitafloxacin and gemifloxacin, to overcome fluoroquinolone resistance needs to be validated in further studies.

Bismuth Quadruple Therapy, Including Furazolidone-Containing Regimens

Classic bismuth quadruple regimen has also been proposed in international guidelines as a rescue therapy.[11] In a recent review, its weighted efficacy was 77% (including different durations, drug doses, and interval dosing).[60] Concerns with this therapy are complexity, patient compliance, and availability. Meta-analyses comparing fluoroquinolone-based triple therapy and bismuth quadruple therapies for rescue therapy did not find significant differences between both therapies regarding efficacy, albeit fluoroquinolone therapy was significantly better tolerated and induced significantly fewer side effects.[60–62] Importantly, the results with both regimens were likely unacceptably low because of the poor choices of doses, duration, and the presence of resistance.

Bismuth quadruple therapy, however, is the regimen with the most unanswered questions regarding what the optimal doses are and the frequencies of drug administration. A recent study from China has evaluated the efficacy of 14-day bismuth quadruple therapies (PPI, bismuth salts, and 2 antibiotics) with different antibiotic combinations in patients with previous eradication treatment failure.[58] They used for all 4 evaluated regimens twice-a-day bismuth (220 mg twice a day) and full doses and adequate dosing intervals for the antibiotics (amoxicillin 1 g 3 times a day, tetracycline 500 mg 4 times a day, metronidazole 400 mg 3 times a day, furazolidone 100 mg 3 times a day). Cure rates were excellent (>90%), regardless of the presence of clarithromycin, levofloxacin, or metronidazole resistance, with the best results for furazolidone-containing regimens. Of note, these bismuth quadruple regimens were equally effective for patients allergic to penicillin, combining tetracycline with either metronidazole or furazolidone. However, furazolidone is seldom available in developed countries; concerns about possible genotoxic and carcinogenetic effects may prevent its implementation. This study, however, importantly highlights that both efficacy and compliance with bismuth quadruple therapy can be improved through optimization of therapy.

Rifabutin-Containing Therapy

Rifabutin is a rifamycin-S derivative, which shares many of the properties of rifampin (rifampicin). Rifabutin is commonly used to treat *Mycobacterium avium* and *Mycobacterium intracellulare*; it has shown utility against *H pylori* seeing as the in vitro sensitivity is high and prevalence rate of rifabutin resistance is very low, only about 1%. A recent systematic review disclosed the mean *H pylori* eradication rate with rifabutin-containing rescue regimens was 73%.[66] Respective cure rates for second-, third- and fourth/fifth-line rifabutin therapies were 79%, 66%, and 70%. The most prescribed regimen has been a triple therapy combining PPI, amoxicillin, and rifabutin. The most effective dose is 300 mg/d; the ideal length remains unclear, although 10- to 14 day-regimens are generally recommended. The most successful cure rates (≥90%) have been reported using high-dose PPI (60 mg twice a day, 80 mg 3 times a day), high-dose amoxicillin (1.0 or 1.5 g 3 times a day), and rifabutin (150 mg twice a day) for 7 to 12 days.[67,68] The main disadvantages of this drug are its high cost, uncommon but relevant adverse effects (mainly myelotoxicity and hepatotoxicity), and the potential development of resistance to *M tuberculosis* in populations with a high prevalence of tuberculosis. Owing to all these reasons, it should be kept as the last therapeutic resort.

PROBIOTICS

Probiotics are live microorganisms or produced substances that are orally administrated, usually in addition to conventional antibiotic therapy for *H pylori* infection. They may modulate the human microbiota, stimulate the immune response, and directly compete with pathogenic bacteria, besides preventing antibiotic side effects.[69] Indeed, probiotics have exhibited inhibitory activity against *H pylori* in vitro and in vivo.[70,71] Now 10 meta-analyses have been published addressing the specific benefit of *Lactobacillus and Bifidobacterium*,[72,73] bovine lactoferrin,[74,75] fermented milk-based,[76] *Lactobacillus*,[77,78] and *Saccharomyces boulardii*[79] probiotic formulations as well as probiotics as a whole therapeutic group.[80–82] Available evidence collectively points toward a benefit of using probiotic for decreasing antibiotic-related side effects and, to a much lesser extent, increasing cure rates.

However, several considerations should be taking into consideration when it comes to probiotic supplementation. To begin with, they add complexity as they mean a fourth or fifth drug, depending on dealing with triple and quadruple therapies, and it may increase the risk of poor compliance with therapy. Furthermore, probiotics are over-the-counter medications; the cost of eradication therapy may notably increase. Unlike meta-analyses, several studies have failed to find any advantage by adding probiotics to *H pylori* therapy.[83–85] Most likely, the discordant results are probably related to the different products used and their different concentrations, probiotic strain, dose, and the length of duration. Further studies, refining the most effective probiotic and the patient profile that will most benefit from probiotic supplementation are needed before a general recommendation in clinical practice can be made.

SUMMARY

H pylori infection has proven challenging to eradicate because of several bacteria-, environmental-, host-, and drug-associated factors. An effective therapy is defined as one achieving at least a 90% eradication rate with the first attempt. Cure rates of *H pylori* with triple therapy have declined to unacceptable levels worldwide, mostly because of increasing clarithromycin resistance rates. Therefore, novel first-line treatments are required and should be chosen on local prevalence of *H pylori* antimicrobial resistance or, if unavailable, empirically based on a combination using only regimens that have proven to be reliably excellent locally and knowledge of prior use of antibiotics by patients. The preferred empirical choices are currently 14-day concomitant therapy and 14-day bismuth quadruple therapy. Optimization of eradication schemes should always be ensured to maximize their efficacy. Rescue therapy after failure eradication regimens should be tailored based on antimicrobial susceptibility testing and, if not available, chosen on which treatments used initially (eg, bismuth or nonbismuth quadruple therapy) and the prevalence of fluoroquinolone resistance locally. Where available, furazolidone- and rifabutin-containing therapies are likely to be successful as a rescue therapy. Probiotics may reduce side effects and improve adherence to increasingly complex regimens. Whether probiotics can also increase eradication rates should be further elucidated. On large variations in *H pylori* resistance patterns, the golden rule for choice of treatment is only to use what works locally (>90%–95% success) and to closely monitor its effectiveness over time.

REFERENCES

1. Marshall BJ, Warren JR. Unidentified curved bacilli in the stomach of patients with gastritis and peptic ulceration. Lancet 1984;1:1311–5.
2. Graham DY. History of *Helicobacter pylori*, duodenal ulcer, gastric ulcer and gastric cancer. World J Gastroenterol 2014;20:5191–204.
3. Infection with *Helicobacter pylori*. In: IARC monographs on the evaluation of the carcinogenic risks to humans. Vol. 61. Schistosomes, liver flukes and *Helicobacter pylori*. Lyon (France): International Agency for Research on Cancer; 1994. p. 177–240.
4. Shiotani A, Cen P, Graham DY. Eradication of gastric cancer is now both possible and practical. Semin Cancer Biol 2013;23:492–501.
5. Graham DY, Fischbach L. *Helicobacter pylori* treatment in the era of increasing antibiotic resistance. Gut 2010;59:1143–53.
6. Graham DY, Lee YC, Wu MS. Rational *Helicobacter pylori* therapy: evidence based medicine rather than medicine based evidence. Clin Gastroenterol Hepatol 2014;12:177–86.
7. Megraud F. The challenge of *Helicobacter pylori* resistance to antibiotics: the comeback of bismuth-based quadruple therapy. Therap Adv Gastroenterol 2012;5:103–9.
8. Graham DY, Lu H, Yamaoka Y. A report card to grade *Helicobacter pylori* therapy. Helicobacter 2007;12:275–8.
9. Zhao F, Wang J, Yang Y, et al. Effect of CYP2C19 genetic polymorphisms on the efficacy of proton pump inhibitor based triple therapy for *Helicobacter pylori* eradication: a meta-analysis. Helicobacter 2008;13:532–41.
10. Tang HL, Li Y, Hu YF, et al. Effects of CYP2C19 loss-of function variants on the eradication of *H. pylori* infection in patients treated with proton pump inhibitor-based triple therapy regimens: a meta analysis of randomized clinical trials. PLoS One 2013;8:e62162.
11. Malfertheiner P, Megraud F, O'Morain CA, et al, European Helicobacter Study Group. Management of *Helicobacter pylori* infection–the Maastricht IV/Florence Consensus Report. Gut 2012;61:646–64.
12. Molina-Infante J, Gisbert JP. Optimizing clarithromycin-containing therapy for *Helicobacter pylori* in the era of antibiotic resistance. World J Gastroenterol 2014;10:10338–47.
13. Yuan Y, Ford AC, Khan KJ, et al. Optimum duration of regimens for *Helicobacter pylori* eradication. Cochrane Database Syst Rev 2013;(12):CD008337.
14. Megraud F, Coenen S, Versporten A, et al, Study Group participants. *Helicobacter pylori* resistance to antibiotics in Europe and its relationship to antibiotic consumption. Gut 2013;62:34–42.
15. Vilaichone RK, Gumnarai P, Ratanachu-Ek T, et al. Nationwide survey of *Helicobacter pylori* antibiotic resistance in Thailand. Diagn Microbiol Infect Dis 2013; 77:346–9.
16. Prasertpetmanee S, Mahachai V, Vilaichone RK. Improved efficacy of proton pump inhibitor - amoxicillin - clarithromycin triple therapy for *Helicobacter pylori* eradication in low clarithromycin resistance areas or for tailored therapy. Helicobacter 2013;18:270–3.
17. Dolapcioglu C, Koc-Yesiltoprak A, Ahishali E, et al. Sequential therapy versus standard triple therapy in *Helicobacter pylori* eradication in a high clarithromycin resistance setting. Int J Clin Exp Med 2014;7:2324–8.
18. Toros AB, Ince AT, Kesici B, et al. A new modified concomitant therapy for *Helicobacter pylori* eradication in Turkey. Helicobacter 2011;16:225–8.

19. Lim JH, Lee DH, Choi C, et al. Clinical outcomes of two-week sequential and concomitant therapies for *Helicobacter pylori* eradication: a randomized pilot study. Helicobacter 2013;18:180–6.

20. Oh DH, Lee DH, Kang KK, et al. The efficacy of hybrid therapy as first line regimen for *Helicobacter pylori* infection compared with sequential therapy. J Gastroenterol Hepatol 2014;29:1171–6.

21. Zullo A, Rinaldi V, Winn S, et al. A new highly effective short-term therapy schedule for *Helicobacter pylori* eradication. Aliment Pharmacol Ther 2000;14: 715–8.

22. De Francesco V, Zullo A, Hassan C, et al. Two new treatment regimens for *Helicobacter pylori* eradication: a randomised study. Dig Liver Dis 2001;33:676–9.

23. Zullo A, De Francesco V, Hassan C, et al. The sequential therapy regimen for *Helicobacter pylori* eradication: a pooled-data analysis. Gut 2007;56:1353–7.

24. Jafri NS, Hornung CA, Howden CW. Meta-analysis: sequential therapy appears superior to standard therapy for *Helicobacter pylori* infection in patients naive to treatment. Ann Intern Med 2008;148:923–31.

25. Tong JL, Ran ZH, Shen J, et al. Sequential therapy vs standard triple therapies for *Helicobacter pylori* infection: a meta-analysis. J Clin Pharm Ther 2009;34:41–53.

26. Gatta L, Vakil N, Leandro G, et al. Sequential therapy or triple therapy for *Helicobacter pylori* infection: systematic review and meta-analysis of randomized controlled trials in adults and children. Am J Gastroenterol 2009;104:3069–79.

27. Horvath A, Dziechciarz P, Szajewska H. Meta-analysis: sequential therapy for *Helicobacter pylori* eradication in children. Aliment Pharmacol Ther 2012;36:534–41.

28. Yoon H, Lee DH, Kim N, et al. Meta-analysis: is sequential therapy superior to standard triple therapy for *Helicobacter pylori* infection in Asian adults? J Gastroenterol Hepatol 2013;28:1801–9.

29. Zullo A, Hassan C, Ridola L, et al. Standard triple and sequential therapies for *Helicobacter pylori* eradication: an update. Eur J Intern Med 2013;24:16–9.

30. Kate V, Kalayarasan R, Ananthakrishnan N. Sequential therapy versus standard triple-drug therapy for *Helicobacter pylori* eradication: a systematic review of recent evidence. Drugs 2013;73:815–24.

31. Gatta L, Vakil N, Vaira D, et al. Global eradication rates for *Helicobacter pylori* infection: systematic review and meta-analysis of sequential therapy. BMJ 2013;28:1801–9.

32. Liou JM, Chen CC, Chen MJ, et al, Taiwan Helicobacter Consortium. Sequential versus triple therapy for the first-line treatment of *Helicobacter pylori*: a multicentre, open-label, randomised trial. Lancet 2013;381:205–13.

33. Essa AS, Kramer JR, Graham DY, et al. Meta-analysis: four-drug, three-antibiotic, non-bismuth-containing "concomitant therapy" versus triple therapy for *Helicobacter pylori* eradication. Helicobacter 2009;14:109–18.

34. Gisbert JP, Calvet X. Update on non-bismuth quadruple (concomitant) therapy for eradication of *Helicobacter pylori*. Clin Exp Gastroenterol 2012;5:23–34.

35. Greenberg ER, Anderson GL, Morgan DR, et al. 14-day triple, 5-day concomitant, and 10-day sequential therapies for *Helicobacter pylori* infection in seven Latin American sites: a randomised trial. Lancet 2011;378:507–14.

36. Kongchayanun C, Vilaichone RK, Pornthisarn B, et al. Pilot studies to identify the optimum duration of concomitant *Helicobacter pylori* eradication therapy in Thailand. Helicobacter 2012;17:282–5.

37. Yanai A, Sakamoto K, Akanuma M, et al. Non-bismuth quadruple therapy for first-line *Helicobacter pylori* eradication: a randomized study in Japan. World J Gastrointest Pharmacol Ther 2012;3:1–6.

38. Wu DC, Hsu PI, Wu JY, et al. Sequential and concomitant therapy with 4 drugs are equally effective for eradication of *H. pylori* infection. Clin Gastroenterol Hepatol 2010;8:36–41.
39. Hsu PI, Wu DC, Chen WC, et al. Randomized controlled trial comparing 7-day triple, 10-day sequential, and 7-day concomitant therapies for *Helicobacter pylori* infection. Antimicrob Agents Chemother 2014;58:5936–42.
40. Huang YK, Wu MC, Wang SS, et al. Lansoprazole-based sequential and concomitant therapy for the first-line *Helicobacter pylori* eradication. J Dig Dis 2012;13: 232–8.
41. Kim SY, Lee SW, Hyun JJ, et al. Comparative study of *Helicobacter pylori* eradication rates and 7-day standard triple therapy with 5-day quadruple "concomitant" therapy. J Clin Gastroenterol 2013;47:21–4.
42. Heo J, Jeon SW, Jung JT, et al. A randomised clinical trial of 10-day concomitant therapy and standard triple therapy for *Helicobacter pylori* eradication. Dig Liver Dis 2014;46:1980–4.
43. Molina-Infante J, Pazos-Pacheco C, Vinagre-Rodriguez G, et al. Nonbismuth quadruple (concomitant) therapy: empirical and tailored efficacy versus standard triple therapy for clarithromycin susceptible *Helicobacter pylori* and versus sequential therapy for clarithromycin-resistant strains. Helicobacter 2012;17:269–76.
44. Molina-Infante J, Romano M, Fernandez-Bermejo M, et al. Optimized nonbismuth quadruple therapies cure most patients with *Helicobacter pylori* infection in populations with high rates of antibiotic resistance. Gastroenterology 2013;145:121–8.
45. McNicholl AG, Marin AC, Molina-Infante J, et al. Randomised clinical trial comparing sequential and concomitant therapies for *Helicobacter pylori* eradication in routine clinical practice. Gut 2014;63:244–9.
46. Georgopoulos S, Papastergiou V, Xirouchakis E, et al. Evaluation of a four-drug, three-antibiotic, nonbismuth-containing "concomitant" therapy as first-line *Helicobacter pylori* eradication regimen in Greece. Helicobacter 2012;17:49–53.
47. Georgopoulos SD, Xirouchakis E, Martinez-Gonzalez B, et al. Clinical evaluation of a ten-day regimen with esomeprazole, metronidazole, amoxicillin, and clarithromycin for the eradication of *Helicobacter pylori* in a high clarithromycin resistance area. Helicobacter 2013;18:459–67.
48. Zullo A, Scaccianoce G, De Francesco V, et al. Concomitant, sequential, and hybrid therapy for *H. pylori* eradication: a pilot study. Clin Res Hepatol Gastroenterol 2013;37:647–50.
49. De Francesco V, Hassan C, Ridola L, et al. Sequential, concomitant and hybrid first-line therapies for *H. pylori* eradication: a prospective, randomized study. J Med Microbiol 2014;63:748–52.
50. Sharara AI, Sarkis FS, El-Halabi MM, et al. Challenging the dogma: a randomized trial of standard vs half-dose concomitant nonbismuth quadruple therapy for *Helicobacter pylori* infection. United European Gastroenterol J 2014;2:179–88.
51. Georgopoulos SD, Xirouchakis E, Mentris A. Is there a nonbismuth quadruple therapy that can reliably overcome bacterial resistance? Gastroenterology 2013;145:1496–7.
52. Hsu PI, Wu DC, Wu YC, et al. Modified sequential *Helicobacter pylori* therapy: proton pump inhibitor and amoxicillin for 14 days with clarithromycin and metronidazole added as a quadruple (hybrid) therapy for the final 7 days. Helicobacter 2011;16:139–45.
53. Wu JY, Hsu PI, Wu DC, et al. Feasibility of shortening 14-day hybrid therapy while maintaining an excellent *Helicobacter pylori* eradication rate. Helicobacter 2014; 19:207–13.

54. Sardarian H, Fakheri H, Hosseini V, et al. Comparison of hybrid and sequential therapies for *Helicobacter pylori* eradication in Iran: a prospective randomized trial. Helicobacter 2013;18:129–34.

55. Wang B, Wang YH, Lv ZF, et al. Efficacy and safety of hybrid therapy for *helicobacter pylori* infection: a systematic review and meta-analysis. Helicobacter 2015;20(2):79–88.

56. Salazar CO, Cardenas VM, Reddy RK, et al. Greater than 95% success with 14-day bismuth quadruple anti- *Helicobacter pylori* therapy: a pilot study in US Hispanics. Helicobacter 2012;17:382–90.

57. Dore MP, Farina V, Cuccu M, et al. Twice-a-day bismuth-containing quadruple therapy for *Helicobacter pylori* eradication: a randomized trial of 10 and 14 days. Helicobacter 2011;16:295–300.

58. Liang X, Xu X, Zheng Q, et al. Efficacy of bismuth containing quadruple therapies for clarithromycin-, metronidazole-, and fluoroquinolone resistant *Helicobacter pylori* infections in a prospective study. Clin Gastroenterol Hepatol 2013;11:802–7.

59. Delchier JC, Malfertheiner P, Thieroff-Ekerdt R. Use of a combination formulation of bismuth, metronidazole and tetracycline with omeprazole as a rescue therapy for eradication of *Helicobacter pylori*. Aliment Pharmacol Ther 2014;40:171–7.

60. Marín AC, McNicholl AG, Gisbert JP. A review of rescue regimens after clarithromycin-containing triple therapy failure (for *Helicobacter pylori* eradication). Expert Opin Pharmacother 2013;14:843–61.

61. Gisbert JP, Morena F. Systematic review and meta-analysis: levofloxacin-based rescue regimens after *Helicobacter pylori* treatment failure. Aliment Pharmacol Ther 2006;23:35–44.

62. Saad RJ, Schoenfeld P, Kim HM, et al. Levofloxacin-based triple therapy versus bismuth-based quadruple therapy for persistent *Helicobacter pylori* infection: a meta-analysis. Am J Gastroenterol 2006;101:488–96.

63. Gisbert JP, Pérez-Aisa A, Bermejo F, et al, H. pylori Study Group of the Asociación Española de Gastroenterología (Spanish Gastroenterology Association). Second-line therapy with levofloxacin after failure of treatment to eradicate *helicobacter pylori* infection: time trends in a Spanish multicenter study of 1000 patients. J Clin Gastroenterol 2013;47:130–5.

64. Chuah SK, Tai WC, Hsu PI, et al. The efficacy of second-line anti-*Helicobacter pylori* therapy using an extended 14-day levofloxacin/amoxicillin/proton-pump inhibitor treatment–a pilot study. Helicobacter 2012;17:374–81.

65. Liao J, Zheng Q, Liang X, et al. Effect of fluoroquinolone resistance on 14-day levofloxacin triple and triple plus bismuth quadruple therapy. Helicobacter 2013;18:373–7.

66. Gisbert JP, Calvet X. Review article: rifabutin in the treatment of refractory *Helicobacter pylori* infection. Aliment Pharmacol Ther 2012;35:209–21.

67. Borody TJ, Pang G, Wettstein AR, et al. Efficacy and safety of rifabutin-containing 'rescue therapy' for resistant *Helicobacter pylori* infection. Aliment Pharmacol Ther 2006;23:481–8.

68. Lim HC, Lee YJ, An B, et al. Rifabutin-based high-dose proton-pump inhibitor and amoxicillin triple regimen as the rescue treatment for *Helicobacter pylori*. Helicobacter 2014;19:455–61.

69. Vitor JM, Vale FF. Alternative therapies for *Helicobacter pylori* infection: probiotics and phytomedicine. FEMS Immunol Med Microbiol 2011;63:153–64.

70. Aiba Y, Suzuki N, Kabir AM, et al. Lactic acid-mediated suppression of *Helicobacter pylori* by the oral administration of *Lactobacillus salivarius* as a probiotic in a gnotobiotic murine model. Am J Gastroenterol 1998;93:2097–101.

71. Pinchuk IV, Bressollier P, Verneuil B, et al. In vitro anti-*Helicobacter pylori* activity of the probiotic strain *Bacillus subtilis 3* is due to secretion of antibiotics. Antimicrob Agents Chemother 2001;45:3156–61.

72. Tong JL, Ran ZH, Shen J, et al. Meta-analysis: the effect of supplementation with probiotics on eradication rates and adverse events during *Helicobacter pylori* eradication therapy. Aliment Pharmacol Ther 2007;25:155–68.

73. Wang ZH, Gao QY, Fang JY. Meta-analysis of the efficacy and safety of *Lactobacillus*-containing and *Bifidobacterium*-containing probiotic compound preparation in *Helicobacter pylori* eradication therapy. J Clin Gastroenterol 2013;47: 25–32.

74. Sachdeva A, Nagpal J. Meta-analysis: efficacy of bovine lactoferrin in *Helicobacter pylori* eradication. Aliment Pharmacol Ther 2009;29:720–30.

75. Zou J, Dong J, Yu XF. Meta-analysis: the effect of supplementation with lactoferrin on eradication rates and adverse events during *Helicobacter pylori* eradication therapy. Helicobacter 2009;14:119–27.

76. Sachdeva A, Nagpal J. Effect of fermented milk-based probiotic preparations on *Helicobacter pylori* eradication: a systematic review and meta-analysis of randomized-controlled trials. Eur J Gastroenterol Hepatol 2009;21:45–53.

77. Zou J, Dong J, Yu X. Meta-analysis: Lactobacillus containing quadruple therapy versus standard triple first-line therapy for *Helicobacter pylori* eradication. Helicobacter 2009;14:97–107.

78. Zheng X, Lyu L, Mei Z. Lactobacillus-containing probiotic supplementation increases *Helicobacter pylori* eradication rate: evidence from a meta-analysis. Rev Esp Enferm Dig 2013;105:445–53.

79. Szajewska H, Horvath A, Piwowarczyk A. Meta-analysis: the effects of Saccharomyces boulardii supplementation on *Helicobacter pylori* eradication rates and side effects during treatment. Aliment Pharmacol Ther 2010;32:1069–79.

80. Zhu R, Chen K, Zheng YY, et al. Meta-analysis of the efficacy of probiotics in *Helicobacter pylori* eradication. World J Gastroenterol 2014;20:18013 21.

81. Li S, Huang XL, Sui JZ, et al. Meta-analysis of randomized controlled trials on the efficacy of probiotics in *Helicobacter pylori* eradication therapy in children. Eur J Pediatr 2014;173:153–61.

82. Dang Y, Reinhardt JD, Zhou X, et al. The effect of probiotics supplementation on *Helicobacter pylori* eradication rates and side effects during eradication therapy: a meta-analysis. PLoS One 2014;9:e111030.

83. Navarro-Rodriguez T, Silva FM, Barbuti RC, et al. Association of a probiotic to a *Helicobacter pylori* eradication regimen does not increase efficacy or decreases the adverse effects of the treatment: a prospective, randomized, double-blind, placebo-controlled study. BMC Gastroenterol 2013;13:56.

84. Mirzaee V, Rezahosseini O. Randomized control trial: comparison of triple therapy plus probiotic yogurt vs standard triple therapy on *Helicobacter pylori* eradication. Iran Red Crescent Med J 2012;14:657–66.

85. Medeiros JA, Gonçalves TM, Boyanova L, et al. Evaluation of *Helicobacter pylori* eradication by triple therapy plus Lactobacillus acidophilus compared to triple therapy alone. Eur J Clin Microbiol Infect Dis 2011;30:555–9.

How to Effectively Use Bismuth Quadruple Therapy: The Good, the Bad, and the Ugly

David Y. Graham, MD[a],*, Sun-Young Lee, MD, PhD[b]

KEYWORDS

- *Helicobacter pylori* • Therapy • Bismuth • Tetracycline • Metronidazole
- Proton pump inhibitors • Side effects • Adherence

KEY POINTS

- Bismuth quadruple therapy, consisting of a proton pump inhibitor, bismuth, metronidazole, and tetracycline, is a good alternative first-line therapy and is especially useful when penicillin cannot be used or when clarithromycin and metronidazole resistance is common.
- The literature is confusing because bismuth quadruple therapy is used to denote regimens that differ greatly in terms of duration, doses, and administration in relation to meals.
- Proton pump inhibitors can help negate the deleterious effects of metronidazole resistance in bismuth quadruple therapy. The optimum dose of proton pump inhibitor is unclear. A double dose twice a day is recommended.
- In the presence of metronidazole resistance, the optimum duration is 14 days along with 1500 to 1600 mg of metronidazole in divided dosages. The optimum doses and dosing intervals for tetracycline and bismuth are as yet unclear.

Continued

Author Contributions: Each of the authors has been involved equally and has read and approved the final article. Each meets the criteria for authorship established by the International Committee of Medical Journal Editors and verifies the validity of the results reported.
Supportive Foundations: Dr D.Y. Graham is supported in part by the Office of Research and Development Medical Research Service Department of Veterans Affairs, Public Health Service grants DK067366 and DK56338, which funds the Texas Medical Center Digestive Diseases Center. The contents are solely the responsibility of the authors and do not necessarily represent the official views of the Veterans Affairs or National Institutes of Health.
Potential Conflicts: Dr D.Y. Graham is an unpaid consultant for Novartis in relation to vaccine development for treatment or prevention of *H pylori* infection. Dr D.Y. Graham is also a paid consultant for RedHill Biopharma regarding novel *H pylori* therapies, for Otsuka Pharmaceuticals regarding diagnostic testing, and for BioGaia regarding use of probiotics for *H pylori* infections. Dr D.Y. Graham has received royalties from Baylor College of Medicine patents covering materials related to ^{13}C-urea breath test. Dr S.-Y. Lee has nothing to declare.

[a] Department of Medicine, Michael E. DeBakey Veterans Affairs Medical Center & Baylor College of Medicine, 2002 Holcombe Boulevard, Houston, TX 77030, USA; [b] Department of Internal Medicine, Konkuk University School of Medicine, 120-1 Neungdong-ro, Seoul 143-729, Korea
* Corresponding author.
E-mail address: dgraham@bcm.edu

Gastroenterol Clin N Am 44 (2015) 537–563
http://dx.doi.org/10.1016/j.gtc.2015.05.003
0889-8553/15/$ – see front matter Published by Elsevier Inc.

gastro.theclinics.com

Continued

- Poor patient adherence is a major issue with bismuth quadruple therapy. Patient education and counseling regarding the goals of therapy, the side effects, and the necessity to complete the full 14 days should be provided.
- As with all therapies, the decision to use bismuth quadruple therapy should be guided by the regional, local, and patient-specific antimicrobial resistance patterns and knowledge about effectiveness locally.
- Twice-a-day dosing may provide a high cure rate with fewer side effects, accomplishes a reduction in total antibiotic dose, and improves adherence. However, its effectiveness in relation to metronidazole resistance remains unclear.

BACKGROUND

Eberle, in 1834, noted that bismuth, primarily as the white oxide, was introduced into medicine in 1697 by Jacobi and that its use was later popularized by Drs Odier of Geneva and De la Roche, of Paris.[1] Throughout the nineteenth century, bismuth salts were widely and successfully used in gastroenterology.[2] Bismuth continued to be used as a primary or adjuvant therapy for dyspepsia and peptic ulcer until being replaced successively by antacids, histamine-2 receptor antagonists, and proton pump inhibitors (PPIs). Bismuth also had a long history of use as an antimicrobial especially for the treatment of syphilis.[3] In the United States, bismuth subsalicylate (eg, as Pepto-Bismol) was also used for dyspepsia and diarrhea and later to treat and prevent travelers' diarrhea.[4] In travelers' diarrhea, bismuth was shown to function as a topical antimicrobial, thus linking its use as an anti-infective to its subsequent use for treatment of *Helicobacter pylori*-related peptic ulcer disease.[5–7]

The most widely used forms of bismuth in use for gastroenterology at the time of the discovery of *H pylori* were bismuth subnitrate, subsalicylate, and subcitrate. In the 1970s, Gist-Brocades introduced a proprietary preparation of colloidal bismuth subcitrate (De-Nol) as an antiulcer therapy. The original De-Nol formulation was a colloidal suspension in ammonia water and had the very pungent odor of ammonia. The 1970s were also a time of great interest in ulcer pathogenesis and ulcer treatments. Many groups were also active in the study of ulcer in experimental animals. Colloidal bismuth subcitrate was shown to be able to coat and thus potentially protect the ulcer base, a property not seen with other bismuth preparations.[8–11] Over time, the list of its properties potentially important in the treatment of peptic ulcer grew large (**Box 1**).[12]

BISMUTH IN THE ERA OF NEW CONCEPTS REGARDING PATHOGENESIS AND TREATMENT OF PEPTIC ULCER

In the mid-twentieth century, peptic ulcer and its complications were a major medical problem in western countries. The importance of peptic ulcer was illustrated by the awarding of a Nobel prize to James Black in 1988 for the discovery of the histamine-2 receptor antagonists (in 1972) and for β-blockers (in 1964). The late 1970s and early 1980s saw the introduction of many new antiulcer agents (eg, sucralfate, histamine-2 receptor antagonists, synthetic prostaglandins, a tablet formulation of De-Nol, and finally, the PPIs). An epidemic of bismuth neurotoxicity occurred in France, which led to the removal of bismuth from many countries.[3,13] However, in

> **Box 1**
> **Pharmacodynamic properties reported for bismuth subcitrate**
>
> - Bactericidal effect on *H pylori*
> - Binding to the ulcer base
> - Inactivation of pepsin
> - Binding of bile acids
> - Stimulation of prostaglandin biosynthesis
> - Suppression of leukotriene biosynthesis
> - Stimulation of complexation with mucus
> - Inhibition of various enzymes
> - Binding of epithelial growth factor
> - Stimulation of lateral epithelial growth

Europe, considerable interest in colloidal bismuth subcitrate continued based on studies showing that both endoscopically and histologically ulcer healing was more complete and recurrences less frequent following treatment with De-Nol compared with other agents. One particularly important comparison of liquid colloidal bismuth subcitrate and cimetidine randomized 46 patients with active duodenal ulcers.[14] Forty patients (25 cimetidine, 15 bismuth) had symptomatic follow-up and 39 had endoscopic follow-up for up to 1 year. Ulcer relapse confirmed by endoscopy occurred in 79% of the cimetidine group compared with 27% of those receiving bismuth. Most importantly, *H pylori* was present at follow-up in 100% of those who received cimetidine, whereas 10 of the 15 receiving bismuth (43%) showed healing of gastritis, elimination of *H pylori*, and no ulcer relapse at the 1-year follow-up. At that time, peptic ulcer disease was thought to be incurable; "once an ulcer, always an ulcer" was the current dogma. Those results showed that the natural history of ulcer might be changed and provided a potential biologic basis for observation of a reduced rate of ulcer relapse following ulcer healing with bismuth subcitrate.[15–22] It also was a harbinger of the results of subsequently published randomized studies proving that *H pylori* eradication prevented duodenal and gastric ulcer recurrences among those not also taking nonsteroidal anti-inflammatory drugs.[23]

The initial trials of bismuth as an antimicrobial therapy for *H pylori* eradication reported *H pylori* eradication rates ranging from 10% to 30%.[12] However, the duration of those early experiments were typically short and subsequent experience has suggested that these were possibly overestimated or changes in the formulation of bismuth subcitrate (eg, from liquid to tablet) may have reduced its effectiveness. Because the liquid formulation was not well accepted by patients, it was replaced by a swallow tablet produced by spray drying the liquid preparation. The fact that long-term follow-up of duodenal ulcer recurrence identified late recurrences and loss of statistical significance compared with H_2-receptor antagonists[18] is consistent with current notions that bismuth alone rarely cures *H pylori* infections and that all currently available preparations are similar in anti-*H pylori* effect. However, head-to-head comparisons of bismuth preparation alone or part of multidrug therapy are generally lacking. As noted above, following the epidemic of bismuth neurotoxicity in France,[3] many countries removed all bismuth preparations from their pharmacopeias, and thus, bismuth compounds are not universally available for the treatment of *H pylori* infections. When used short term as for anti-*H pylori* therapy, bismuth therapy has proven to be both safe and effective.

BISMUTH QUADRUPLE THERAPY FOR *H PYLORI* ERADICATION

Starting in the mid to late 1980s, there were numerous clinical trials attempting to cure *H pylori* infections.[12] When a single antibiotic proved ineffective, dual- and triple-drug therapies were tried, and eventually an effective regimen consisting of bismuth subcitrate, tetracycline, and metronidazole was identified by Tom Borody and colleagues[24] in Australia.[12,25] That original study used bismuth subcitrate 120 mg and tetracycline 500 mg, both 4 times a day, for 28 days and metronidazole 200 mg 4 times a day for 14 days. They reported a success rate of 94 of 100 subjects. Subsequently, metronidazole resistance was found to reduce the regimen's effectiveness. However, the addition of a PPI proved to enhance its effectiveness irrespective of the presence or absence of metronidazole resistance.[26,27] The regimen, often called bismuth quadruple therapy, consists of a PPI, a bismuth, metronidazole, and tetracycline. The dosages, duration of therapy, and administration in relation to meals differ as discussed later.

Antimicrobial resistance generally renders that particular antibiotic ineffective for resistant infections (eg, it functionally drops out of the regimen). The fact that the addition of a PPI appeared to negate the effect of metronidazole resistance suggested that metronidazole was possibly unnecessary and that the combination of a PPI, bismuth, and tetracycline components might suffice. That hypothesis was examined in 44 patients with peptic ulcer disease who received either tetracycline 500 mg and bismuth subsalicylate (Pepto-Bismol) 2 tablets both 4 times a day with or without omeprazole 40 mg in the AM for 14 days. The overall cure rate was 48%, which was clinically unacceptably low. However, the addition of omeprazole was able to approximately double the efficacy of tetracycline and bismuth dual therapy (**Fig. 1**).[28]

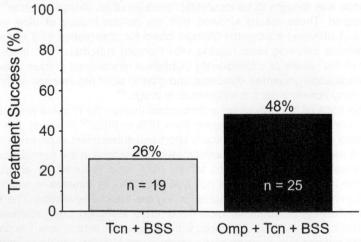

Fig. 1. Effect of removing the metronidazole or the PPI from bismuth quadruple therapy. Peptic ulcer patients received either TCN tetracycline HCl 500 mg, 4 times a day or BSS (bismuth subsalicylate [Pepto-Bismol] 2 tablets 4 times a day) with or without Omp (omeprazole 40 mg in the AM) for 14 days. (*Data from* Al-Assi MT, Genta RM, Graham DY. Short report: omeprazole-tetracycline combinations are inadequate as therapy for *Helicobacter pylori* infection. Aliment Pharmacol Ther 1994;8:259–62.)

Even today, it remains unclear how the PPI helps overcome metronidazole resistance. Metronidazole is a prodrug activated by enzymes within the bacterial cell. Resistance as assessed in vitro is associated with inactivation of one or more of those enzymes. Part of its effectiveness may be topical, and the concentration of metronidazole present in the stomach is very high, suggesting that as yet recognized enzyme pathways in the bacterial cell remain or become active at increased pH. The ability to partially overcome resistance is both metronidazole-dose and treatment-duration dependent.[29–33] It is also unclear whether the ability to overcome the effect of metronidazole resistance is largely restricted to bismuth-containing regimens or even to bismuth–tetracycline-containing regimens. The HOMER study examined omeprazole, metronidazole, and amoxicillin (ie, no bismuth) and also showed an overall effect of dose and duration on effectiveness, but the benefit was not directly related to improved outcomes with resistant strains.[34]

When *H pylori*-infected subjects with pretreatment-confirmed metronidazole-resistant infections received a 14-day bismuth quadruple regimen consisting of tetracycline 500 mg and bismuth subsalicylate (Pepto-Bismol) 2 tablets both 4 times a day with meals, plus metronidazole 500 mg 3 times a day and omeprazole 20 mg in the AM, the cure rate was 92% (**Fig. 2**),[29] which was approximately what was expected in a metronidazole-susceptible population (there was no control group). This direct experiment confirms that the addition of a PPI could partially or possibly completely negate the deleterious effects of metronidazole resistance in bismuth quadruple therapy. Another experiment with 43 metronidazole-resistant strains (77% with minimal inhibitory concentration [MIC] ≥256 by Etest) reported a per-protocol cure rate of 92.1% (81.4% intertion to treat [ITT]).[35] Two subjects dropped out after 7 days and both failed therapy. A large study from China found a large population of subjects with multidrug-resistant *H pylori* (susceptible to amoxicillin and tetracycline) and reported that among

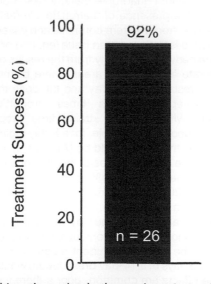

Fig. 2. Effect of 14-day bismuth quadruple therapy in patients with pretreatment-proven metronidazole-resistant infections. Therapy consisted of tetracycline HCl 500 mg and bismuth subsalicylate (Pepto-Bismol) 2 tablets both 4 times a day with meals, plus metronidazole 500 mg 3 times a day and omeprazole 20 mg in the AM. (*Data from* Graham DY, Osato MS, Hoffman J, et al. Metronidazole containing quadruple therapy for infection with metronidazole resistant *Helicobacter pylori*: a prospective study. Aliment Pharmacol Ther 2000;14:745–50.)

101 patient with metronidazole-resistant strains 14-day bismuth quadruple therapy cured 93.1% per protocol, which was similar to the effectiveness of bismuth quadruple therapy, where amoxicillin was substituted for metronidazole (ie, 94.6% of 93 subjects per protocol).[36]

THE EFFECT OF METRONIDAZOLE RESISTANCE AS EXAMINED BY META-ANALYSIS

Several meta-analyses involving bismuth quadruple therapy have focused on understanding the results in terms of antimicrobial resistance (eg,[31–33,37]). The beneficial effect of adding a PPI in relation to metronidazole resistance was confirmed in an analysis of 93 studies (10,178 participants) that showed that metronidazole resistance reduced efficacy of bismuth, metronidazole, and tetracycline therapy (of different durations and dosing) on average by 26%. The reduction was only 14% following the addition of a gastric acid inhibitor, and it was concluded that even in areas with a high prevalence of metronidazole resistance, the quadruple regimen plus a PPI eradicated more than 85% of H pylori infections when given for 10 to 14 days.[37]

CALCULATION OF THE EFFECTIVENESS OF BISMUTH QUADRUPLE THERAPY

In most western countries and in Korea and China, the an unsatisfactory outcome with bismuth quadruple therapy (eg, <90% or <85% treatment success per protocol) can be identified if one examines the duration of therapy, the doses used, patient adherence to the regimen, and whether metronidazole resistance was present. With clarithromycin-containing triple and quadruple therapies, the outcome can be reliably predicted provided one has data concerning the effectiveness of that therapy in relation to antimicrobial resistance (ie, with susceptible strains and with resistance with each individual antimicrobial and with combinations of antimicrobials).[38,39] Similar calculations can theoretically be made for bismuth quadruple therapy based on the duration and the effectiveness of therapy in the presence of metronidazole resistance. Unfortunately, there is a paucity of data even from western countries and essentially none from areas where tetracycline resistance is likely to be an issue (eg, Iran or Turkey).

The data for **Fig. 3** were derived empirically from the results of clinical trials but provides a reasonably accurate estimation in areas where bismuth quadruple therapy produces 90% or greater results with 14-day and full-dose therapy. The formula is ([success rate with susceptible strains times proportion with susceptible strains] + [success rate with resistant strains time proportion with resistant strains] = outcome per protocol). For example, for a 7-day regimen with 25% resistant strains (ie, 75% susceptible), the result would be (75 × 93%) + (25 × 70%) or ~87% per protocol. It shows that the population result (per protocol) is expected to drop to less than 90% with 10-day therapy with 40% metronidazole resistance or less than 90% with 7-day therapy with 20% metronidazole resistance. Intention-to-treat results would be expected to be somewhat lower. The cure rate of those individuals with resistant strains receiving 7- and 10-day therapy would be approximately 70% and 80%, respectively, suggesting that if metronidazole resistance is possibly present and 14-day therapy would be the most prudent recommendation. Poor adherence (eg, the patient taking only 5 days of a 14-day prescription) would have a marked effect on outcome and, as side effects are common, poor adherence is a major issue with bismuth quadruple therapy. Another factor that would influence the outcome is the method used to assess metronidazole resistance. Assessment by Etest tends to overestimate the presence of metronidazole resistance. For example, in one study, 20 of the 37 subjects tested (54%) were judged to be metronidazole resistant by Etest and only 12 were confirmed by agar dilution.[40] In a large study, the change in

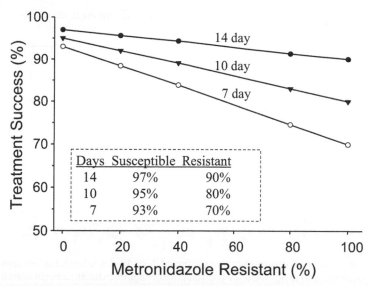

Fig. 3. Empirically derived estimation of effectiveness of 14-day bismuth quadruple therapy in regions where success is known to be dependent on doses, duration, metronidazole resistance, and adherence. The formula is ([success rate with susceptible strains times proportion with susceptible strains] + [success rate with resistant strains time proportion with resistant strains] = outcome per protocol).

susceptibility result was approximately 17%.[41] The authors recommend that for clinical trials, all resistance results with Etest be confirmed with agar dilution.[40]

ADHERENCE (COMPLIANCE) WITH BISMUTH QUADRUPLE THERAPY
Adherence to the Protocol

Many anti-*H pylori* regimens are somewhat complicated and require taking drugs 2 to 4 times daily. In order to achieve the high degrees of success reported in clinical studies, it is important that both the clinician and the patient adhere to the details of successful protocols. Arbitrary changes in the protocol (eg, dose, duration, formulation) are similar to making arbitrary changes in a published recipe for French bread and then being surprised when the product is less than anticipated. **Fig. 4** shows the outcome (ITT) of the bismuth quadruple therapy arms of recent comparative trials with legacy triple therapy.[42] When one examines the details of the studies, one finds that what was called bismuth quadruple therapy often differed in terms of doses given. These studies used either 7 or 10 days to be the same as the triple therapy despite the evidence that all of these regimens do better with 14 days.

From the first part of this article, one would expect outstanding results from bismuth quadruple therapy, and here, neither 7- nor 10-day regimens provided acceptably high intention-to-treat success. An example is a 14-day treatment trial using a formulation in which the antibiotics and bismuth are contained within the same capsules (ie, Pylera) and omeprazole 20 mg 2 times a day.[43] Forty-seven subjects were entered and 12 (25.5%) failed to take the planned 14 days of therapy. The most common reason for early stopping was the presence of an adverse event. As would be expected, treatment success increased as the duration of therapy increased (**Fig. 5, Table 1**).[43] The cure rate ITT was 70% and per protocol (PP) was greater than 95%. All those with metronidazole-resistant strains who completed therapy were cured.

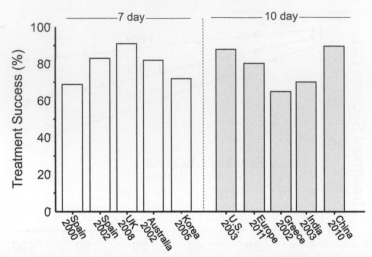

Fig. 4. Intention-to-treat results of recent studies of 7- or 10-day bismuth quadruple therapy with various doses and drugs used for the comparison against clarithromycin-containing triple therapy generally in areas of high clarithromycin and variable metronidazole resistance. (*Data from* Malfertheiner P, Bazzoli F, Delchier JC, et al. *Helicobacter pylori* eradication with a capsule containing bismuth subcitrate potassium, metronidazole, and tetracycline given with omeprazole versus clarithromycin-based triple therapy: a randomised, open-label, non-inferiority, phase 3 trial. Lancet 2011;377:905–13; and original study publications.)

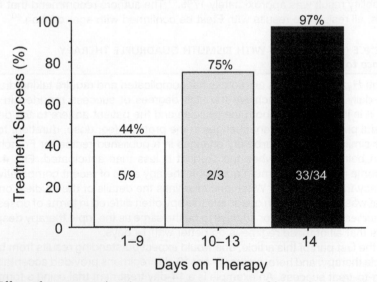

Fig. 5. Effect of treatment duration on treatment success of bismuth quadruple therapy. Therapy consisted of bismuth quadruple therapy (Pylera) plus omeprazole 20 mg 2 times a day for 14 days. Thirty-nine percent of strains cultured were metronidazole resistant. All (100%) of those receiving therapy for 14 days with resistant strains were cured. The duration of therapy was patient-determined based on withdrawal for side effects or other reasons. The number and success for each duration are shown. (*Data from* Salazar CO, Cardenas VM, Reddy RK, et al. Greater than 95% success with 14-day bismuth quadruple anti-*Helicobacter pylori* therapy: a pilot study in US Hispanics. Helicobacter 2012;17:382–9.)

Table 1
Duration of therapy and treatment success

Days Therapy Completed	Status Infected	Status Eradicated	Total	Reason Stopped
2	2[a,b]	0	2	Adverse events
3	1[a]	0	1	—
6	0	2	2	Adverse event
7	1[b]	0	1	Adverse event
8	0	2	2	—
9	1[a]	0	1	Adverse event
10	0	0	0	—
11	1[b]	0	1	Protocol violation
12	0	1	1	—
13	0	2	2	—
14	1[a]	33	34	Completed study
Total	7	40	47	—

[a] Susceptible.
[b] Resistant.

Soon after the introduction of bismuth, metronidazole, and tetracycline therapy, it became apparent that side effects were common; side effects tend to cause a reduced adherence to the regimen prescribed. With the exception of temporary discoloration of the tongue, bismuth is generally an innocuous medication when used for term use therapy. In contrast, tetracycline and metronidazole either separately or together frequently are associated with complaints. As part of the initial development of the regimen, Borody and colleagues[44] examined whether increasing the frequency of administration without increasing the dosages would improve adherence. They compared two 14-day regimens of 4 versus 5 drug administrations per day (between 7 AM and 11 PM). The doses used were 108 mg of bismuth subcitrate in both arms, 500 mg of tetracycline 4 times a day versus 250 mg 5 times daily, and 250 mg of metronidazole 4 times a day versus 200 mg 5 times per day (ie, the total amount of tetracycline was reduced from 2 g to 1.25 g; the dose of metronidazole was 1 g but was less per dose. The antisecretory agent was ranitidine 300 mg at night; resistance was presumably rare). The per-protocol cure rate was slightly higher with the 5-day regimen (96% vs 92%, $P = .07$) (**Fig. 6**).[44] More importantly, side effects were significantly reduced ($P<.001$), suggesting that it is possible to provide a more acceptable regimen. de Boer, who performed many of the initial Dutch trials examining dose, duration, and the use of PPIs, used a 7-point approach of patient education/ motivation starting with taking time to talk to the patient and explaining the rationale. He then went on to explain the potential difficulties and side effects that might occur and provided details about how to take the medications.[45] He and Borody had good but not perfect adherence. It was previously shown that structured counseling and follow-up resulted in improved outcomes with clarithromycin triple therapy.[46] Their results are likely applicable to all H pylori therapies.

One approach to enhance compliance is to enhance convenience. Triple therapy has long been available in dose packs. The US commercial formulation of bismuth quadruple therapy was also formulated in a convenience pack (Helidac) and the newer formulation Pylera is prepackaged into capsules containing bismuth subcitrate potassium, metronidazole, and tetracycline.[42,43] None of these packs have proven to

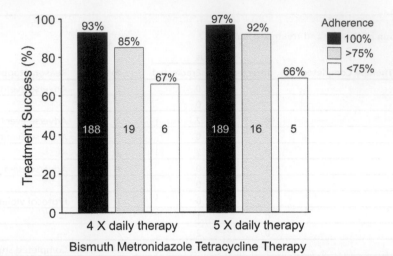

Fig. 6. Results of changing the doses and timing of administration and adherence on outcome of bismuth triple therapy plus ranitidine. Therapy consisted of two 14-day regimens of 4 versus 5 drug administrations per day (between 7 AM and 11 PM). The doses used were 108 mg of bismuth subcitrate in both arms, 500 mg of tetracycline 4 times a day versus 250 mg 5 times daily, and 250 mg of metronidazole 4 times a day versus 200 mg 5 times per day (ie, the total amount of tetracycline was reduced from 2 g to 1.25 g, the dose of metronidazole was 1 g but was less per dose plus ranitidine 300 mg at night). (*Data from* Borody TJ, Brandl S, Andrews P, et al. Use of high efficacy, lower dose triple therapy to reduce side effects of eradicating *Helicobacter pylori*. Am J Gastroenterol 1994;89:33–8.)

improve adherence or result in a clear reduction in side effects. Studies of compliance have not shown that reduced adherence was related to the number of tablets per day required for *H pylori* quadruple therapy.[32,37] The number of tablets or capsules per day can also be reduced in traditional therapy by using 500 mg per capsule of tetracycline and of metronidazole and bismuth 2 times a day (eg,[36]) to be equal to or less than that needed for current prepackaged quadruple therapy products.

All *H pylori* regimens are associated with side effects. A meta-analysis recently compared the side effects of bismuth quadruple therapy with other common *H pylori* regimens and reported that side effects were not greater with the exception of the cosmetic event, black stools. This meta-analysis confirmed the results of prior meta-analyses.[31,32,37,47–49] Despite these encouraging words, those taking care of patients with *H pylori* recognized that all the regimens have a high incidence of side effects and that failure to motivate the patients regarding finishing the regimen often results in dropouts, and in clinical studies, loss to follow-up[42,43] that can likely be reduced by patient education.[50]

HOW TO MAKE BISMUTH QUADRUPLE THERAPY MORE ACCEPTABLE

As noted previously, Borody and colleagues[44] attempted to reduce the side effects by changing the frequency of dose administration and the doses with some success. The current standard regimen consists of a PPI 2 times a day, tetracycline 500 mg 4 times a day, at least 1500 of metronidazole, and bismuth 4 times a day. Shorter durations have been recommended, but this is generally a marketing ploy because bismuth quadruple therapy is generally reserved for patients in whom metronidazole resistance is likely, and duration and doses are important for excellent outcome.[51] Although

14 days of full-dose therapy might be ideal, duration and dose of metronidazole have not been systematically examined in relation to metronidazole resistance. There are in fact some data suggesting that the doses considered ideal may be more than necessary. For example, there are several trials in which bismuth quadruple therapy was administered twice rather than 3 or 4 times a day (**Table 2**).[40,52–58] The authors show data from 11 arms and 9 studies (see **Table 2**). Cure rates for 10- to 14-day studies were more than 86% PP except in one instance, where a low-dose PPI was used. Seven days appeared to be possibly inferior to 10 or 14 days. Drugs included bismuth subcitrate and bismuth subsalicylate, 1 to 1.5 g of tetracycline, and 800 to 1000 mg of metronidazole along with full-dose PPI except in the one instance, where lansoprazole 15 mg 2 times a day was used. Studies were done in high (China, Turkey, and Italy [Sardinia]) and moderate metronidazole resistance areas (Unites States). Clearly, comparative studies are needed to assess efficacy as well as side effects in comparison to 3 and 4 times daily bismuth quadruple therapy and to address whether AM and PM and noon and PM administrations are equivalent. In these studies, drugs were given with or after meals. The was also one study of 2 times a day omeprazole 20 mg, amoxicillin 1 g as a substitute for tetracycline, tinidazole 500 mg, and bismuth subcitrate 240 mg given every 12 hours for only 7 days that achieved a PP cure rate of 86% (84.1% ITT) that was not followed up with another study of longer duration.[59]

These results cannot be considered generalizable until the results can be correlated with metronidazole susceptibility; further studies without concomitant susceptibility testing should be strongly discouraged. Twice-a-day therapy offers the potential of effectiveness, less cost, and fewer side effects.

DOXYCYCLINE

The original experience with doxycycline was that it could not substitute successfully for tetracycline in bismuth triple therapy.[60] Since that time, it has been recommended not to substitute doxycycline for tetracycline. However, randomized trials comparing tetracycline and doxycycline in full-dose 14-day traditional bismuth quadruple therapy are lacking. In the United States, tetracycline has often become largely unavailable, and many pharmacies attempted to substitute doxycycline for tetracycline HCl. In the authors' experience, that substitution led to unsatisfactory results. Most available doxycycline data relate to substitution of doxycycline for tetracycline and amoxicillin for metronidazole all given 2 times a day[61–63] (**Table 3**). The 3 studies from Italy suggest that this might be an effective regimen, whereas the one from China did not. The study from China, a high metronidazole resistance country, also compared 10-day therapy with doxycycline or tetracycline and the results were poor.[64] Further studies with 14-day therapy and with 200 mg of doxycycline 2 times a day are needed. However, to be useful, they must also provide susceptibility testing so that the results can be correlated with metronidazole susceptibility/resistance. Before doxycycline can be recommended as part of traditional bismuth quadruple therapy, studies that include susceptibility data are needed; until then, doxycycline is probably best avoided.

EXAMINATION OF OUTCOME IN REGIONS WHERE BISMUTH QUADRUPLE THERAPY FREQUENTLY FAILS (EG, TURKEY AND IRAN)

In the west, in China, and in Korea, the results with bismuth triple therapy generally follow expectations, and poor results can be understood when one takes into account the doses used, the duration of therapy, and patient adherence. However, even when these factors are taken into account, the results with bismuth quadruple therapy have often been unsatisfactory in Turkey and Iran[65–74] (**Table 4**). Data from Turkey are

Table 2
Summary of twice-a-day bismuth-containing traditional quadruple therapies

Year	Location	Bismuth[a]	Tetracyc	Metro	Meals	PPI**	Days	No.	PP%	ITT%	Ref.
1997	USA	BSS 524 b.i.d.	500 b.i.d.	500 b.i.d.	AM, PM	L 15 b.i.d.	10	46	75	70	56
2002	Italy	BSC 240 b.i.d.	500 b.i.d.	500 b.i.d.	Noon, PM	P 20 b.i.d.	14	118	98	95	52
2003	Italy	BSC 240 b.i.d.	500 b.i.d.	500 b.i.d.	Noon, PM	P 20 b.i.d.	14	71	97	93	53
2004	USA	BSS 524 b.i.d.	500 b.i.d.	500 b.i.d.	AM, PM	R 20 b.i.d.	14	37	92.3	92.3	56
2006	Italy	BSC 240 b.i.d.	500 b.i.d.	500 b.i.d.	AM, PM	E 20 b.i.d.	10	95	95	91	55
2009	China	BSC 220 b.i.d.	750 b.i.d.	400 b.i.d.	AM, PM	P 40 b.i.d.	7	43	82.9	79.1	57
2009	China[a]	BSC 220 b.i.d.	750 b.i.d.	400 b.i.d.	AM, PM	P 40 b.i.d.	10	45	90.9	88.9	57
2010	China[a]	BSC 220 b.i.d.	750 b.i.d.	400 b.i.d.	AM, PM	P 40 b.i.d.	10	85	91.6.	89.9	58
2011	Italy	BSC 240 b.i.d.	500 b.i.d.	500 b.i.d.	Noon, PM	P 20 b.i.d.	14	202	98	92	109
2011	Italy	BSC 240 b.i.d.	500 b.i.d.	500 b.i.d.	Noon, PM	P 20 b.i.d.	10	215	95	92	109
2013	Turkey	BSC 600 b.i.d.	500 b.i.d.	500 b.i.d.	AM, PM	O 20 b.i.d.	14	38	86.8	73.3	110
2005	Iran	BSC 240 b.i.d.	500 b.i.d.	500 b.i.d.	AM, PM	O 20 b.i.d.	14	76	-	76.3	111
2006	Iran[a]	BSC 240 b.i.d.	750 b.i.d.	500 b.i.d.	AM, PM	O 20 b.i.d.	3	40	54	50	75
2006	Iran[a]	BSC 240 b.i.d.	750 b.i.d.	500 b.i.d.	AM, PM	O 20 b.i.d.	7	41	45.9	41.4	75
2006	Iran[a]	BSC 240 b.i.d.	750 b.i.d.	500 b.i.d.	AM, PM	O 20 b.i.d.	14	40	40	35	75

Doses are in milligrams.

Abbreviations: BSC, bismuth subcitrate; BSS, bismuth subsalicylate; L, lansoprazole; Metro, metronidazole; O, omeprazole; P, pantoprazole; R, rabeprazole; Tetracyc, tetracycline.

[a] Extension of the same study.

** Proton pump inhibitor.

Table 3

Summary of twice-a-day proton pump inhibitor, bismuth, doxycycline, and amoxicillin containing quadruple therapies

Year	Location	Bismuth	Doxycyc	Amox	Meals	PPI**	Days	No.	PP	ITT	Ref.
2004	Italy	BSC 240 b.i.d.	100 b.i.d.	1000 b.i.d.	AM, PM	O 20 b.i.d.	7	89	92	91	61
2009	Turkey	RBC 400 b.i.d.	100 b.i.d.	1000 b.i.d.	AM, PM	Ranit b.i.d.	14	57	45.7	36.9	112
2012	China	BSC 220 b.i.d.	100 b.i.d.	1000 b.i.d.	AM, PM	E 20 b.i.d.	10	43	72.5	64.1	64
2015	Italy	BSC 240 b.i.d.	100 b.i.d.	1000 b.i.d.	AM, PM	E 20 b.i.d.	10	52	90.1	88.5	63
2015	Italy	BSC 240 b.i.d.	200 b.i.d.	1000 b.i.d.	AM, PM	E 20 b.i.d.	10	51	94	92.1	63

Doses are in milligrams.

Abbreviations: Amox, amoxicillin; BSC, bismuth subcitrate; Doxycyc, doxycycline; L, larsoprazole; O, omeprazole; P, pantoprazole; R, rabeprazole; Ranit, ranitidine bismuth citrate.

** Proton pump inhibitor.

Table 4
Summary of bismuth and metronidazole containing quadruple therapies in Turkey and Iran

Year	Location	Bismuth	Tetracyc	Metro	PPI**	Days	No.	PP	ITT	Ref.
2004	Turkey	BSC 300 q.i.d.	500 q.i.d.	500 q.i.d.	O 20 b.i.d.	14	32	63.5	63.5	65
2004	Turkey	RBC 400 b.i.d.	1000 b.i.d.	500 t.i.d.	None	14	27	44.4	44.4	66
2007	Turkey	BSS 200 q.i.d.	500 q.i.d.	500 t.i.d.	L 30 b.i.d.	14	120	82.3	70	67
2009	Turkey	BSC 300 q.i.d.	500 q.i.d.	500 b.i.d.	L 30 b.i.d.	10	104	54.9	47.1	68
2010	Turkey	BSC 400 b.i.d.	500 q.i.d.	500 t.i.d.	P 40 b.i.d.	14	92	86.5	83.6	69
2011	Turkey	BSS 200 q.i.d.	500 q.i.d.	500 t.i.d.	L 30 b.i.d.	14	100	82.3	70	70
2013	Turkey	BSC 300 q.i.d.	500 q.i.d.	500 t.i.d.	L 30 b.i.d.	14	25	92	92	71
2014	Turkey	BSC 120 q.i.d.	500 q.i.d.	500 t.i.d.	R 20 b.i.d.	14	40	76.5	77.5	72
2014	Iran	BSC 240 q.i.d	500 q.i.d.	500 q.i.d.	O 20 b.i.d.	14	18	89	89	73
2014	Iran	BSC 240 b.i.d.	500 q.i.d.	250 q.i.d.	O 20 b.i.d.	14	55	72	?	74

Doses are in milligrams.
Abbreviations: BSC, bismuth subcitrate; BSS, bismuth subsalicylate; L, lansoprazole; Metro, metronidazole; O, omeprazole; P, pantoprazole; R, rabeprazole; Tetracyc, tetracycline.
** Proton pump inhibitor.

especially interesting because there have been several studies that used full-dose 14-day duration and yet the results have been poor (see **Table 4**). The recent study by Songur and colleagues[68] is particularly interesting. They treated approximately 100 subjects with bismuth quadruple therapy. The study was randomized and used standard dose PPI, full-dose tetracycline, but only 1 g of metronidazole (500 mg 2 times a day) and for only 10 days despite this being a high metronidazole-resistance area. They reported acceptable compliance but achieved a cure rate of only 54.9% PP.[68] Importantly, another group was randomized to receive PPI and antibiotics but no bismuth and achieved essentially the same result (60%) as when the regimen included bismuth (**Fig. 7**, see **Table 4**).[68] Bismuth provided no additional benefit to antibiotics, and PPI suggested the bismuth preparation used might have been biologically inactive. Fortunately, they also randomized a group to receive traditional PPI-BMT (bismuth metronidazole tetracycline) plus a second bismuth preparation, ranitidine bismuth citrate 400 mg 2 times a day (ie, the 5-drug regimen PPI-BMT-RBC [ranitidine bismuth citrate]) again with no significant additional benefit (ie, 64% cured) (see **Fig. 7**).[68] Unfortunately, no susceptibility testing was done to assess metronidazole resistance, tetracycline resistance, and combined metronidazole and tetracycline resistance. The drugs were as follows: the bismuth was DE-NOL, obtained from Genesis/Zentiva; the tetracycline HCl was in 500-mg capsules from Mustafa Nevzat, and the metronidazole was tablets from Eczacibasi (Yildiran Songur, personal communication, 2014).

There are few publications regarding antimicrobial susceptibility to metronidazole and tetracycline available from Turkey.[75] However, a good number are available from Iran.[64,76–86] In both countries, metronidazole resistance is high and widespread.

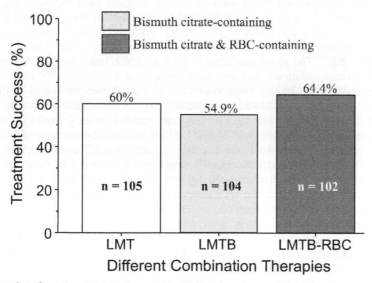

Fig. 7. Results of randomized 14-day trial in Turkey showing poor results irrespective of the addition of bismuth. Therapy consisted of 10-day regimens consisting of lansoprazole 30 mg 2 times a day metronidazole 500 mg 2 times a day, tetracycline 500 mg 4 times a day (LMT) with more traditional bismuth quadruple therapy (LMTB) and that regimen with the addition of ranitidine bismuth subcitrate 400 mg 2 times a day (LMTB-RBC). (*Data from* Songur Y, Senol A, Balkarli A, et al. Triple or quadruple tetracycline-based therapies versus standard triple treatment for *Helicobacter pylori* treatment. Am J Med Sci 2009;338:50–3.)

In contrast to most other regions, tetracycline resistance is relatively common (eg, ~10%). Although there are essentially no data regarding the effects of tetracycline resistance on bismuth quadruple therapy, the authors suspect it might be a critical variable. The general rule of antimicrobial therapy is that when the same drugs are used, the results are similar everywhere such that knowledge from one region is transferable to any other region. The general lack of pretreatment susceptibility testing worldwide has been the major factor preventing tailoring therapy based on the local or regional pattern of antimicrobial susceptibility. Unexplained and unexplainable treatment failures or successes add data but not useful knowledge. Studies of antimicrobial therapy for *H pylori*, especially comparative studies that do not include the information needed to explain the results, are likely not ethical because no generalizable conclusions are possible.

BISMUTH, TETRACYCLINE, AMOXICILLIN, PROTON PUMP INHIBITORS QUADRUPLE THERAPY

Amoxicillin was found not be inferior to metronidazole in bismuth triple therapy.[32,87] Its role in quadruple therapy has not been extensively studied[88–90] (**Table 5**). As noted previously, in China the combination of bismuth subcitrate 2 times a day, tetracycline 500 mg 4 times a day, and high-dose amoxicillin (1000 mg 3 times a day) for 14 days cured 94.6% of 93 subjects per protocol.[36] Additional studies of 14-day therapy are needed before a reliable estimation of its value can be rendered.

BISMUTH SEQUENTIAL THERAPIES

Sequentially administered drugs were attempted in some early regimens (eg, Logan and colleagues[91] in 1994); however, the first true sequential therapy was a bismuth-containing regimen used to treat a patient who had failed therapy with then standard bismuth, metronidazole, tetracycline triple therapy (n = 31) or dual PPI plus amoxicillin therapy (n = 88).[92] The study was done in Greece, which has a high background rate of metronidazole resistance and was typically an outlier in terms of cure rates from BMT triple therapy.[32] The regimen consisted of 60 mg of omeprazole and 2 g of amoxicillin days 1 through 10, followed by metronidazole 1.5 g and bismuth citrate 120 mg 4 times a day for 10 days with the bismuth being continued for 6 weeks (ie, until day 52). The cure rate per protocol was 95% (113/119). Seven subjects were lost to follow-up and 5 withdrew because of side effects (4%) and thus ITT analysis yielded 85%. More recently, Uygun and colleagues[93] proposed a different bismuth sequential regimen consisting of pantoprazole 40 mg and bismuth subcitrate 300 mg 2 times a day both for 14 days, amoxicillin 1 g 2 times a day for the first 7 days, and tetracycline 500 mg 4 times a day and metronidazole 500 mg 3 times a day, both for the last 7 days. One hundred forty-two subjects entered, and the per-protocol cure rate was 92% (ITT 81%, largely due to loss of follow-up). A prior study by the same group of 14-day PPI, bismuth, amoxicillin, tetracycline concomitant regimen from Turkey with 100 subjects achieved a per-protocol cure rate of 89.7%.[90]

INFORMATION NEEDED TO OBTAIN GENERALIZABLE RESULTS

As a general rule, data needed to explain poor results should be collected and published. When unexpected poor results occur, one should provide results in relation to antimicrobial susceptibility/resistance. In this era of generic drugs, one should also provide details about the manufacture of the drugs used because fake and inferior drugs are now widely available, especially in developing countries. In the past, when

Table 5
Summary of bismuth, tetracycline, and amoxicillin containing quadruple therapies

Year	Location	Bismuth[a]	Tetracy	Amox	PPI**	Days	No.	PP	ITT	Ref.
2003	Taiwan	BSC 120 t.i.d.	500 q.i.d.	1000 b.i.d.	O 20 b.i.d.	7	50	88.6	78	88
2009	Turkey	RBC 400 b.i.d.	500 q.i.d.	1000 b.i.d.	Ranit b.i.d.	14	58	40.5	34.5	112
2011	Taiwan	BSC 120 q.i.d.	500 q.i.d.	500 q.i.c.	E 40 b.i.d.	7	58	64	62	113
2006	Korea	BSC 300 q.i.d.	500 q.i.d.	1000 b.i.d.[a]	P 40 b.i.d.	7	29	17.4	16	89
2011	Turkey	BSS 300 q.i.d.	500 q.i.d.	1000 b.id.	E 40 b.i.d.	14	100	89.7	79	90

Doses are in milligrams.
Abbreviations: Amox, amoxicillin; BSC, bismuth subcitrate; E, esomeprazole; O, omeprazole; P, pantoprazole; Ranit, ranitidine bismuth citrate; Tetracy, tetracycline.
[a] Amoxicillin-claulanate.
** Proton pump inhibitor.

faced with unexpectedly poor results, the authors have confirmed the potency of the antibiotics used before publishing the results. They propose a checklist for planning and reporting bismuth quadruple studies to ensure that the results will be interpretable and generalizable (**Box 2**). **Table 6** shows the results of the use of a checklist to study why there was considerable variability in results from Korea.[30,94–103]

ISSUES RIPE FOR SYSTEMATIC STUDY
Relation of Drug Administration and Meals

The relation between treatment outcome and drug administration in relation to meals remains largely unstudied. This issue encompasses the proportion of the benefit derived from the topical action of the drugs versus the systemic antimicrobial activity. It has been proposed that administration with meals will enhance retention within the stomach and distribution of the drugs over the surface of the stomach. These potential benefits come with dilution of the drug concentration by the food and liquids ingested as well as potential binding of the drugs to food components or drug components (eg, bismuth and tetracycline). Pharmacists will often warn patients to separate the ingestion of tetracycline from food or milk. Those who advocate taking the drugs with meals must also caution patients to ignore that warning. Although the use of intravenously administered drugs has not been studied systematically, at a minimum, it has not shown any advantage, and 1-hour topical therapy in which the duodenum was blocked with a balloon proved effective in most patients.[104] Often the relation of drug administration and meals is not reported. However, success and failures have been reported with many different combinations of before, during, and after meals but not in relation to the presence of metronidazole susceptibility. Similarly, the effectiveness of formulation has achieved little attention. With amoxicillin-PPI dual therapy, there seemed to be no advantage to administration of capsules before meals; however, there seemed to be an advantage of using a liquid formulation of amoxicillin.[105,106] This observation has not been followed up or systematically examined

---

Box 2
Checklist for bismuth quadruple treatment trials

- Pretreatment susceptibility results for metronidazole and tetracycline
- Confirmation of Etest-determined metronidazole resistance by agar dilution
- Treatment failures in relation to the number of days of full doses of medicine taken
- Effect of the MIC of metronidazole on treatment failure
- Effect of the MIC of tetracycline on treatment failure
- Names and location of manufacturer of each component of the treatment regimen
- Dosing for each drug in relation to meals and time of day
- Treatment results in relation to resistance for each antibiotic and combination of antibiotics
- Results should include several different subgroups, including:
  - Intention to treat (all who received at least one dose)
  - Modified intention to treat (all those with a determination of outcome)
  - Per protocol (all those who completed the study)
  - Per protocol per adherence (results for those taking drugs for different number of days such as <7, >7 but <10, 10, >10 but <14, and 14 days).

Table 6
Use of a checklist to identify possible reasons for lower than expected results in some clinical trials in Korea

	Factors that Affect the Eradication Rate	Possibility of Affecting the Results in Koreans
Regimen	Drugs used (manufacturer)	Low (to be considered as less important factor because there are not that many manufacturers. Most of the Korean studies used similar quadruple drugs provided by the same company.)
	Dose, frequency (interval), formulation (tablet, capsule), duration	Low: dose, interval, formulation High: duration (Korean papers with 14 d showed better eradication rates than those with 7 d, although few studies showed similar eradication rates.)
	Relation to meals	Low (most of the studies recommended after the meals)
	PPI, mucolytics, probiotics	High: PPI (type of PPI differs greatly between the studies) Uncertain: other medications (insufficient data in Korea)
Study	Diagnosis methods used before and after eradication	High (due to the risk of false urea breath test [UBT] results)
	Antimicrobial resistance	High (resistance rates differ between the provinces)
	Odds of reinfection	Low (most of the reinfections might be recrudescences)
Patient	Compliance with instructions	High (although most of the patients followed the instructions, approximately 10%–20% skipped due to busy schedule or side effects of the drug)
	Side effects of medications	High
	Genetic polymorphisms that affect drug metabolism	Low (most of the Korean genetic studies show that there is not that much difference among Koreans)

for other regimens. Nonetheless, drug administration should be specified, and the issue is worthy of further study.

Reduction of Side Effects with Bismuth Quadruple Therapy

Possibilities include administration in relation to meals, dose reduction of the more noxious components (tetracycline and metronidazole) directly, or altering the frequency of administration. As noted above, there are data that twice-a-day dosing may provide a high cure rate with fewer side effects and accomplishes a reduction in total antibiotic dose. An advance would need to be proven in the presence of metronidazole resistance and could be most efficiently examined in randomized trials in patients with proven metronidazole resistance as confirmed by agar dilution susceptibility tests. Ideally, the subjects should be treatment naïve because it is as yet unclear whether metronidazole resistance arising from recent treatment failure with a metronidazole-containing regimen is identical in outcome to treatment-naïve subjects. At least, the analysis should also look at the 2 groups separately and in addition in relation to the MIC (eg, <256 or >256 µg/mL).

Studies that are needed are morning and evening versus noon and evening twice-a-day therapy, the best twice-a-day regimen versus 4 times a day, and depending on the results, possibly 3 times a day versus 4 times a day therapy. For 4 times a day therapy, it appears likely that one can reduce the dosage of tetracycline to approximately 1 g without loss of effectiveness, whereas at least 1.5 g of metronidazole appears best. Because twice-a-day therapy has only 1 g of metronidazole and 1 g of tetracycline, it would seem that lower-dose metronidazole should suffice, but the current data suggest otherwise. Only randomized studies in metronidazole-resistant infection can address the question. Studies from China and elsewhere have clearly confirmed that twice-a-day bismuth therapy is sufficient.[107]

PROTON PUMP INHIBITORS DOSAGE

With PPI, amoxicillin, clarithromycin triple therapy, higher-dose PPI therapy (eg, double dose) typically improves outcome. The effectiveness of both amoxicillin and clarithromycin is greater at higher pH. If the pH is consistently greater than 6, the clarithromycin is often no longer needed. However, tetracycline and metronidazole are relatively pH-insensitive antimicrobials. The interaction of bismuth salts with acid leads to the formation of bismuth oxychloride, which some think is the antimicrobially active form. The fact that PPI adjuvant therapy helps overcome metronidazole suggests that higher doses may be better. Systematic studies are needed.

EFFICIENT STUDY DESIGN

Efficient study design implies that the variables are controlled as much as possible and that stopping rules are in place to limit exposure when it becomes clear that a regimen cannot succeed.[108] The use of stopping rules allows most efficient use of resources and has been used successfully with bismuth quadruple therapy.[63]

RECOMMENDATIONS

All therapy should be guided by the regional, local, and patient-specific antimicrobial resistance patterns and knowledge about the effectiveness of anti-*H pylori* regimens available locally. Patient-specific information is obtained from knowledge of about resistance patterns and the patient's history of antimicrobial use or by testing directly (eg, by culture) or indirectly (by molecular testing of stool or biopsy samples) for resistance. Bismuth quadruple therapy is an excellent alternate first-line regimen in regions where it has proven to be effective. However, generally 14-day therapy with a PPI, amoxicillin, and clarithromycin or metronidazole or concomitant therapy with all 4 drugs is better tolerated. The primary indications for bismuth quadruple therapy are intolerance to amoxicillin (eg, allergy) and prior failure with a PPI-amoxicillin-containing triple therapy.[38,39]

If the infection is susceptible to metronidazole, a 10-day course is satisfactory; however, in low metronidazole-resistant areas, triple therapy with a PPI, amoxicillin, and metronidazole for 14 days is effective and generally better tolerated. The main role of bismuth quadruple therapy is for those intolerant to penicillin derivatives or the presence of modest to high levels of metronidazole and clarithromycin resistance. In the presence of metronidazole resistance, doses and duration are critical for good treatment success. Recommended therapy is a double-dose PPI (40 mg of omeprazole or equivalent) at least 1500 mg of metronidazole, 1500 to 2000 mg of tetracycline 4 times a day, and a bismuth salt at least twice a day for 14 days. Unless proven effective in the local population, doxycycline is not recommended as a substitute for tetracycline hydrochloride.

The decision to treat an *H pylori* infection carries with it an obligation to provide specific patient education and counseling regarding the goals of therapy, the side effects possibly anticipated (eg, abdominal pain, nausea, black stools with bismuth), and the necessity to complete the full 14 days. Bismuth quadruple therapy still remains to be optimized but this must be done in relation to metronidazole and, for some regions, tetracycline resistance.

In most of the world, resistance to amoxicillin or tetracycline is rare and, in contrast to metronidazole, clarithromycin, and fluoroquinolones, resistance to amoxicillin or tetracycline rarely develops after failed therapy. As such, treatment failure does not preclude using either or both again after treatment failure with bismuth quadruple therapy.[97]

REFERENCES

1. Eberle J. A treatise of the materia medica and therapeutics. 4th edition. Philadelphia: Crigg & Elliot; 1834.
2. Brinton W. Ulcer of the stomach successfully treated. Assoc Med J 1855;3: 1125–6.
3. Salvador JA, Figueiredo SA, Pinto RM, et al. Bismuth compounds in medicinal chemistry. Future Med Chem 2012;4:1495–523.
4. DuPont HL. Bismuth subsalicylate in the treatment and prevention of diarrheal disease. Drug Intell Clin Pharm 1987;21:687–93.
5. Graham DY, Estes MK, Gentry LO. Double-blind comparison of bismuth subsalicylate and placebo in the prevention and treatment of enterotoxigenic Escherichia coli-induced diarrhea in volunteers. Gastroenterology 1983;85:1017–22.
6. Graham DY, Klein PD, Opekun AR, et al. In vivo susceptibility of *Campylobacter pylori*. Am J Gastroenterol 1989;84:233–8.
7. Graham DY, Evans DG. Prevention of diarrhea caused by enterotoxigenic Escherichia coli: lessons learned with volunteers. Rev Infect Dis 1990; 12(Suppl 1):S68–72.
8. Hall DW. Review of the modes of action of colloidal bismuth subcitrate. Scand J Gastroenterol Suppl 1989;157:3–6.
9. Koo J, Ho J, Lam SK, et al. Selective coating of gastric ulcer by tripotassium dicitrato bismuthate in the rat. Gastroenterology 1982;82:864–70.
10. Sandha GS, LeBlanc R, van Zanten SJ, et al. Chemical structure of bismuth compounds determines their gastric ulcer healing efficacy and anti-*Helicobacter pylori* activity. Dig Dis Sci 1998;43:2727–32.
11. Wieriks J, Hespe W, Jaitly KD, et al. Pharmacological properties of colloidal bismuth subcitrate (CBS, DE-NOL). Scand J Gastroenterol Suppl 1982;80:11–6.
12. Borsch GM, Graham DY. Helicobacter pylori. Handbook of Experimental Pharmacology. In: Collen MJ, Benjamin SB, editors. Pharmacology of peptic ulcer disease, vol. 99. Berlin: Springer-Verlag; 1991. p. 107–48.
13. Lambert JR. Pharmacology of bismuth-containing compounds. Rev Infect Dis 1991;13(Suppl 8):S691–5.
14. Coghlan JG, Gilligan D, Humphries H, et al. *Campylobacter pylori* and recurrence of duodenal ulcers–a 12-month follow-up study. Lancet 1987;2:1109–11.
15. Martin DF, Hollanders D, May SJ, et al. Difference in relapse rates of duodenal ulcer after healing with cimetidine or tripotassium dicitrato bismuthate. Lancet 1981;1:7–10.
16. Vantrappen G, Schuurmans P, Rutgeerts P, et al. A comparative study of colloidal bismuth subcitrate and cimetidine on the healing and recurrence of duodenal ulcer. Scand J Gastroenterol Suppl 1982;80:23–30.

17. Miller JP, Hollanders D, Ravenscroft MM, et al. Likelihood of relapse of duodenal ulcer after initial treatment with cimetidine or colloidal bismuth subcitrate. Scand J Gastroenterol Suppl 1982;80:39–42.

18. Kang JY, Piper DW. Cimetidine and colloidal bismuth in treatment of chronic duodenal ulcer. Comparison of initial healing and recurrence after healing. Digestion 1982;23:73–9.

19. Shreeve DR, Klass HJ, Jones PE. Comparison of cimetidine and tripotassium dicitrato bismuthate in healing and relapse of duodenal ulcers. Digestion 1983;28: 96–101.

20. Bianchi PG, Lazzaroni M, Petrillo M, et al. Relapse rates in duodenal ulcer patients formerly treated with bismuth subcitrate or maintained with cimetidine. Lancet 1984;2:698.

21. Hamilton I, O'Connor HJ, Wood NC, et al. Healing and recurrence of duodenal ulcer after treatment with tripotassium dicitrato bismuthate (TDB) tablets or cimetidine. Gut 1986;27:106–10.

22. Bianchi PB, Lazzaroni M, Parente F, et al. The influence of colloidal bismuth subcitrate on duodenal ulcer relapse. Scand J Gastroenterol Suppl 1986;122:35–8.

23. Graham DY, Lew GM, Klein PD, et al. Effect of treatment of *Helicobacter pylori* infection on the long-term recurrence of gastric or duodenal ulcer. A randomized, controlled study. Ann Intern Med 1992;116:705–8.

24. Borody TJ, Cole P, Noonan S, et al. Recurrence of duodenal ulcer and *Campylobacter pylori* infection after eradication. Med J Aust 1989;151:431–5.

25. George LL, Borody TJ, Andrews P, et al. Cure of duodenal ulcer after eradication of *Helicobacter pylori*. Med J Aust 1990;153:145–9.

26. Borody TJ, Andrews P, Fracchia G, et al. Omeprazole enhances efficacy of triple therapy in eradicating *Helicobacter pylori*. Gut 1995;37:477–81.

27. de Boer W, Driessen W, Jansz A, et al. Effect of acid suppression on efficacy of treatment for *Helicobacter pylori* infection. Lancet 1995;345:817–20.

28. Al-Assi MT, Genta RM, Graham DY. Short report: omeprazole-tetracycline combinations are inadequate as therapy for *Helicobacter pylori* infection. Aliment Pharmacol Ther 1994;8:259–62.

29. Graham DY, Osato MS, Hoffman J, et al. Metronidazole containing quadruple therapy for infection with metronidazole resistant *Helicobacter pylori*: a prospective study. Aliment Pharmacol Ther 2000;14:745–50.

30. Lee BH, Kim N, Hwang TJ, et al. Bismuth-containing quadruple therapy as second-line treatment for *Helicobacter pylori* infection: effect of treatment duration and antibiotic resistance on the eradication rate in Korea. Helicobacter 2010;15:38–45.

31. Fischbach LA, Goodman KJ, Feldman M, et al. Sources of variation of *Helicobacter pylori* treatment success in adults worldwide: a meta-analysis. Int J Epidemiol 2002;31:128–39.

32. Fischbach LA, van ZS, Dickason J. Meta-analysis: the efficacy, adverse events, and adherence related to first-line anti-*Helicobacter pylori* quadruple therapies. Aliment Pharmacol Ther 2004;20:1071–82.

33. van der Wouden EJ, Thijs JC, van Zwet AA, et al. The influence of in vitro nitroimidazole resistance on the efficacy of nitroimidazole-containing anti-*Helicobacter pylori* regimens: a meta-analysis. Am J Gastroenterol 1999;94:1751–9.

34. Bardhan K, Bayerdorffer E, Veldhuyzen van Zanten SJ, et al. The HOMER study: the effect of increasing the dose of metronidazole when given with omeprazole and amoxicillin to cure *Helicobacter pylori* infection. Helicobacter 2000;5: 196–201.

35. Miehlke S, Kirsch C, Schneider-Brachert W, et al. A prospective, randomized study of quadruple therapy and high-dose dual therapy for treatment of *Helicobacter pylori* resistant to both metronidazole and clarithromycin. Helicobacter 2003;8:310–9.

36. Liang X, Xu X, Zheng Q, et al. Efficacy of bismuth-containing quadruple therapies for clarithromycin-, metronidazole-, and fluoroquinolone-resistant *Helicobacter pylori* infections in a prospective study. Clin Gastroenterol Hepatol 2013;11:802–7.

37. Fischbach L, Evans EL. Meta-analysis: the effect of antibiotic resistance status on the efficacy of triple and quadruple first-line therapies for *Helicobacter pylori*. Aliment Pharmacol Ther 2007;26:343–57.

38. Graham DY, Lee YC, Wu MS. Rational *Helicobacter pylori* therapy: evidence-based medicine rather than medicine-based evidence. Clin Gastroenterol Hepatol 2014;12:177–86.

39. Wu JY, Liou JM, Graham DY. Evidence-based recommendations for successful *Helicobacter pylori* treatment. Expert Rev Gastroenterol Hepatol 2014;8:21–8.

40. Graham DY, Belson G, Abudayyeh S, et al. Twice daily (mid-day and evening) quadruple therapy for *H. pylori* infection in the United States. Dig Liver Dis 2004;36:384–7.

41. Osato MS, Reddy R, Reddy SG, et al. Comparison of the Etest and the NCCLS-approved agar dilution method to detect metronidazole and clarithromycin resistant *Helicobacter pylori*. Int J Antimicrob Agents 2001;17:39–44.

42. Malfertheiner P, Bazzoli F, Delchier JC, et al. *Helicobacter pylori* eradication with a capsule containing bismuth subcitrate potassium, metronidazole, and tetracycline given with omeprazole versus clarithromycin-based triple therapy: a randomised, open-label, non-inferiority, phase 3 trial. Lancet 2011;377:905–13.

43. Salazar CO, Cardenas VM, Reddy RK, et al. Greater than 95% success with 14-day bismuth quadruple anti-*Helicobacter pylori* therapy: a pilot study in US Hispanics. Helicobacter 2012;17:382–9.

44. Borody TJ, Brandl S, Andrews P, et al. Use of high efficacy, lower dose triple therapy to reduce side effects of eradicating *Helicobacter pylori*. Am J Gastroenterol 1994;89:33–8.

45. de Boer WA. How to achieve a near 100% cure rate for *H. pylori* infection in peptic ulcer patients. A personal viewpoint. J Clin Gastroenterol 1996;22:313–6.

46. Al-Eidan FA, McElnay JC, Scott MG, et al. Management of *Helicobacter pylori* eradication–the influence of structured counselling and follow-up. Br J Clin Pharmacol 2002;53:163–71.

47. Ford AC, Malfertheiner P, Giguere M, et al. Adverse events with bismuth salts for *Helicobacter pylori* eradication: systematic review and meta-analysis. World J Gastroenterol 2008;14:7361–70.

48. Gene E, Calvet X, Azagra R, et al. Triple vs quadruple therapy for treating *Helicobacter pylori* infection: a meta-analysis. Aliment Pharmacol Ther 2003;17:1137–43.

49. Hojo M, Miwa H, Nagahara A, et al. Pooled analysis on the efficacy of the second-line treatment regimens for *Helicobacter pylori* infection. Scand J Gastroenterol 2001;36:690–700.

50. Delchier JC, Malfertheiner P, Thieroff-Ekerdt R. Use of a combination formulation of bismuth, metronidazole and tetracycline with omeprazole as a rescue therapy for eradication of *Helicobacter pylori*. Aliment Pharmacol Ther 2014;40:171–7.

51. Graham DY, Dore MP. Variability in the outcome of treatment of *Helicobacter pylori* infection: a critical analysis. In: Hunt RH, Tytgat GNJ, editors. *Helicobacter*

pylori basic mechanisms to clinical cure 1998. Dordrecht (Netherlands): Kluwer Academic Publishers; 1998. p. 426–40.

52. Dore MP, Graham DY, Mele R, et al. Colloidal bismuth subcitrate-based twice-a-day quadruple therapy as primary or salvage therapy for *Helicobacter pylori* infection. Am J Gastroenterol 2002;97:857–60.

53. Dore MP, Marras L, Maragkoudakis E, et al. Salvage therapy after two or more prior *Helicobacter pylori* treatment failures: the super salvage regimen. Helicobacter 2003;8:307–9.

54. Dore MP, Farina V, Cuccu M, et al. Twice-a-day bismuth-containing quadruple therapy for *Helicobacter pylori* eradication: a randomized trial of 10 and 14 days. Helicobacter 2011;16:295–300.

55. Dore MP, Maragkoudakis E, Pironti A, et al. Twice-a-day quadruple therapy for eradication of *Helicobacter pylori* in the elderly. Helicobacter 2006;11:52–5.

56. Graham DY, Hoffman J, El-Zimaity HM, et al. Twice a day quadruple therapy (bismuth subsalicylate, tetracycline, metronidazole plus lansoprazole) for treatment of *Helicobacter pylori* infection. Aliment Pharmacol Ther 1997;11:935–8.

57. Zheng Q, Dai J, Li X, et al. Comparison of the efficacy of pantoprazole-based triple therapy versus quadruple therapy in the treatment of *Helicobacter pylori* infections: a single-center, randomized, open and parallel-controlled study. Chin J Gastroenterol 2009;14:8–11.

58. Zheng Q, Chen WJ, Lu H, et al. Comparison of the efficacy of triple versus quadruple therapy on the eradication of *Helicobacter pylori* and antibiotic resistance. J Dig Dis 2010;11:313–8.

59. Garcia N, Calvet X, Gene E, et al. Limited usefulness of a seven-day twice-a-day quadruple therapy. Eur J Gastroenterol Hepatol 2000;12:1315–8.

60. Borody TJ, George LL, Brandl S, et al. *Helicobacter pylori* eradication with doxycycline-metronidazole-bismuth subcitrate triple therapy. Scand J Gastroenterol 1992;27:281–4.

61. Cammarota G, Martino A, Pirozzi G, et al. High efficacy of 1-week doxycycline- and amoxicillin-based quadruple regimen in a culture-guided, third-line treatment approach for *Helicobacter pylori* infection. Aliment Pharmacol Ther 2004;19:789–95.

62. Wang Z, Wu S. Doxycycline-based quadruple regimen versus routine quadruple regimen for rescue eradication of *Helicobacter pylori*: an open-label control study in Chinese patients. Singapore Med J 2012;53:273–6.

63. Ciccaglione A, Cellini L, Grossi L, et al. A triple and quadruple therapy with doxycycline and bismuth for first-line treatment of *Helicobacter pylori* infection: a pilot study. Helicobacter 2015. [Epub ahead of print].

64. Kohanteb J, Bazargani A, Saberi-Firoozi M, et al. Antimicrobial susceptibility testing of *Helicobacter pylori* to selected agents by agar dilution method in Shiraz-Iran. Indian J Med Microbiol 2007;25:374–7.

65. Gumurdulu Y, Serin E, Ozer B, et al. Low eradication rate of *Helicobacter pylori* with triple 7–14 days and quadruple therapy in Turkey. World J Gastroenterol 2004;10:668–71.

66. Altintas E, Ulu O, Sezgin O, et al. Comparison of ranitidine bismuth citrate, tetracycline and metronidazole with ranitidine bismuth citrate and azithromycin for the eradication of *Helicobacter pylori* in patients resistant to PPI based triple therapy. Turk J Gastroenterol 2004;15:90–3.

67. Uygun A, Kadayifci A, Safali M, et al. The efficacy of bismuth containing quadruple therapy as a first-line treatment option for *Helicobacter pylori*. J Dig Dis 2007;8:211–5.

68. Songur Y, Senol A, Balkarli A, et al. Triple or quadruple tetracycline-based therapies versus standard triple treatment for *Helicobacter pylori* treatment. Am J Med Sci 2009;338:50–3.
69. Demir M, Gokturk S, Ozturk NA, et al. Bismuth-based first-line therapy for *Helicobacter pylori* eradication in type 2 diabetes mellitus patients. Digestion 2010; 82:47–53.
70. Uygun A, Kadayifci A, Yesilova Z, et al. Comparison of sequential and standard triple-drug regimen for *Helicobacter pylori* eradication: a 14-day, open-label, randomized, prospective, parallel-arm study in adult patients with nonulcer dyspepsia. Clin Ther 2008;30:528–34.
71. Onal IK, Gokcan H, Benzer E, et al. What is the impact of *Helicobacter pylori* density on the success of eradication therapy: a clinico-histopathological study. Clin Res Hepatol Gastroenterol 2013;37:642–6.
72. Sapmaz F, Kalkan IH, Guliter S, et al. Comparison of *Helicobacter pylori* eradication rates of standard 14-day quadruple treatment and novel modified 10-day, 12-day and 14-day sequential treatments. Eur J Intern Med 2014;25:224–9.
73. Hosseini SM, Sharifipoor F, Nazemian F, et al. *Helicobacter pylori* eradication in renal recipient: triple or quadruple therapy? Acta Med Iran 2014;52:271–4.
74. Talaie R. Efficacy of standard triple therapy versus bismuth-based quadruple therapy for eradication of *Helicobacter pylori* infection. J Paramedical Sci 2014;5:9–14.
75. Goral V, Zeyrek FY, Gul K. Antibiotic resistance in *Helicobacter pylori* infection. T Klin J Gastroenterohepatol 2000;11:87–92.
76. Abadi AT, Taghvaei T, Mobarez AM, et al. Frequency of antibiotic resistance in *Helicobacter pylori* strains isolated from the northern population of Iran. J Microbiol 2011;49:987–93.
77. Fallahi GH, Maleknejad S. *Helicobacter pylori* culture and antimicrobial resistance in Iran. Indian J Pediatr 2007;74:127–30.
78. Farshad S, Alborzi A, Japoni A, et al. Antimicrobial susceptibility of *Helicobacter pylori* strains isolated from patients in Shiraz, Southern Iran. World J Gastroenterol 2010;16:5746–51.
79. Khademi F, Faghri J, Poursina F, et al. Resistance pattern of *Helicobacter pylori* strains to clarithromycin, metronidazole, and amoxicillin in Isfahan, Iran. J Res Med Sci 2013;18:1056–60.
80. Milani M, Ghotaslou R, Akhi MT, et al. The status of antimicrobial resistance of *Helicobacter pylori* in Eastern Azerbaijan, Iran: comparative study according to demographics. J Infect Chemother 2012;18:848–52.
81. Mohammadi M, Doroud D, Mohajerani N, et al. *Helicobacter pylori* antibiotic resistance in Iran. World J Gastroenterol 2005;11:6009–13.
82. Shokrzadeh L, Jafari F, Dabiri H, et al. Antibiotic susceptibility profile of *Helicobacter pylori* isolated from the dyspepsia patients in Tehran, Iran. Saudi J Gastroenterol 2011;17:261–4.
83. Siavoshi F, Safari F, Doratotaj D, et al. Antimicrobial resistance of *Helicobacter pylori* isolates from Iranian adults and children. Arch Iran Med 2006;9:308–14.
84. Siavoshi F, Saniee P, Latifi-Navid S, et al. Increase in resistance rates of *H. pylori* isolates to metronidazole and tetracycline—comparison of three 3-year studies. Arch Iran Med 2010;13:177–87.
85. Talebi Bezmin AA, Ghasemzadeh A, Taghvaei T, et al. Primary resistance of *Helicobacter pylori* to levofloxacin and moxifloxacine in Iran. Intern Emerg Med 2012;7:447–52.
86. Zendedel A, Moradimoghadam F, Almasi V, et al. Antibiotic resistance of *Helicobacter pylori* in Mashhad, Iran. J Pak Med Assoc 2013;63:336–9.

87. van der Hulst RW, Keller JJ, Rauws EA, et al. Treatment of *Helicobacter pylori* infection: a review of the world literature. Helicobacter 1996;1:6–19.
88. Chi CH, Lin CY, Sheu BS, et al. Quadruple therapy containing amoxicillin and tetracycline is an effective regimen to rescue failed triple therapy by overcoming the antimicrobial resistance of *Helicobacter pylori*. Aliment Pharmacol Ther 2003;18:347–53.
89. Cheon JH, Kim SG, Kim JM, et al. Combinations containing amoxicillin-clavulanate and tetracycline are inappropriate for *Helicobacter pylori* eradication despite high in vitro susceptibility. J Gastroenterol Hepatol 2006;21:1590–5.
90. Kadayifci A, Uygun A, Polat Z, et al. Comparison of bismuth-containing quadruple and concomitant therapies as a first-line treatment option for *Helicobacter pylori*. Turk J Gastroenterol 2012;23:8–13.
91. Logan RP, Gummett PA, Misiewicz JJ, et al. One week's anti-*Helicobacter pylori* treatment for duodenal ulcer. Gut 1994;35:15–8.
92. Tzivras M, Balatsos V, Souyioultzis S, et al. High eradication rate of *Helicobacter pylori* using a four-drug regimen in patients previously treated unsuccessfully. Clin Ther 1997;19:906–12.
93. Uygun A, Ozel AM, Sivri B, et al. Efficacy of a modified sequential therapy including bismuth subcitrate as first-line therapy to eradicate *Helicobacter pylori* in a Turkish population. Helicobacter 2012;17:486–90.
94. Chung JW, Lee JH, Jung HY, et al. Second-line *Helicobacter pylori* eradication: a randomized comparison of 1-week or 2-week bismuth-containing quadruple therapy. Helicobacter 2011;16:289–94.
95. Chung JW, Lee GH, Han JH, et al. The trends of one-week first-line and second-line eradication therapy for *Helicobacter pylori* infection in Korea. Hepatogastroenterology 2011;58:246–50.
96. Jang HJ, Choi MH, Kim YS, et al. Effectiveness of triple therapy and quadruple therapy for *Helicobacter pylori* eradication. Korean J Gastroenterol 2005;46:368–72.
97. Lee SK, Lee SW, Park JY, et al. Effectiveness and safety of repeated quadruple therapy in *Helicobacter pylori* infection after failure of second-line quadruple therapy: repeated quadruple therapy as a third-line therapy. Helicobacter 2011;16:410–4.
98. Park SC, Chun HJ, Jung SW, et al. Efficacy of 14 day OBMT therapy as a second-line treatment for *Helicobacter pylori* infection. Korean J Gastroenterol 2004;44:136–41.
99. Cheon JH, Kim N, Lee DH, et al. Long-term outcomes after *Helicobacter pylori* eradication with second-line, bismuth-containing quadruple therapy in Korea. Eur J Gastroenterol Hepatol 2006;18:515–9.
100. Yoon JH, Baik GH, Kim YS, et al. Comparison of the eradication rate between 1- and 2-week bismuth-containing quadruple rescue therapies for *Helicobacter pylori* eradication. Gut Liver 2012;6:434–9.
101. Yoon JH, Baik GH, Sohn KM, et al. Trends in the eradication rates of *Helicobacter pylori* infection for eleven years. World J Gastroenterol 2012;18:6628–34.
102. Chung SJ, Lee DH, Kim N, et al. Eradication rates of *Helicobacter pylori* infection with second-line treatment: non-ulcer dyspepsia compared to peptic ulcer disease. Hepatogastroenterology 2007;54:1293–6.
103. Lee ST, Lee DH, Lim JH, et al. Efficacy of 7-day and 14-day bismuth-containing quadruple therapy and 7-day and 14-day moxifloxacin-based triple therapy as second-line eradication for *Helicobacter pylori* infection. Gut Liver 2015.
104. Kimura K, Ido K, Saifuku K, et al. A 1-h topical therapy for the treatment of *Helicobacter pylori* infection. Am J Gastroenterol 1995;90:60–3.

105. Atherton JC, Hudson N, Kirk GE, et al. Amoxycillin capsules with omeprazole for the eradication of *Helicobacter pylori*. Assessment of the importance of antibiotic dose timing in relation to meals. Aliment Pharmacol Ther 1994;8:495–8.
106. Atherton JC, Cullen DJ, Kirk GE, et al. Enhanced eradication of *Helicobacter pylori* by pre- versus post- prandial amoxycillin suspension with omeprazole: implications for antibiotic delivery. Aliment Pharmacol Ther 1996;10:631–5.
107. Lu H, Zhang W, Graham DY. Bismuth-containing quadruple therapy for *Helicobacter pylori*: lessons from China. Eur J Gastroenterol Hepatol 2013;25:1134–40.
108. Graham DY. Efficient identification and evaluation of effective *Helicobacter pylori* therapies. Clin Gastroenterol Hepatol 2009;7:145–8.
109. Dong Q, Hyde D, Herra C, et al. Identification of genes regulated by prolonged acid exposure in *Helicobacter pylori*. FEMS Microbiol Lett 2001;196:245–9.
110. Koksal AS, Onder FO, Torun S, et al. Twice a day quadruple therapy for the first-line treatment of *Helicobacter pylori* in an area with a high prevalence of background antibiotic resistance. Acta Gastroenterol Belg 2013;76:34–7.
111. Amini M, Khedmat H, Yari F. Eradication rate of *Helicobacter pylori* in dyspeptic patients. Med Sci Monit 2005;11:CR193–5.
112. Akyildiz M, Akay S, Musoglu A, et al. The efficacy of ranitidine bismuth citrate, amoxicillin and doxycycline or tetracycline regimens as a first line treatment for *Helicobacter pylori* eradication. Eur J Intern Med 2009;20:53–7.
113. Hu TH, Chuah SK, Hsu PI, et al. Randomized comparison of two nonbismuth-containing rescue therapies for *Helicobacter pylori*. Am J Med Sci 2011;342:177–81.

Is There a Role for Probiotics in *Helicobacter pylori* Therapy?

Maria P. Dore, MD[a,b], Elisabetta Goni, MD[c],
Francesco Di Mario, MD[d],*

KEYWORDS

• *Helicobacter pylori* • Probiotics • *Lactobacillus reuteri*

KEY POINTS

• Probiotics are live bacteria that may confer a health benefit to the host.
• Several studies provided evidence that probiotics may also compete directly with *Helicobacter pylori*, interfering with other pathogens colonization or by the production of antimicrobial molecules.
• The effectiveness of many commonly recommended treatments has declined to unacceptably low levels for the increasing antimicrobial resistance and compliance reduction.
• *Lactobacillus reuteri* has been shown to inhibit *H pylori* in vitro and in vivo and may play a role in eradication therapy.
• The goals of this therapy could be to eradicate *H pylori*, reduce the inflammation associated with the infection, and enhance therapy by improving treatment success.

WHAT PROBIOTICS ARE

Microbial communities are present on all mucosal surfaces. The intestinal tract is the host to a vast microbe community that plays an important role in the integrity and function of the gastrointestinal tract. They also provide a relevant contribution in the maturation and induction of gut-associated lymphoid system (innate immunity), and stimulation of specific systemic and local immune responses (acquired immunity). The gut-associated lymphoid system is a major component of the immune system, accounting for more than 70% of lymphoid tissue.[1]

We have any commercial or financial conflict of interest and any founding sources.
[a] Dipartimento di Medicina Clinica e Sperimentale, University of Sassari, Viale San Pietro n 8, Sassari 07100, Italy; [b] Department of Medicine, Michael E. DeBakey VAMC, Baylor College of Medicine, 2002 Holcombe Boulevard, Houston, TX 77030, USA; [c] Department of Gastroenterology, Hepatology and Infectious Diseases, Otto-von-Guericke University, Magdeburg 39106, Germany; [d] Department of Clinical and Experimental Medicine, University of Parma, School of Medicine, Via Gramsci 14, Parma 43125, Italy
* Corresponding author.
E-mail address: francesco.dimario@unipr.it

Gastroenterol Clin N Am 44 (2015) 565–575
http://dx.doi.org/10.1016/j.gtc.2015.05.005
0889-8553/15/$ – see front matter © 2015 Elsevier Inc. All rights reserved.

In addition, the gut microbiome consumes, stores, and redistributes energy allowing humans to extract calories from otherwise indigestible carbohydrates. In humans, the contribution of microbial fermentation to the host's energy balance is usually around 10% to 30%. Short chain fatty acids promote colonocyte proliferation, acidification of the intracolonic environment, enhancement of colonic contraction, stimulation of colonic blood flow, and absorption of salt and water.[2] Moreover, these microbial communities serve as an important barrier against pathogen colonization by competing for attachment sites and for available nutrients, as well as by directly inhibiting pathogen growth by altering the intraluminal pH, reducing redox potential, and producing inhibitory molecules such as bacteriocins.[3,4] Disturbances of the intestinal epithelial barrier function can result in increased uptake of microbial and food antigens, stimulating the mucosal immune system and triggering an inflammatory response.[5–7]

However, the gut microbiome also has the potential to contribute to the development of diseases by a variety of mechanisms. Conditions affecting gastric acid barrier, such as use of antisecretory drugs, gastric atrophy, surgery, autoimmune disease, and aging, or local mucosal and systemic immune diseases, such as selective immunoglobulin A deficit, human immunodeficiency virus infection, immunosenescence, and/or intestinal clearance modifications may result in qualitative and quantitative alterations of gastric, digiuno-ileal, and colonic flora dysbiosis (ie, specific bacteria overgrowth/reduction).[8–10]

PROBIOTICS

The role for intestinal microbes in health and disease has been recognized in alternative and complementary forms of medicine for many years. The Russian Nobel Prize recipient Eli Metchnikoff, professor at the Pasteur Institute in Paris, in 1907 states that "senility is due to poisoning of the body by the products of certain of these intestinal bacteria.... The multiplication of these organisms could be prevented by a diet containing milk fermented by bacilli which produce large amounts of lactic acid."[11]

Manipulation of the intestinal microflora with therapeutic intention is the subject of intensive and ongoing research. The methods by which the intestinal microflora can be altered include administration of antibiotics, prebiotics (dietary components able to promote the growth and metabolic activity of beneficial bacteria), and probiotics. Probiotics are microorganisms that have beneficial properties for the host. This definition has been made more precise over time. For example, Fuller[12] described probiotics as "live microbial feed supplement which beneficially affects the host animal by improving its intestinal microbial balance". He stressed 2 important factors: the viable nature of probiotics and the capacity to help with intestinal balance. In 2001, an Expert Consultation of international scientists working on behalf of the Food and Agriculture Organization of the United Nations and the World Health Organization defined probiotics as, "live microorganisms which when administered in adequate amounts confer a health benefit on the host".[13] The International Scientific Association for Probiotics and Prebiotics organized a meeting of clinical and scientific experts on probiotics (with specialties in gastroenterology, pediatrics, family medicine, gut microbiome, microbiology of probiotic bacteria, microbial genetics, immunology, and food science) in 2013 to reexamine the concept of probiotics and suggested a more grammatically correct definition: "live microorganisms that, when administered in adequate amounts, confer a health benefit on the host." Overall, the definition includes the essence of the term, *microbial*, namely, viable and beneficial to health.[14]

The European Commission advised the Food Safety Authority of Ireland that where terms like 'live' or 'active' are used to describe bacteria and imply a probiotic function, they are considered to be health claims. Because no health claims have been approved for 'probiotic,' terms that imply a probiotic function are not permitted. For this reason, currently any terms that imply probiotic activity (ie, imply that the bacteria in the product may be beneficial for health) are considered health claims and are thus not permitted.[15]

In contrast, in Italy there is a long tradition of consuming "beneficial bacteria" administered as food supplements or food ingredients. Their use in the food sector has been under the regulation of the Italian Ministry of Health for more than 13 years. Recently, the use of the word *probiotic* for food and food supplements was updated, requiring certain conditions, including a minimum number of viable cells (1×10^9 colony-forming unit [CFU]) administered per day, a full genetic characterization of the probiotic strain, and a demonstrable history of safe use in the Italian market.[16]

Sardinia, a Mediterranean Italian island, is the site of a hot spot of exceptional longevity, called the Longevity Blue Zone, located on the mountain. This observation has stimulated a strong interest in traditional food as one of the potential causal factors of the exceptional longevity. It has been shown that consumption of dairy products, both from goats and sheep, especially a sort of fresh sour cheese called *casuajedu*, which is rich in *Lactobacilli*, was abundant in this region.[17] Another important source of *Lactobacilli* in this special Sardinian population is a bread prepared from whole grains with 'homemade' microbial starters. It has been demonstrated that this type of bread is associated with a reduction in postprandial glucose and insulin blood levels of up to 25% compared with regular bread and thus is potentially able to preserve the function of pancreatic insulin-secreting cells and prevent obesity and diabetes.[18]

Use of Probiotics Clinically

The complexity of the microbial community is not yet completely understood; however, there is strong scientific interest in proving the benefits of probiotics in the therapeutic armamentarium. The available literature includes well-designed clinical trials, systematic reviews, and metaanalyses ascribing beneficial medical effects with several well-studied probiotic microbial species.[19]

The list of these microorganisms includes strains of lactic acid bacilli such as *Lactobacillus* and *Bifidobacterium*, a nonpathogenic strain of *Escherichia coli*, "*E coli* Nissle 1917," *Clostridium butyricum*, *Streptococcus salivarius*, and *Saccharomyces boulardii*, a nonpathogenic strain of yeast. There are also strains that have been genetically engineered to have specific properties, such as to stimulate secretion of specific cytokines and thus to modulate the immune system.

Specific probiotic species, alone or in combination, have suggested potential efficacy in several gastrointestinal illnesses. The best studied to date include inflammatory bowel diseases, antibiotic-related diarrhea, *Clostridium difficile* colitis, infectious diarrhea, hepatic encephalopathy, irritable bowel syndrome, and allergy. Therapeutic benefit has also been suggested in several other disorders including the use of probiotics in the treatment of *Helicobacter pylori* infection.

PROBIOTICS AS ADJUVANT THERAPY FOR *HELICOBACTER PYLORI* ERADICATION

In recent years the use of probiotics as adjuvant therapies in *H pylori* eradication has been extensively studied and its role is still debated. The Maastricht IV guidelines emphasize that certain prebiotics and probiotics show promising results as an adjuvant treatment in reducing side effects (evidence level 5, grade of recommendation D).[20]

Lactoferrin has been used to improve *H pylori* treatment. Two metaanalyses obtained the same results and showed that lactoferrin increases the efficacy of proton pump inhibitors and clarithromycin-containing triple therapies.[21,22] However, the poor quality of many trials and the limited number of centers involved should be emphasized and preclude giving a positive recommendation.

Metaanalyses on the studies where *Lactobacilli* were used are heterogeneous, because they mixed different species and strains. For this reason, additional work needs to be performed to determine the strain, dose and administration to be used.[23,24] A metaanalysis on the use of *S boulardii* as adjuvant to triple therapy showed not conclusive results.[25]

All these treatments are most likely to lead to a decrease of adverse events, especially diarrhea, and only indirectly may help to improve the eradication rate by an improvement in the compliance.[20]

Recently, O'Connor and associates observed that some probiotics, such as *Lactobacilli* and *Bifidobacteria*, exert an anti–*H pylori* effect in vitro and were helpful in reducing antibiotic-related side effects.[26] The most frequently studied agents have been *Lactobacillus sp. strains.* In 1 study where 70 naïve patients were treated, *Lactobacillus reuteri* increased eradication rate by 8.6% and reduced the reported side effects when compared with placebo-supplemented triple therapy.[27] A metaanalysis of 9 studies on probiotic use as an adjunct to triple therapy found that when specific *Lactobacillus* strains were used, eradication rates increased significantly by 17%, but when multistrain probiotics were used, eradication rates enhanced by only 2.8%.[28] This also was reflected in 2 other trials from Iran and Brazil where multistrain probiotics as adjunct therapy failed to show a benefit for eradication.[29,30]

Bifidobacterium infantis has also been proposed as having anti–*H pylori* activity, and in a recent study from Asia, it was observed that adding it to standard triple therapy increased the cure rate from 69% to 83% and when pretreatment with 2 weeks of *B infantis* was given as well, the success rate of eradication increased to 91%.[31]

If eradication regimens take into account local and regional resistance patterns and use optimized acid suppressant therapy, adjunct probiotic therapy seems add little to treatment efficacy.[29,30] In scenarios characterized by low *H pylori* eradication rates, the addition of *L reuteri* may lead to a therapeutic gain of 10%.[27] The strength of probiotics as add-on therapy, however, is their ability to reduce antibiotic side effects and thereby improve adherence.[27,32,33]

In contrast, Navarro-Rodriguez and colleagues[30] concluded that the use of probiotic compound (*Lactobacillus acidophilus, Lactobacillus rhamnosus, Bifido bacterium,* and *Streptococcus faecium*) compared with placebo in the regimen in Brazilian patients with peptic ulcer or functional dyspepsia showed no difference in efficacy or adverse effects rate. In this double-blind study, patients with peptic ulcer or functional dyspepsia infected by *H pylori* were randomized to receive a triple therapy with furazolidone, tetracycline, and lansoprazole regimen twice a day for 7 days. Patients received placebo or a probiotic compound in capsules twice a day for 30 days. A symptoms questionnaire was administered at baseline, after completion of antibiotic therapy, after the probiotic, use and 8 weeks after the end of the treatment. Upper digestive endoscopy, histologic assessment, rapid urease test, and breath test were performed before and 8 weeks after eradication treatment. One hundred seven patients were enrolled: 21 men with active probiotic and 19 with placebo plus 34 women with active probiotic and 33 with placebo for a total of 55 patients receiving active probiotic and 52 receiving placebo. The per protocol (PP) eradication rate with active probiotic was 89.8% and with placebo 85.1% ($P = .49$); intention to treat 81.8% and 79.6%, respectively ($P = .53$). The rate of adverse effects at 7 days with the active probiotic was 59.3% and 71.2% with placebo (*P* = .20). At 30 days, it was 44.9% and 60.4%, respectively (*P* = .08).

Four recent meta-analyses have tried to better clarify the role of probiotics in the treatment of *H pylori* infection. Szajewska and colleagues[25] selected 5 randomized, controlled trials comparing *Saccaromyces boulardii* given along with triple therapy compared with placebo or no intervention. They found that *S boulardii* significantly increased the eradication rate with a relative risk [RR] of 1.13 (95% CI, 1.05–1.21) and reduced the risk of overall related adverse effects with a RR of 0.46 (95% CI, 0.3–0.7), especially with regard to diarrhea (RR, 0.47; 95% CI, 0.32–0.69).

Wang and colleagues[34] performed a metaanalysis of 10 clinical trials. They included all parallel controlled trials comparing *Lactobacillus*-containing and *Bifidobacterium*-containing probiotic compound preparation supplementation or not during *H pylori* eradication therapy. Eradication odds ratio (OR) was available for 1469 patients (708 in the probiotic supplementation group and 761 in the control group). The pooled OR by intention to treat and by PP analysis in the probiotics supplementation versus no probiotics was 2.06 (95% CI, 1.40–3.06) and 2.32 (95% CI 1.72–3.14), respectively. The pooled OR of incidence of total side effects was significantly decreased in the probiotics supplementation group (OR, 0.3; 95% CI, 0.1–0.8) by the random model without significant publication bias. The authors concluded that *Lactobacillus*-containing and *Bifidobacterium*-containing probiotic compound preparation during *H pylori* eradication therapy in the adult may have beneficial effects on eradication rate and incidence of total side effects.

Zheng and colleagues[28] in another metaanalysis evaluated 9 randomized, controlled trials containing *Lactobacilli* performed on adult and children showing a significantly increasing in the eradication rate with a RR of 1.4 (95% CI, 1.06–1.22), but without a significant decrease in overall side effects (RR, 0.88, 95% CI, 0.73–1.06).

Finally, Dang and associates[35] included eligible randomized, controlled trials examining effects of probiotics supplementation on eradication rates and side effects, published up to May 2014. Subgroup analysis was performed to compare different probiotic strains and antibiotic therapies with different effectiveness in controls (eradication rates of 80% vs 80%). The quality of the trials was assessed with the Cochrane risk of bias tool. The pooled data suggest that supplementation with specific strains of probiotics compared with eradication therapy may be considered an option for increasing eradication rates, particularly when antibiotic therapies are relatively ineffective. The impact on side effects remains unclear and more high-quality trials on specific probiotic strains and side effects are thus needed. **Table 1** summarizes the overall results.

PROBIOTICS AS CURE FOR *HELICOBACTER PYLORI* INFECTION

The effect of *Lactobacilli* in patients with *H pylori* infection has been studied, although not extensively. *Lactobacillus* species are rod-shaped, Gram-positive bacteria able to produce lactic acid resulting in acidification of the microenvironment,[36] which can inhibit the growth of *H pylori* at concentrations of 50 to 156 mmol/L in vitro.[37] The effect of 17 different *Lactobacillus* strains on *H pylori* activity confirmed that the bactericidal effect of lactobacilli results from acid production. However strains such as *L acidophilus* CRL 639, showed other specific anti–*H pylori* activities, including the release of antibacterial products such as autolysins.[38]

The majority of available data are concerned with whether the probiotics will reduce the density of *H pylori* bacteria and thus the inflammatory response. For example, Michetti and colleagues[39] in an uncontrolled study, tested whether *L acidophilus*

Table 1
Probiotics as adjuvant therapy for *Helicobacter pylori* eradication

Author, Year	Study Design	Probiotic	Results
Zou et al,[21] 2009	Metaanalysis	*Lactobacilli strains*	+
Szajewska et al,[25] 2010	Metaanalysis	*Saccaromyces boulardii*	NS
O'Connor et al,[26] 2014	Review	*Lactobacilli, Bifidobacteria*	+
Emara et al,[27] 2014	Double-blind placebo	*Lactobacillus reuteri*	+
Zheng et al,[28] 2013	Metaanalysis	*Lactobacilli strains*	+
Shavakhi et al,[29] 2013	Triple-blind placebo	Lactobacillus, *Bifidobacterium* strains and *Streptococcus thermophiles*	+
Dajani et al,[31] 2013	Open label randomized	*Bifidus infantis*	+
Malfartheiner & Selgrad,[33] 2014	Review	*Lactobacillus reuteri*	+
Navarro-Rodriguez et al,[30] 2013	Double-blind placebo	*L acidophilus, L rhamnosus, Bifido bacterium* and *Streptococcus faecium*	NS
Wang et al,[34] 2013	Metaanalysis	*Lactobacillus* and *Bifidobacterium*	+
Dang et al,[35] 2014	Metaanalysis	*L acidophilus, L casei* DN-114001, *L gasseri* and *Bifidobacterium infantis* 2036	NS

(*johnsonii*) La1 culture supernatant was able to downregulate *H pylori* infection. The outcome was assessed in terms of a decrease in urease activity assessed by urea breath test (UBT) and was seen in 80% of patients with *H pylori* infections. In that study, patients were treated for 2 weeks with 50 mL of *L johnsonii* (La1) supernatant combined with either omeprazole 20 mg 4 times a day or with placebo.[39] Coconnier and colleagues[40] in a similar study analyzed the in vitro and in vivo effects of a culture supernatant of *L acidophilus* strain LB and showed that the anti–*H pylori* effects were independent of pH and lactic acid levels.

Based on previous results, showing that *Lactobacillus gasseri* (LG21) was able to bind to gastric epithelium and resist gastric acidity, it was tested in an open label crossover study in 31 *H pylori* positive Japanese subjects. They also reported a slight but significant decrease in urease activity after consumption of 90 g of yogurt containing *L gasseri* OLL 2716 (LG 21) twice a day for 8 weeks (ie, excess $13CO_2$ [%0]; 26.6 ± 13 decreased to 20.9 ± 11; $P = .05$).[41,42] An in vitro study by Kabir and colleagues[43] showed that *Lactobacillus salivarius* WB 1004 could inhibit the attachment of *H pylori* to both murine and human gastric epithelial cells. This was also associated with a reduction in interleukin-8 release. In addition they provided in vivo data using a gnotobiotic murine model, and showed that *L salivarius* was able to protect these mice from an *H pylori* infection.

Mukai and colleagues[44] studied *L reuteri*, and showed that selected strains (JCM1081 and TM105) could hinder *H pylori* binding to its putative glycolipid receptors (asialo-GM1 and sulfatide), suggesting a possible role for these strains as probiotics. A double-blind, randomized, placebo-controlled, cross-over clinical study from Japan administered a different strain of *L reuteri* (strain ATCC 55730), 4 times daily for 8 weeks and reported a significant decrease in urease activity consistent with a decrease in bacterial density.[45] Similar results were obtained by Francavilla and co-workers in Italy in a placebo-controlled study where *L reuteri* ATCC55730 1 × 10^8 CFU given alone for 4 weeks.[46] *L reuteri* was able to reduce *H pylori* load, assessed by both 13C-UBT delta-value and *H pylori* stool antigen quantification after 4 weeks of treatment (P<.05). In patients receiving placebo, no change was observed. In addition, *L reuteri* administration was associated with a significant decrease in dyspeptic symptoms.[46]

Overall, these studies suggested that various Lactobacilli were able to affect *H pylori* colonization, but few subjects were actually cured.

In contrast, Saggioro and colleagues[47] studied 30 dyspeptic patients with *H pylori* infections in a randomized, placebo-controlled pilot study. They were randomly and blindly assigned to either omeprazole 20 mg plus *L reuteri* 1 × 10^8 CFU twice a day before breakfast and dinner or omeprazole 20 mg plus placebo twice a day for 30 days. The *H pylori* status was established by UBT, rapid urease test, and histology 4 weeks after the end of therapy. *L reuteri* plus omeprazole was able to eradicate *H pylori* infection in 9 of 15 treated patients (60%) versus no eradication in the control population (omeprazole alone; $P = .0001$).

Another prospective, double-blind, randomized, placebo-controlled study in an Italian tertiary care setting evaluated 100 *H pylori*-positive treatment naive patients who received either *L reuteri* strain (2 × 10 CFU) or placebo during a 3-phase study (pre-eradication, eradication, and follow-up). In all patients 13C-UBT, blood assessments of gastrin-17, and upper endoscopy were performed. Eradication was confirmed by 13C-UBT after 8 weeks from the completion of therapy. The 13C-UBT delta decreased by 13% in *L reuteri* combination group compared with an increase of 4% in the placebo group (P≤.03). However, there was a significant improvement in gastrin-17 levels in patients receiving *L reuteri* compared with those receiving

Table 2
Clinical experiences by using *L reuteri* for cure of *Helicobacter pylori*

Author, Year	Patients (n)	Study Design	Results	Statistics
Imase et al,[45] 2007	33	Double-blind placebo 8 wk	The decrease in UBT owing to medication with *L reuteri* was 69.7% ± 4.0%	P<.05
Francavilla et al,[46] 2008	40	Double-blind placebo 4 wk	*L reuteri* reduces *H pylori* load (P<.05); no difference in eradication rates was observed	P = NS
Saggioro et al,[47] 2005	30	Double-blind placebo 4 wk	*L reuteri* eradication rate 60%	P<.0001
Francavilla et al,[48] 2014	100	Double-blind placebo 4 wk	Eradication rate was 75% in *L reuteri* and 65.9% in placebo	P = NS
Dore et al,[49] 2014	22	Open pilot 8 wk	Urease activity showed a significant reduction with a difference of mean of 38.8 vs 25.4 *L reuteri* plus pantoprazole cured 13.6% of patients by ITT analysis	P = .002

Abbreviations: ITT, intention to treat; UBT, urea breath test.

placebo consistent with improvement in mucosal inflammation ($P \leq .02$). Eradication rate was greater in the *L reuteri* combination groups (75% vs 65.9%).[48]

Finally, Dore and colleagues[49] performed an open pilot to study the effects of pantoprazole 20 mg plus *L reuteri* DSM17938 10^8 CFU twice a day in adult *H pylori*-infected patients. Treatment duration was 60 days. Urease activity assessed before and 4 to 6 weeks after therapy showed a significant reduction with a difference of means of 38.8 versus 25.4 by 1-tailed test ($P = .002$). More important, *L reuteri* plus pantoprazole twice a day cured 13.6% of patients (3/22; 95% CI, 2.9%–34.9%) with *H pylori* infection by intention to treat analysis and 14.2% (3/21; 95% CI, 3.0%–36%) by PP analysis. The cured patients included 1 patient with a history of several previous unsuccessfully therapies. **Table 2** summarizes the overall results.

SUMMARY

Although lactobacilli can be shown to inhibit *H pylori* in vitro, the most relevant antibacterial mechanism of action seems to be related to acid production. However, some strains of lactobacilli may also exert specific antimicrobial effects which are strain specific (ie, *L acidophilus* LB was more active than *Lactobacillus* GG, and *L johnsonii* La1 more than La10 3). to date there is no strong evidence of a benefit on eradication rate when probiotics are added to more complex regimen (sequential or concomitant). Despite some promising results obtained by using compounds of *L reuteri* and *S boulardii*, overall no exhaustive data are available and multicenter, high-quality, double-blind, randomized, controlled trials are needed to better define the role of probiotics as adjuvant therapy in *H pylori* eradication. Variables that remain to be studied with *L reuteri*, currently the most promising strain, include dosage, frequency of administration, administration in relation to meals, and duration of therapy.

REFERENCES

1. Hooper LV, Wong MH, Thelin A, et al. Molecular analysis of commensal host-microbial relationships in the intestine. Science 2001;291:881–4.
2. Tannock GW. Molecular assessment of intestinal microflora. Am J Clin Nutr 2001; 73(2 Suppl):410S–4S.
3. Jones ML, Ganopolsky JG, Martoni CJ, et al. Emerging science of the human microbiome. Gut Microbes 2014;5:446–57.
4. Staib L, Fuchs TM. From food to cell: nutrient exploitation strategies of enteropathogens. Microbiology 2014;160:1020–39.
5. Nieuwdorp M, Gilijamse PW, Pai N, et al. Role of the microbiome in energy regulation and metabolism. Gastroenterology 2014;146:1525–33.
6. Caricilli AM, Castoldi A, Câmara NO. Intestinal barrier: a gentlemen's agreement between microbiota and immunity. World J Gastrointest Pathophysiol 2014;5:18–32.
7. Putignani L, Del Chierico F, Petrucca A, et al. The human gut microbiota: a dynamic interplay with the host from birth to senescence settled during childhood. Pediatr Res 2014;76:2–10.
8. Kostic AD, Xavier RJ, Gevers D. The microbiome in inflammatory bowel disease: current status and the future ahead. Gastroenterology 2014;146:1489–99.
9. Walker MM, Talley NJ. Review article: bacteria and pathogenesis of disease in the upper gastrointestinal tract–beyond the era of *Helicobacter pylori*. Aliment Pharmacol Ther 2014;39:767–79.
10. Grace E, Shaw C, Whelan K, et al. Review article: small intestinal bacterial overgrowth–prevalence, clinical features, current and developing diagnostic tests, and treatment. Aliment Pharmacol Ther 2013;38:674–88.

11. Metchnikoff E. Essaisoptimistes. Paris. In: Chalmers Mitchell P, editor. The prolongation of life. Optimistic studies. London: Heinemann; 1907. p. 161–83.
12. Fuller R. Probiotics in human medicine. Gut 1991;32:439–42.
13. Food and Agricultural Organization of the United Nations and World Health Organization. Health and nutritional properties of probiotics in food including powder milk with live lactic acid bacteria. Cordoba, Argentina: World Health Organization; 2001 [online].
14. Hill C, Guarner F, Reid G, et al. Expert consensus document: the international scientific association for probiotics and prebiotics consensus statement on the scope and appropriate use of the term probiotic. Nat Rev Gastroenterol Hepatol 2014;11:506–14.
15. Food Safety Authority of Ireland. Probiotic health claims. Food Safety Authority of Ireland; 2013. Available at: www.fsai.ie/science_and_health/nutrition_and_health_claims.html.
16. Ministero della Salute. Commissione unica per la nutrizione e la dietetica. Guidelines on probiotics and prebiotics. Italy: Ministero della Salute; 2013.
17. Pes GM, Tolu F, Dore MP, et al. Male longevity in Sardinia, a review of historical sources supporting a causal link with dietary factors. Eur J Clin Nutr 2015;69(4): 411–8.
18. Maioli M, Pes GM, Sanna M, et al. Sourdough-leavened bread improves postprandial glucose and insulin plasma levels in subjects with impaired glucose tolerance. Acta Diabetol 2008;45:91–6.
19. Rowland I, Capurso L, Collins K, et al. Current level of consensus on probiotic science–report of an expert meeting–London, 23 November 2009. Gut Microbes 2010;1:436–9.
20. Malfertheiner P, Megraud F, O'Morain CA, et al, European Helicobacter Study Group. Management of *Helicobacter pylori* infection–the Maastricht IV/Florence Consensus Report. Gut 2012;61:646–64.
21. Zou J, Dong J, Yu X. Meta-analysis: lactobacillus containing quadruple therapy versus standard triple first-line therapy for *Helicobacter pylori* eradication. Helicobacter 2009;14:97–107.
22. Sachdeva A, Nagpal J. Meta-analysis: efficacy of bovine lactoferrin in *Helicobacter pylori* eradication. Aliment Pharmacol Ther 2009;29:720–30.
23. Tong JL, Ran ZH, Shen J, et al. Meta-analysis: the effect of supplementation with probiotics on eradication rates and adverse events during *Helicobacter pylori* eradication therapy. Aliment Pharmacol Ther 2007;25:155–68.
24. Sachdeva A, Nagpal J. Effect of fermented milk-based probiotic preparations on *H pylori* eradication: a systematic review and meta-analysis of randomized-controlled trials. Eur J Gastroenterol Hepatol 2009;1:45–53.
25. Szajewska H, Horvath A, Piwowarczyk A. Meta-analysis: the effects of *Saccharomyces boulardii* supplementation on *Helicobacter pylori* eradication rates and side effects during treatment. Aliment Pharmacol Ther 2010;32: 1069–79.
26. O'Connor A, Vaira D, Gisbert JP, et al. Treatment of *Helicobacter pylori* infection 2014. Helicobacter 2014;19(Suppl 1):38–45.
27. Emara MH, Mohamed SY, Abdel-Aziz HR. *Lactobacillus reuteri* in management of *Helicobacter pylori* infection in dyspeptic patients: a double-blind placebo-controlled randomized clinical trial. Therap Adv Gastroenterol 2014;7:4–13.
28. Zheng X, Lyu L, Mei Z. Lactobacillus-containing probiotic supplementation increases *Helicobacter pylori* eradication rate: evidence from a meta-analysis. Rev Esp Enferm Dig 2013;105:445–53.

29. Shavakhi A, Tabesh E, Yaghoutkar A, et al. The effects of multistrain probiotic compound on bismuth-containing quadruple therapy for Helicobacter pylori infection: a randomized placebo-controlled triple-blind study. Helicobacter 2013;18:280–4.

30. Navarro-Rodriguez T, Silva FM, Barbuti RC, et al. Association of a probiotic to a Helicobacter pylori eradication regimen does not increase efficacy or decreases the adverse effects of the treatment: a prospective, randomized, double-blind, placebo-controlled study. BMC Gastroenterol 2013;13:56.

31. Dajani AI, Abu Hammour AM, Yang DH, et al. Do probiotics improve eradication response to Helicobacter pylori on standard triple or sequential therapy? Saudi J Gastroenterol 2013;19:113–20.

32. Passariello A, Agricole P, Malfertheiner P. A critical appraisal of probiotics (as drugs or food supplements) in gastrointestinal diseases. Curr Med Res Opin 2014;30:1055–64.

33. Malfertheiner P, Selgrad M. Helicobacter pylori. Curr Opin Gastroenterol 2014;30: 589–95.

34. Wang ZH, Gao QY, Fang JY. Meta-analysis of the efficacy and safety of Lactobacillus-containing and Bifidobacterium-containing probiotic compound preparation in Helicobacter pylori eradication therapy. J Clin Gastroenterol 2013;47:25–32.

35. Dang Y, Reinhardt JD, Zhou X, et al. The effect of probiotics supplementation on Helicobacter pylori eradication rates and side effects during eradication therapy: a meta-analysis. PLoS One 2014;9:e111030.

36. Carr FJ, Chill D, Maida N. The lactic acid bacteria: a literature survey. Crit Rev Microbiol 2002;28:281–370.

37. Midolo PD, Lambert JR, Hull R, et al. In vitro inhibition of Helicobacter pylori NCTC 11637 by organic acids and lactic acid bacteria. J Appl Bacteriol 1995; 79:475–9.

38. Lorca GL, Wadstrom T, Valdez GF, et al. Lactobacillus acidophilus autolysins inhibit. Helicobacter pylori in vitro. Curr Microbiol 2001;42:39–44.

39. Michetti P, Dorta G, Wiesel PH, et al. Effect of whey-based culture supernatant of Lactobacillus acidophilus (johnsonii) La1 on Helicobacter pylori infection in humans. Digestion 1999;60:203–9.

40. Coconnier MH, Lievin V, Hemery E, et al. Antagonistic activity against Helicobacter infection in vitro and in vivo by the human Lactobacillus acidophilus strain LB. Appl Environ Microbiol 1998;64:4573–80.

41. Sakamoto I, Igarashi M, Kimura K, et al. Suppressive effect of Lactobacillus gasseri OLL 2716 (LG21) on Helicobacter pylori infection in humans. J Antimicrob Chemother 2001;47:709–10.

42. Aiba Y, Suzuki N, Kabir AM, et al. Lactic acid-mediated suppression of Helicobacter pylori by the oral administration of Lactobacillus salivarius as a probiotic in a gnotobiotic murine model. Am J Gastroenterol 1998;93:2097–101.

43. Kabir AM, Aiba Y, Takagi A, et al. Prevention of Helicobacter pylori infection by lactobacilli in a gnotobiotic murine model. Gut 1997;41:49–55.

44. Mukai T, Asasaka T, Sato E, et al. Inhibition of binding of Helicobacter pylori to the glycolipid receptors by probiotic Lactobacillus reuteri. FEMS Immunol Med Microbiol 2002;32:105–10.

45. Imase K, Tanaka A, Tokunaga K, et al. Lactobacillus reuteri tablets suppress Helicobacter pylori infection—a double-blind randomised placebo-controlled cross-over clinical study. Kansenshogaku Zasshi 2007;81:387–93.

46. Francavilla R, Lionetti E, Castellaneta SP, et al. Inhibition of *Helicobacter pylori* infection in humans by *Lactobacillus reuteri* ATCC 55730 and effect on eradication therapy: a pilot study. Helicobacter 2008;13:127–34.
47. Saggioro A, Caron M, Pasini M, et al. *Helicobacter pylori* eradication with *Lactobacillus reuteri*. A double-blind-placebo-controlled study. Dig Liver Dis 2005; 37(Suppl 1):S88 [abstract: P01.49].
48. Francavilla R, Polimeno L, Demichina A, et al. *Lactobacillus reuteri* strain combination in *Helicobacter pylori* infection: a randomized, double-blind, placebo-controlled study. J Clin Gastroenterol 2014;48:407–13.
49. Dore MP, Cuccu M, Pes GM, et al. *Lactobacillus reuteri* in the treatment of *Helicobacter pylori* infection. Intern Emerg Med 2014;9:649–54.

Molecular Approaches to Identify *Helicobacter pylori* Antimicrobial Resistance

CrossMark

Francis Mégraud, MD*, Lucie Bénéjat, MS,
Esther Nina Ontsira Ngoyi, MD, Philippe Lehours, Pharm, PhD

KEYWORDS

- Macrolides • Fluoroquinolones • Tetracyclines • Rifampins
- Polymerase chain reaction • Fluorescent in situ hybridization
- Real-time polymerase chain reaction • Dual priming oligonucleotide

KEY POINTS

- Detection of antimicrobial resistance of *Helicobacter pylori* is important to tailor the treatment and obtain the best outcome of eradication.
- Molecular methods that detect mutations in genes relevant to antimicrobial resistance can be applied, especially for the most important antibiotic (ie, clarithromycin).
- Numerous molecular methods have been proposed to detect the main 3 mutations associated with clarithromycin resistance of *H pylori*, the most commonly used being real-time polymerase chain reaction protocols.
- The correlation between molecular detection of resistance via mutations and antimicrobial susceptibility testing by Etest is not perfect, because the former is better for detecting heteroresistance, but which method correlates the best with eradication is not known.
- Molecular methods can also be applied to detect *H pylori* resistance to fluoroquinolones, tetracycline, and rifampin, although they are not so commonly used.
- The advantage of molecular methods is their rapidity, lack of stringent transport conditions, and standardization.
- Their limit is that they cannot be used for all antibiotics and they do not detect resistance caused by mutations other than those already known or other resistance mechanisms.

There are several reasons for failure of the treatments aiming to eradicate *Helicobacter pylori*. They include a poor compliance to the regimen and a high gastric acidity, which is not overcome by the recommended dose of proton pump inhibitor (PPI) that increases the minimal inhibitory concentration (MIC) of the antibiotics used. In the

Conflicts of interest: the authors do not declare any conflict of interest.
Disclosure: the authors received research grants from Aptalis Pharma and Biocodex.
Bacteriology Laboratory, INSERM U853, University of Bordeaux, Bordeaux F-33000, France
* Corresponding author. Laboratoire de Bactériologie, Inserm U853, Université de Bordeaux, 146 rue Leo Saignat, Bordeaux Cedex 33076, France.
E-mail address: francis.megraud@chu-bordeaux.fr

past, different conditions, such as an important bacterial load, infection by CagA (cytotoxin-associated gene A)-positive versus CagA-negative *H pylori* strains, and the presence of intracellular bacteria and some immunologic deficiencies have been suggested to influence eradication[1] but seem less important when susceptibility and compliance are taken into consideration.

H pylori may become resistant to all the antibiotics used for eradication in the various regimens proposed, essentially according to the same mechanism (ie, acquisition of point mutations).[2] Point mutations occur by chance, and increase the MIC of the bacteria. Those organisms with point mutations are then selected by the corresponding antibiotics when prescribed. Another mechanism that sometimes occurs is an efflux mechanism of resistance (ie, efflux pumps, which tend to eliminate the antibiotic having penetrated into the bacterial cell).

Acquisition of resistance in *H pylori* is important essentially for macrolides (clarithromycin) and fluoroquinolones (levofloxacin). It rarely occurs for β-lactams (amoxicillin), tetracyclines, and for rifampin (rifabutin). To the contrary, although they seem to be frequent for 5-nitroimidazoles (metronidazole), they can be overcome in vivo.[3]

As for any infection, it seems crucial to detect *H pylori* resistance before prescribing a treatment, the efficacy of which would be jeopardized by the presence of resistant organisms.

The standard detection method consists of performing an antibiogram, usually or MIC determination, using Etest. Although this procedure has the advantage of offering testing of all of the antibiotics of interest, it also has some drawbacks. It requires living organisms, and culturing *H pylori* is sometimes challenging because of the special transport conditions necessary for gastric biopsies, as well as special care in the laboratory; several days are necessary for primary culture and then performing the antibiogram. For these reasons, alternative methods to this phenotypic approach have been proposed, including various molecular approaches.

The aim of this article is to review these methods, focusing on the determination of *H pylori* resistance to macrolides and fluoroquinolones, which are the most important, and mentioning also the methods used for tetracycline and rifampin.

MOLECULAR DETERMINATION OF *HELICOBACTER PYLORI* RESISTANCE TO MACROLIDES
Mechanisms

Macrolides target the 23S ribosomal RNA (rRNA). There are in particular 2 nucleotide positions at the domain V level of the peptidyl transferase loop, which can lead to resistant organisms, because they induce a change in the ribosome conformation and decrease macrolide binding. These positions are 2142 and 2143. A transition can be found at both positions, whereas a transversion is found only at the former (**Fig. 1**).[4,5] Other mutations that could theoretically occur are not found in nature, possibly because they lead to nonviable organisms. Some reports of other mutations associated with clarithromycin resistance have been made but could not be confirmed.[6]

However, a recent study questions this dogma. Comparing phenotypic and genotypic resistance to clarithromycin, De Francesco and colleagues[7] found a high rate of discrepancy. Of 42 clarithromycin-resistant strains, only 23 harbored the 3 known mutations, whereas 19 did not. These investigators identified the following mutations in 14 of 19 cases: A2115G, G2141A, and A2144T.

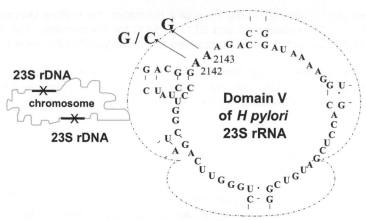

Fig. 1. Mutations in domain V of *H pylori* 23S rRNA, leading to clarithromycin resistance via decrease binding to the target.

Confirmation of such findings has not yet been made. In our recent experience (2014), there were only 3 discrepancies between genotypic and phenotypic methods out of 400 strains tested (Mégraud, 2015).

Others mechanisms that could be involved in clarithromycin resistance concern efflux pumps, as was found in campylobacters.[8]

Methods

There are various molecular methods to detect these mutations, essentially polymerase chain reaction (PCR)-based methods as well as a non-PCR-based method, fluorescent in situ hybridization (FISH).

One of the most efficient methods is real-time PCR. This method is described first. The other techniques are also reviewed.

Real-time polymerase chain reaction for detection of Helicobacter pylori resistance to macrolides

The beauty of this method is that it is first able to detect the presence of *H pylori* with a better sensitivity than other methods, including culture. In our experience, 3% to 5% of true positives detected by PCR cannot be cultured probably because of preanalytical problems.

Principle The first step consists of designing primers specific for *H pylori* on the 23S rRNA gene used as the target gene, on both sides of the mutation site. The second step is to design probes inside the fragment to be amplified: a 3′ anchor probe labeled with a fluorochrome (eg, fluorescein) and a 5′ sensor probe labeled with another fluorochrome (eg, LC-Red640), which must be located close to the other (3 bases upstream) to allow an energy transfer from the former to the latter. This is the principle of so-called fluorescence resonance energy transfer (FRET), performed in a Light-Cycler thermocycler (Roche Diagnostics, Neuilly sur Seine, France), which allows the amplicon formation to be followed in real time.

If the 23S rRNA gene of *H pylori* is present in the mixture, a curve is obtained after 35 cycles, allowing the identification of an *H pylori*–positive specimen.

Then, a melting curve analysis (MCA) is performed (ie, the temperature of the mixture is increased to determine the temperature at which dissociation of the double amplicon strands occurs). In the case of a wild-type, the melting temperature is the highest (62°C), whereas in the case of a mismatch, the melting temperature is lower: 58°C for the transversion and 53°C to 54°C for the transition (**Fig. 2**).[9] This approach was also performed by Matsumura and colleagues[10] with different primers and probes.

Historically, this method was first proposed using SYBR green, a fluorophore specific for double-stranded DNA and used as a quencher, which transfers its energy to a second fluorophore Cy5 fixed on a probe specific to *H pylori*.[11,12]

Advantages of this procedure

- It is not necessary to have viable organisms, so the transport conditions are not as strict as for culture, because DNA remains unaltered even at ambient temperature during long periods.
- The procedure can be performed within a few hours. DNA must be extracted: this can be done in various ways, including the use of commercial kits, and it can also be automatized. Then, the amplification reaction is performed within 2 hours.
- Mixed populations made of resistant and susceptible bacteria can be better detected than by traditional-based culture methods.
- There are commercially available PCR kits that offer a standardized procedure: ClariRes Assay (Ingenetix, Vienna, Austria), MutaReal (Immundiagnostic, Bensheim, Germany). Another interesting point is that this methodology can be applied not only to fresh biopsy specimens but also to archival material (eg, fixed material on histologic preparations), as well as on other specimens in which culture is seldom positive (ie, stool specimens).[13,14] However, the accuracy of the results of *H pylori* detection in stools is still controversial.[15,16] The amount of *H pylori* DNA in stools is not important, and inhibitors of the Taq polymerase may decrease the sensitivity of the method unless a long DNA extraction procedure is performed.

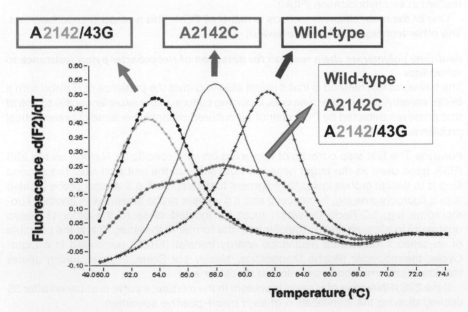

Fig. 2. Detection of clarithromycin resistance in *H pylori* by real-time PCR using a biprobe according to the FRET-MCA principle. The different melting temperatures allow the mutation to be detected.

A variation of the method proposed by Lascols and colleagues[17] consists of a quantitative detection of *H pylori* in gastric biopsy specimens followed, in the event of a positive result, by the performance of another hybridization with a different biprobe, followed by an MCA.

Variants of the method

The TaqMan format For each of the 3 known mutations (A2142C, A2142G, and A2143G) and the wild-type of the 23S rRNA gene, 4 TaqMan-MGB (Minor Groove Binder) probes are designed.[18] A first probe having the fluorochrome VIC allows the detection of the wild-type, a second labeled with fluorochrome FAM detects the mutated form A2142C, a third FAM probe the A2142G mutation, and a fourth FAM probe the A2143G mutation. It is necessary to perform several amplifications for each specimen and test the corresponding probes.

The fluorescence emitted by the activated fluorochrome hydrolyzed probe is then detected.

Advantages and limitations The absence of melting curve requires different amplifications to be performed for each sample and the use of 4 TaqMan probes, which increases the cost.

The scorpion format An alternative method described by Burucoa and colleagues[19] is based on a single-vessel multiplex real-time PCR that detects *H pylori* infection and the wild-type sequence and the 3 mutations conferring clarithromycin resistance using allele-specific scorpion primers directly on biopsy specimens. The scorpion primers combine a primer and a probe in a single molecule and are able to distinguish between single nucleotide polymorphisms. Fluorescent signals produced when the probes are annealed are read in 4 channels by a SmartCycler thermocycler (Cepheid, Sunnyval, CA, USA).

Multiplex polymerase chain reaction followed by strip hybridization
The principle is the same as for real-time PCR (ie, the mixture contains primers to specifically amplify *H pylori* and others targeting the 23S rRNA gene). Once the PCR is carried out, there is a second step of DNA strip hybridization. Strips coated with different oligonucleotides (DNA probes) are commercially available. The probes are designed to hybridize with the sequences of the wild-type alleles or the mutated alleles.

To assess positive and negative bands, the strips are pasted to an evaluation sheet after hybridization, and a template is aligned with the conjugate control band of the respective strip. Control bands of the conjugate control and amplification control should appear positive (**Fig. 3**). Using the commercially available GenoType HelicoDR (Hain LifeScience, Nehren, Germany) a concordance score of 0.96 was found with real-time PCR for clarithromycin resistance.[20] The sensitivity and specificity in the published studies are presented in **Table 1**.

A similar prototype named line probe assay was developed earlier, in which oligonucleotide probes were immobilized on a strip (Innogenetics now Fujirebio Europe, Gent, Belgium).[21,22]

Advantages and limits As with real-time PCR, this method does not require specific transport conditions and can be performed rapidly. However, it is technically more demanding, because the procedures are not automated. Furthermore, the result is based on human interpretation, and it is sometimes difficult to identify weak bands present on the strip.

Because standard PCR is performed, a risk of amplicon contamination exists, and therefore, strict pre and post PCR conditions are imperative.

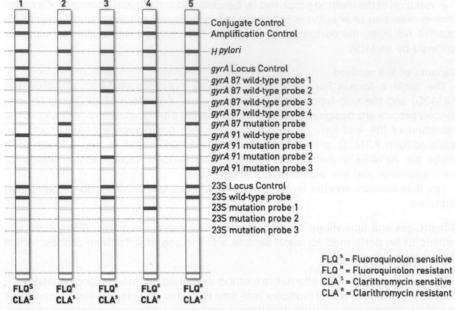

FLQ ^{S} = Fluoroquinolon sensitive
FLQ ^{R} = Fluoroquinolon resistant
CLA ^{S} = Clarithromycin sensitive
CLA ^{R} = Clarithromycin resistant

Fig. 3. Prototype of the strip of the GenoType HelicoDR test. Lane 1, gyrA pattern with a wild-type1 codon at position 87, a wt codon at codon 91, and a wild-type rrl pattern; lane 2, gyrA pattern with an MUT codon at position 87, a wt codon at codon 91, and a wild-type rrl pattern; lane 3, gyrA pattern with a wt2 codon at position 87, an MUT2 codon at position 91, and a wild-type rrl pattern; lane 4, gyrA pattern with a wt3 codon at position 87, a wt codon at position 91, and an MUT1 rrl mutation; lane 5, double mutation in gyrA with mutation at both 87 (MUT) and 91 (MUT3) and a wild-type rrl pattern. (Data from Cambau E, Allerheiligen V, Coulon C, et al. Evaluation of a new test, GenoType HelicoDR, for molecular detection of antibiotic resistance in Helicobacter pylori. J Clin Microbiol 2009;47:3600–7.)

Table 1
Determination of H pylori resistance to macrolides and fluoroquinolones by GenoType HelicoDR (Hain LifeScience, Nehren, Germany)

| Country | Specimen | N | Macrolide | | Fluoroquinolone | | Reference |
			Sensitivity (%)	Specificity (%)	Sensitivity (%)	Specificity (%)	
France	Gastric biopsies	105	97.9	100	92.3	97.4	Cambau et al,[20] 2009
	Strains	92	89.6	97.7	82.9	100	—
Belgium	Gastric biopsies	128	100	86.2	82.6	95.1	Miendje Deyi et al,[82] 2011
Korea	Gastric biopsies	101	94.9	87.1	98.2	80	Lee et al,[54] 2005
South Africa	Strains	78	98	100	89	93	Tanih & Ndip,[83] 2013

On the other hand, this method allows the detection of other resistance mutations present, especially those related to fluoroquinolones, as discussed in the corresponding section.

Dual priming oligonucleotide–polymerase chain reaction

This is a multiplex PCR assay that increases specificity and sensitivity of detection compared with conventional PCR, by blocking nonspecific binding sites and then eliminating imperfect primer annealing (**Fig. 4**). The structure of the dual priming oligonucleotide (DPO) primers is basically different from that of conventional primers. The primer is divided into 2 parts by a 5 polydeoxyinosine linker, which allows a more specific hybridization at temperatures between 55°C and 65°C. This linker forms a bubblelike structure, which itself is not involved in priming but delineates the boundary between the 2 parts. It then generates 2 recognition reactions of the primer on the target sequence. According to the manufacturer, the 5′ end (approximately 20 bases) binds preferentially to the matrix and initiates stable annealing acting as a stabilizer. The 3′ end is shorter (approximately 10 bases) and binds afterward to the target site, but only if the first step has taken place without a mismatch. The 3′ end determines a target-specific extension and acts as a determiner. Therefore, although the longer 5′ segment binds to a nontarget site, the shorter segment resists nonspecific extension. The short 3′ portion alone fails to make a priming at an annealing temperature. The latter also binds preferentially to the target and avoids nonspecific binding.[23] This PCR can be performed in any conventional thermocycler, and a kit is commercially available, the Seeplex ClaR-*H. pylori* ACE detection kit (Seegene, Seoul, Korea).

The performances of the DPO-PCR have been evaluated in several studies.[24–26] In the study of Siffre and colleagues, the sensitivity and specificity versus culture were 97.7% and 83.1%, respectively. Like real-time FRET-PCR, DPO-PCR detected 14 positive samples, which were negative by culture. Both methods were concordant in 95% of cases with regard to clarithromycin susceptibility.[26]

Other polymerase chain reaction–based assays

Nested polymerase chain reaction followed by sequencing or standard polymerase chain reaction followed by sequencing or restriction length polymorphism or colorimetric detection of the amplicons In the early days, the method to detect clarithromycin resistance consisted of a standard PCR targeting the 23S RNA gene.[27]

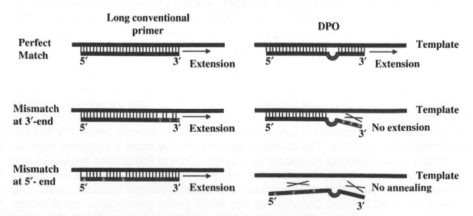

Fig. 4. Long conventional primer-based and DPO-based PCR strategies.

To detect the point mutation, amplicon sequencing can be performed but, for laboratories lacking a sequencing machine, other approaches were proposed. A popular one was to perform a restriction on the DNA fragment. This method is based on the fact that mutations show restriction sites within the amplicon, which are recognized by BsaI for the A2142G mutation and BsbI for the A2143G mutation, leading to the presence of 2 bands on the gel instead of 1.[4] Later, a third enzyme (BceAl) was proposed to detect the A2142C mutation.[5] This method is interesting but has recently been replaced by more rapid real-time PCR-based methods, furthermore eliminating the risk of amplicon contamination.

Another alternative is to detect mutations by a colorimetric hybridization assay in liquid phase. For this purpose, 5′ biotinylated probes were developed to be specific for each genotype (wild-type and the 3 mutants A2143C, A2143G, A2144G). The cutoffs were determined by receiving operating characteristic curves, and a very high accuracy was obtained.[28,29]

The discrimination between allelic sequence variants can also be performed by 2 colorimetric methods: (1) the oligonucleotide ligation assay, which can be automated,[30,31] and (2) the preferential homoduplex formation assay.[32]

It is also possible to detect the mutations by PCR-based denaturing high-performance liquid chromatography, as described by Posteraro and colleagues.[33]

Allele-specific primer polymerase chain reaction Allele-specific primer (ASP)-PCR is especially useful to determine single nucleotide polymorphism in DNA samples, and this technique allows the identification of mutations without direct sequencing or digestion with restriction enzymes. This PCR format is based on the use of forward and reverse primers, which specifically anneal with the 2143G-mutated and 2142G-mutated sequences, respectively, of the 23S rRNA gene of H pylori. These primers are used with another primer pair designed upstream and downstream from the positions 2142 and 2143, respectively, to distinguish the wild-type A2142G and A2143G mutations from each other by amplicon sizes.

Using this method, Trespalacios and colleagues[34] reported a 100% sensitivity and specificity for macrolide resistance in a series of 107 strains.

A modified version of the ASP-PCR was also proposed by Furuta and colleagues.[35]

Primer mismatch polymerase chain reaction This method uses 3′-end mismatch primers with the terminal nucleotide complementary only to the mutated nucleotide on the DNA template.[36]

It was used to detect the A2142G, A2143G, and A2142C mutations in H pylori.[37,38] This PCR was then extended to detect wild-type and 3 mutant genotypes. This method had a slightly better specificity than real-time PCR and a much better specificity than PCR–restriction length polymorphism (RFLP).[39]

Invader assay for single nucleotide polymorphism genotyping The Invader assay (or invasive signal amplification reaction assay) offers a simple diagnostic platform to detect single nucleotide changes with high specificity and sensitivity, originally used with unamplified genomic DNA. The Invader assay uses a structure-specific 5′ nuclease (or flap endonuclease) to cleave sequence-specific structures in each of 2 cascading reactions. The cleavage structure forms when 2 synthetic oligonucleotide probes hybridize in tandem to a target. One of the probes cycles on and off the target and is cut by the nuclease only when the appropriate structure forms. These cleaved probes then participate in a second Invader reaction involving a dye-labeled FRET probe. Cleavage of this FRET probe generates a signal, which can be readily analyzed by fluorescence microtiter plate readers. The 2 cascading reactions amplify the signal significantly; each original target molecule can lead to more than 10^6 cleaved signal probes in 1 hour. This signal amplification permits identification of single base changes directly, even from genomic DNA without previous target amplification. The sequences of the oligonucleotide components of the secondary reaction are independent of the target of interest and allow the development of universal secondary reaction components useful to identify any target.[40]

This method was used by Furuta and colleagues[41] on PCR amplicons (407 bp) of the 23S rRNA gene from gastric biopsies collected for the rapid urease test.

Non–polymerase chain reaction–based assays

Fluorescence in situ hybridization The first report of FISH applied to the detection of *H pylori* resistance to clarithromycin was published by Trebesius and colleagues in 2000.[42] It consists of an rRNA-based whole-cell in situ hybridization using a set of fluorescent-labeled oligonucleotide probes. Labeling of intact fluorescent bacteria is monitored by fluorescence microscopy. Using a 16S rRNA probe labeled with fluorochrome Cy3 (red) allows detection of *H pylori*, and simultaneously, a 23S rRNA probe labeled with fluorescein (green) detects the resistant mutants, which appear yellow by superposition of red and green.

This method proved to be sensitive and specific compared with standard methods of culture and antimicrobial susceptibility testing (AST).

Advantages

- This method does not need DNA extraction or amplification, therefore no apparati are needed, and it allows the bacteria-including coccoidal forms- to be visualized.
- It can be performed reliably on formalin-fixed material and therefore can be performed in a pathology laboratory.[43]
- It allows a quick result.
- A test is commercially available, seaFAST *H. pylori* Combi Kit (SeaPro Theranostics International, Lelystad, The Netherlands).[44]

Limitations are obtaining an observer-dependent result and sometimes it is difficult to read.

Peptide nucleic acid–fluorescence in situ hybridization Peptide nucleic acid (PNA) probes using FISH can be designed to detect bacteria. PNA molecules are DNA mimics that have the negatively charged sugar-phosphate backbone replaced by an achiral, neutral polyamide backbone formed by a repetitive *N*-(2amninoethyl) glycine unit.

Specific hybridization between the PNA sequences and complementary nucleic acid sequences still occurs. The neutral PNA molecule is responsible for a higher thermal stability between PNA and DNA or RNA compared with the traditional DNA probes. Because of this situation, high-affinity PNA probes have sequences relatively smaller (13–18 nucleotides) than DNA sequences (>18 nucleotides) and are more resistant to nucleases and proteases than DNA molecules. They can be labeled by a fluorochrome dye and then detected by fluorescence microscopy or cytometry using the FISH method.

This method has been commonly used to detect *H pylori* in the environment, especially the aquatic environment, but it has also been applied to detect clarithromycin-resistant *H pylori* after culture[45] and in histologic preparations from human gastric biopsies, with a sensitivity of 80% and specificity of 93.8%.[46]

Furthermore, another variant of FISH named fluorescence in vivo hybridization has been developed using oligonucleotide variations comprising locked nucleic acids and 2'-O-methyl RNAs with 2 types of backbone linkages (phosphate or phosphorothioate). These probes hybridize at 37°C, with high sensitivity and specificity for *H pylori*, allowing visualization of these bacteria in biofilms.[47]

Other methods

- Microelectronic chip assay: the assay performs multiple determinations, including identification of *Helicobacter* species (*H pylori* vs *H heilmannii*) and antibiotic resistance (macrolides and tetracycline), on the same microelectronic platform.[48]
- Electrocatalytic detection of DNA sequences: the assay is based on electrocatalytic DNA detection assay, which reports DNA hybridization and resolves single-base changes in the target sequence. For example, an A2143C substitution significantly attenuates hybridization to an immobilized probe corresponding to the wild-type sequence. The single-base mismatch introduced by this mutation slows the kinetics of hybridization and permits discrimination of the 2 sequences when short hybridization times are used.[49]

Correlation with Clinical Outcome

The main reason for discrepancies is essentially that genotypic methods are more accurate than culture plus antibiogram in detecting low numbers of resistant mutants in a population of susceptible bacteria, leading to several so-called heteroresistances (ie, a mixture of susceptible and resistant organisms) (**Table 2**).[9]

Discrepancies were found between genotypic and phenotypic resistance. The concordance was 71.2% in 1 study[50] and 80.6% in another,[51] both using the TaqMan format of real-time PCR. Therefore, the question is: which method is the best predictor of the clinical outcome (ie, eradication of *H pylori*)?

According to De Francesco and colleagues,[50] the best correlation is obtained with phenotypic results (Etest on *H pylori* strains) or with genotypic results not considering heteroresistance (TaqMan real-time PCR on paraffin-embedded gastric biopsies). Because the treatment used in this study was either standard clarithromycin-based triple therapy or sequential therapy, the latter may have a special impact on curing heteroresistant organisms in contrast to the former.

Liou and colleagues[52] in Taiwan reported a result to the contrary in a subgroup of patients from a multicenter study (N = 303) comparing clarithromycin-based standard therapy with levofloxacin-amoxicillin-PPI. AST was performed on *H pylori* strains by agar dilution and a molecular method (PCR followed by sequencing of the 23S rRNA gene) on gastric biopsies. Contrary to what is established, these investigators found that the correlation between clarithromycin genotypic and phenotypic resistance was highest when the cutoff for resistance was set at MIC greater than 2 mg/L (κ correlation = 0.694). In the group of patients receiving clarithromycin, the eradication rates were 7.7% versus 93.5% for those harboring strains with or without 23S rRNA gene mutations (κ = 0.687) and 28.6% versus 90.8% for those harboring strains with MIC greater than 2 mg/L versus 2 mg/L or less, respectively (κ = 0.356).

The result may also depend on the type and the prevalence of the different mutations worldwide. The A2143G mutation may confer a higher risk of treatment failure.[50,53]

Furuta and colleagues[41] found the same proportion of *H pylori* eradication (ie, 87.3%) for susceptible versus 43.3% for resistant strains when resistance was

Table 2
Correlation between *H pylori* eradication rate and the method of determination of resistance, genotypic versus phenotypic

Reference, Country	Treatment Used	N Patients	Genotypic Method	Eradication Susceptibility (%)	Resistance (%)	Phenotypic Method	Eradication Susceptibility (%)	Resistance (%)
De Francesco et al,[18] 2006 Italy	Clari Amox PPI and sequential	146	TaqMan real-time PCR	94.5 (N = 91)	46.1 (N = 13) 78.5 (N = 42)[a]	Etest	92.4 (N = 119)	55.5 (N = 27)
Liou et al,[52] 2011 Taiwan	Clari Amox PPI	303	PCR sequencing	90.8	28.6	Agar dilution	93.5	7.7
Furuta et al,[41] 2005 Japan	Clari Amox PPI	139	Invader assay on amplicon	87.3	43.3	Agar dilution	87.3	43.3
Lee et al,[54] 2005 Korea	Clari Amox PPI	114	PCR-RFLP and sequencing	79.8 (N = 91)	0 (N = 23)	Etest	79.8 (N = 91)	0 (N = 23)

Abbreviations: Amox, amoxicillin; Clari, clarithromycin.
[a] Heteroresistance only.

determined phenotypically (agar dilution method) or genotypically (detection of the mutations by invasive signal amplification assay).

Lee and colleagues[54] also found a perfect agreement between genotypic and phenotypic methods and furthermore a perfect correlation between clarithromycin resistance (or mutation) and lack of eradication and vice versa.

MOLECULAR DETERMINATION OF *HELICOBACTER PYLORI* RESISTANCE TO FLUOROQUINOLONES
Mechanisms

Resistance to fluoroquinolones occurs essentially after mutations at key sites in topoisomerase II (DNA gyrase) or topoisomerase IV, enzymes responsible for the DNA negative supercoiling necessary for DNA replication, which leads to a decreased binding affinity to the antibiotic, reducing its effectiveness.

H pylori possesses only DNA gyrase, which comprises 2 subunits (GyrA and GyrB), and mutations are found in a specific region of GyrA, namely the quinolone resistance-determining region (QRDR). Eleven mutations have already been reported. They are located at codons 86, 87, 88, and 91; however, the principal amino acid positions concerned are 87 and 91.[55,56] Efflux does not play an important role in fluoroquinolone resistance of *H pylori*.

Polymorphism can also be found at the QRDR level, which complicates molecular detection of fluoroquinolone resistance.

Methods

Real-time polymerase chain reaction
Glocker and Kist developed a real-time PCR based on the FRET principle with MCA to differentiate between mutants and wild-type. These investigators designed 2 pairs of hybridization probes to detect aa87 and aa91 mutations instead of membranes. The sensor probes were labeled with 2 different fluorophores: LCRed 705 (for aa 87) and LCRed 640 (for aa91).

This test was applied to 100 strains (35 fluoroquinolone resistant and 65 fluoroquinolone susceptible as determined by sequencing) which could be distinguished. However, the differentiation between aa91 TAT and AAT mutants (combined with an aa 87AAC-wild-type) could not be made, because of their similar melting temperatures. No double mutants were tested in this series.[57]

Multiplex polymerase chain reaction followed by strip hybridization
The commercially available GenoType HelicoDR (Hain LifeScience) allows the detection of mutations associated with fluoroquinolone resistance, in addition to those associated with macrolide resistance.

Because of the polymorphism Asn → Thr observed at aa87, the test includes 4 wild-type probes corresponding to this codon.

In the princeps study of Moore and colleagues, a mutated *gyr*A was observed in 60 (30%) of the *H pylori* strains, 30 with 1 mutation at aa87, 25 with 1 mutation at aa91, 4 with a mutation at both codons, and 1 with 2 mutations at aa91. A concordance of 0.94 was found.

The sensitivity and specificity of GenoType HelicoDR in the published studies is presented in **Table 1**.

Other polymerase chain reaction–based assays
Sequencing of the *gyr*A quinolone resistance-determining region After PCR amplification of 238 bp of the *gyr*A QRDR, sequencing was the method used in the work

of Moore and colleagues.[55] These investigators described 4 classes of mutations with substitutions at aa87 (Asn → Lys), aa88 (Ala → Val), aa91 (Asp → Gly, → Asn, or → Tyr), and a double substitution at aa91 and 97 (Ala → Val). They used PCR amplicons of these resistant strains to transform susceptible H pylori. These mutations were found in 10 of 11 fluoroquinolone-resistant strains, indicating that it was the main resistance mechanism.

This method has been used the most subsequently.[52,58–64]

Allele-specific polymerase chain reaction This method, previously described in the section on macrolides, was first proposed by Nishizawa and colleagues[65] to detect fluoroquinolone resistance in H pylori strains.

It was applied to 107 gastric biopsies in the study of Trespalacios and colleagues[34] in Columbia. Using the primers proposed by Nishizawa and colleagues, the method had a sensitivity and a specificity of 52% and 92.7%, respectively. This low sensitivity was caused by the presence in many cases (44.6%) of the mutation with substitution Asn → Ile in aa87. When new primers were designed and used in addition to the others, sensitivity and specificity reached 100%. The limit of this method is the standardization time when using new primers.

Correlation with Clinical Outcome

Liou and colleagues[52] also studied the correlation in patients receiving levofloxacin-amoxicillin-PPI therapy. These investigators found a better correlation when the genotype method (PCR and sequencing) was used: the eradication rate was 82.7% versus 41.7% when no mutation or a mutation was present, respectively, and 84.1% versus 50% when MICs were 1 mg/L or less versus 1 mg/L. However, this study suffers from the low number of resistant strains found (N = 12).

Detection of H pylori resistance to fluoroquinolones by molecular methods is not as easy as detection of macrolide resistance. There is only 1 commercially available test (GenoType HelicoDR), which has been designed with H pylori strains from Europe, and the pattern of mutations leading to resistance may be different in other parts of the world. It has been recently shown that strains with resistance mutations have a clonal diffusion in some areas, with prevalence varying from 1 country to another.[62] This seems to be the case for South America, where the Asn → Ile at aa87 mutation, absent from the kit, is frequent.

Real-time PCR for fluoroquinolone resistance is also not as straightforward as the detection of macrolide resistance, and no test is commercially available. This situation explains why PCR amplification of the QRDR followed by sequencing is still favored by many bacteriologists.

MOLECULAR DETERMINATION OF HELICOBACTER PYLORI RESISTANCE TO TETRACYCLINE
Mechanisms

Tetracyclines interfere in the protein synthesis at the ribosome level by binding to the 30S subunit. A change in the nucleotide triplet (AGA 926–928 TTC) of the 16S rRNA gene has been associated with resistance to antibiotics in this family because of a lack of binding to the h1 loop, which is the binding site of tetracyclines.[66,67] The need to have these 3 contiguous mutations can explain the rarity of high-level tetracycline resistance. Single or dual mutations at these positions lead to intermediary MICs or no change in MICs.[66,68,69] Another resistant mechanism was described: the efflux mechanism,[70] which also leads to a decreased tetracycline accumulation inside the bacterial cells.

Methods

Real-time polymerase chain reaction

A real-time FRET-PCR with MCA was described by Glocker and colleagues[71] These investigators were able to distinguish between wild-type and resistant strains showing single, double, or triple base-pair mutations in the 16S rRNA gene. Besides the usual probes (anchor probe 3' labeled with fluorescein and AGA sensor probe 5' labeled with LCRed 640), an additional sensor probe, 5' labeled with LCRed 705, which matched the sequence of the TTC mutant and covered the same nucleotides as the other sensor probe, was also used in combination with the anchor probe for a more accurate discrimination of the various mutants. This method, applied to both susceptible and resistant strains with different point mutations, gave excellent results even for single mutations. A similar approach was used by Lawson and colleagues[72] on a large collection of H pylori isolates from England and Wales. Of 1006 isolates, these investigators found 18 (1.6%) with reduced susceptibility to tetracycline (inhibition diameter <30 mm). When tested for MICs, only 3 isolates had an MIC 4 mg/L or greater (0.3%). Ten of the 18 isolates had mutations in the 16S rRNA gene. None had the triple mutation. The triplet GCA led to an MIC of 4 mg/L in 2 of 7 isolates. The other was a double mutation TGC. These different sequences would be identified by the MCA.

Standard polymerase chain reaction followed by sequencing or polymerase chain reaction–restriction length polymorphism

Sequencing of part of the 16S rRNA gene is obviously a good way to detect the triplet or single or dual mutations.

A PCR-RFLP was also developed using the restriction enzyme Hinfl. Tetracycline-susceptible H pylori clinical isolates present a single Hinfl cleavage site within the conserved 535-bp region, thus generating 254-bp and 281-bp Hinfl digestion products. In contrast, mutant strains carrying the AGA 926–928 TTC substitution in both copies of the 16S rRNA genes, which mediates high-level tetracycline resistance, show an additional Hinfl restriction site in the conserved 535-bp region, thus generating 40-bp, 214-bp, and 281-bp digestion products after incubation with the endonuclease. With this assay, mutants bearing single or double DNA substitutions at positions 926 to 928 showed a single cleavage, and all were reported to be associated with low-level tetracycline resistance.[73,74]

MOLECULAR DETERMINATION OF HELICOBACTER PYLORI RESISTANCE TO OTHER ANTIBIOTICS

Rifampins

Rifabutin is the antibiotic essentially used in the group. It inhibits the B subunit of the DNA-dependent RNA polymerase encoded by the rpoB gene. Mutations between codons 525 and 544 or in codon 585 were associated with high-level rifampin resistance. These regions show high homology to the resistance-determining region in E coli and mycobacteria. In particular, 4 residues (codons 527, 530, 540, 545) that harbor more than 80% of all resistant clinical isolates in Mycobacterium tuberculosis also showed the most frequent mutations in H pylori.[75]

For detection of these resistances, no specific method was proposed, and only sequencing can be performed.

Amoxicillin

Amoxicillin interferes with synthesis of the peptidoglycan in the bacterial cell wall.

Resistance is seldom found, and its mechanism is not fully understood, although *pbp*1 gene mutations have been described.[76] For these reasons, molecular tests have not been developed.

5-Nitroimidazoles

5-nitroimidazoles have to be reduced in the bacterial cell to alter DNA. An important gene in this respect is *rdx*A, an oxygen-insensitive nitroreductase. Mutations in *rdx*A can render the protein ineffective.[77,78] The important number of mutations that may arise in the *rdx*A gene, some being independent of *H pylori* resistance to these antibiotics, did not allow the development of molecular methods. In addition, other proteins may also be involved in this reduction process, like the flavin oxidoreductase (*frx*A).[79,80]

Efflux mechanisms may also play a role in the resistance to this drug group.[81]

REFERENCES

1. Megraud F, Lamouliatte H. Review article: the treatment of refractory *Helicobacter pylori* infection. Aliment Pharmacol Ther 2003;17:1333–43.
2. Megraud F. *H. pylori* antibiotic resistance: prevalence, importance, and advances in testing. Gut 2004;53:1374–84.
3. Malfertheiner P, Bazzoli F, Delchier JC, et al. *Helicobacter pylori* eradication with a capsule containing bismuth subcitrate potassium, metronidazole, and tetracycline given with omeprazole versus clarithromycin-based triple therapy: a randomised, open-label, non-inferiority, phase 3 trial. Lancet 2011;377:905–13.
4. Versalovic J, Shortridge D, Kibler K, et al. Mutations in 23S rRNA are associated with clarithromycin resistance in *Helicobacter pylori*. Antimicrob Agents Chemother 1996;40:477 80.
5. Menard A, Santos A, Megraud F, et al. PCR-restriction fragment length polymorphism can also detect point mutation A2142C in the 23S rRNA gene, associated with *Helicobacter pylori* resistance to clarithromycin. Antimicrob Agents Chemother 2002;46:1156–7.
6. Burucoa C, Landron C, Garnier M, et al. T2182C mutation is not associated with clarithromycin resistance in *Helicobacter pylori*. Antimicrob Agents Chemother 2005;49:868 [author reply: 868–70].
7. De Francesco V, Zullo A, Giorgio F, et al. Change of point mutations in *Helicobacter pylori* rRNA associated with clarithromycin resistance in Italy. J Med Microbiol 2014;63:453–7.
8. Mamelli L, Prouzet-Mauleon V, Pages JM, et al. Molecular basis of macrolide resistance in *Campylobacter*: role of efflux pumps and target mutations. J Antimicrob Chemother 2005;56:491–7.
9. Oleastro M, Menard A, Santos A, et al. Real-time PCR assay for rapid and accurate detection of point mutations conferring resistance to clarithromycin in *Helicobacter pylori*. J Clin Microbiol 2003;41:397–402.
10. Matsumura M, Hikiba Y, Ogura K, et al. Rapid detection of mutations in the 23S rRNA gene of *Helicobacter pylori* that confers resistance to clarithromycin treatment to the bacterium. J Clin Microbiol 2001;39:691–5.
11. Gibson JR, Saunders NA, Burke B, et al. Novel method for rapid determination of clarithromycin sensitivity in *Helicobacter pylori*. J Clin Microbiol 1999;37:3746–8.
12. Chisholm SA, Owen RJ, Teare EL, et al. PCR-based diagnosis of *Helicobacter pylori* infection and real-time determination of clarithromycin resistance directly from human gastric biopsy samples. J Clin Microbiol 2001;39:1217–20.

13. Schabereiter-Gurtner C, Hirschl AM, Dragosics B, et al. Novel real-time PCR assay for detection of *Helicobacter pylori* infection and simultaneous clarithromycin susceptibility testing of stool and biopsy specimens. J Clin Microbiol 2004;42: 4512–8.

14. Vecsei A, Innerhofer A, Binder C, et al. Stool polymerase chain reaction for *Helicobacter pylori* detection and clarithromycin susceptibility testing in children. Clin Gastroenterol Hepatol 2010;8:309–12.

15. Lottspeich C, Schwarzer A, Panthel K, et al. Evaluation of the novel *Helicobacter pylori* ClariRes real-time PCR assay for detection and clarithromycin susceptibility testing of *H. pylori* in stool specimens from symptomatic children. J Clin Microbiol 2007;45:1718–22.

16. Makristathis A, Hirschl AM, Russmann H, et al. Detection and clarithromycin susceptibility testing of *Helicobacter pylori* in stool specimens by real-time PCR: how to get accurate test results. J Clin Microbiol 2007;45:2756 [author reply: 2756–7].

17. Lascols C, Lamarque D, Costa JM, et al. Fast and accurate quantitative detection of *Helicobacter pylori* and identification of clarithromycin resistance mutations in *H. pylori* isolates from gastric biopsy specimens by real-time PCR. J Clin Microbiol 2003;41:4573–7.

18. De Francesco V, Margiotta M, Zullo A, et al. Primary clarithromycin resistance in Italy assessed on *Helicobacter pylori* DNA sequences by TaqMan real-time polymerase chain reaction. Aliment Pharmacol Ther 2006;23:429–35.

19. Burucoa C, Garnier M, Silvain C, et al. Quadruplex real-time PCR assay using allele-specific scorpion primers for detection of mutations conferring clarithromycin resistance to *Helicobacter pylori*. J Clin Microbiol 2008;46:2320–6.

20. Cambau E, Allerheiligen V, Coulon C, et al. Evaluation of a new test, GenoType HelicoDR, for molecular detection of antibiotic resistance in *Helicobacter pylori*. J Clin Microbiol 2009;47:3600–7.

21. van Doorn LJ, Debets-Ossenkopp YJ, Marais A, et al. Rapid detection, by PCR and reverse hybridization, of mutations in the *Helicobacter pylori* 23S rRNA gene, associated with macrolide resistance. Antimicrob Agents Chemother 1999; 43:1779–82.

22. van der Ende A, van Doorn LJ, Rooijakkers S, et al. Clarithromycin-susceptible and -resistant *Helicobacter pylori* isolates with identical randomly amplified polymorphic DNA-PCR genotypes cultured from single gastric biopsy specimens prior to antibiotic therapy. J Clin Microbiol 2001;39:2648–51.

23. Chun JY, Kim KJ, Hwang IT, et al. Dual priming oligonucleotide system for the multiplex detection of respiratory viruses and SNP genotyping of CYP2C19 gene. Nucleic Acids Res 2007;35:e40.

24. Woo HY, Park DI, Park H, et al. Dual-priming oligonucleotide-based multiplex PCR for the detection of *Helicobacter pylori* and determination of clarithromycin resistance with gastric biopsy specimens. Helicobacter 2009;14:22–8.

25. Cho AR, Lee MK. A comparison analysis on the diagnosis of *Helicobacter pylori* infection and the detection of clarithromycin resistance according to biopsy sites. Korean J Lab Med 2010;30:381–7 [in Korean].

26. Lehours P, Siffre E, Megraud F. DPO multiplex PCR as an alternative to culture and susceptibility testing to detect *Helicobacter pylori* and its resistance to clarithromycin. BMC Gastroenterol 2011;11:112.

27. Noguchi N, Rimbara E, Kato A, et al. Detection of mixed clarithromycin-resistant and -susceptible *Helicobacter pylori* using nested PCR and direct sequencing of DNA extracted from faeces. J Med Microbiol 2007;56:1174–80.

28. Pina M, Occhialini A, Monteiro L, et al. Detection of point mutations associated with resistance of *Helicobacter pylori* to clarithromycin by hybridization in liquid phase. J Clin Microbiol 1998;36:3285–90.
29. Marais A, Monteiro L, Occhialini A, et al. Direct detection of *Helicobacter pylori* resistance to macrolides by a polymerase chain reaction/DNA enzyme immunoassay in gastric biopsy specimens. Gut 1999;44:463–7.
30. Nickerson DA, Kaiser R, Lappin S, et al. Automated DNA diagnostics using an ELISA-based oligonucleotide ligation assay. Proc Natl Acad Sci U S A 1990;87:8923–7.
31. Stone GG, Shortridge D, Versalovic J, et al. A PCR-oligonucleotide ligation assay to determine the prevalence of 23S rRNA gene mutations in clarithromycin-resistant *Helicobacter pylori*. Antimicrob Agents Chemother 1997;41:712–4.
32. Maeda S, Yoshida H, Matsunaga H, et al. Detection of clarithromycin-resistant *Helicobacter pylori* strains by a preferential homoduplex formation assay. J Clin Microbiol 2000;38:210–4.
33. Posteraro P, Branca G, Sanguinetti M, et al. Rapid detection of clarithromycin resistance in *Helicobacter pylori* using a PCR-based denaturing HPLC assay. J Antimicrob Chemother 2006;57:71–8.
34. Trespalacios AA, Rimbara E, Otero W, et al. Improved allele-specific PCR assays for detection of clarithromycin and fluoroquinolone resistant of *Helicobacter pylori* in gastric biopsies: identification of N87I mutation in GyrA. Diagn Microbiol Infect Dis 2015;81(4):251–5.
35. Furuta T, Soya Y, Sugimoto M, et al. Modified allele-specific primer-polymerase chain reaction method for analysis of susceptibility of *Helicobacter pylori* strains to clarithromycin. J Gastroenterol Hepatol 2007;22:1810–5.
36. Ge Z, Taylor DE. Rapid polymerase chain reaction screening of *Helicobacter pylori* chromosomal point mutations. Helicobacter 1997;2:127–31.
37. Alarcon T, Domingo D, Prieto N, et al. PCR using 3′-mismatched primers to detect A2142C mutation in 23S rRNA conferring resistance to clarithromycin in *Helicobacter pylori* clinical isolates. J Clin Microbiol 2000;38:923–5.
38. Pan ZJ, Su WW, Tytgat GN, et al. Assessment of clarithromycin-resistant *Helicobacter pylori* among patients in Shanghai and Guangzhou, China, by primer-mismatch PCR. J Clin Microbiol 2002;40:259–61.
39. Elviss NC, Lawson AJ, Owen RJ. Application of 3′-mismatched reverse primer PCR compared with real-time PCR and PCR-RFLP for the rapid detection of 23S rDNA mutations associated with clarithromycin resistance in *Helicobacter pylori*. Int J Antimicrob Agents 2004;23:349–55.
40. Fors L, Lieder KW, Vavra SH, et al. Large-scale SNP scoring from unamplified genomic DNA. Pharmacogenomics 2000;1:219–29.
41. Furuta T, Sagehashi Y, Shirai N, et al. Influence of CYP2C19 polymorphism and *Helicobacter pylori* genotype determined from gastric tissue samples on response to triple therapy for *H pylori* infection. Clin Gastroenterol Hepatol 2005;3:564–73.
42. Trebesius K, Panthel K, Strobel S, et al. Rapid and specific detection of *Helicobacter pylori* macrolide resistance in gastric tissue by fluorescent in situ hybridisation. Gut 2000;46:608–14.
43. Juttner S, Vieth M, Miehlke S, et al. Reliable detection of macrolide-resistant *Helicobacter pylori* via fluorescence in situ hybridization in formalin-fixed tissue. Mod Pathol 2004;17:684–9.
44. Morris JM, Reasonover AL, Bruce MG, et al. Evaluation of seaFAST, a rapid fluorescent in situ hybridization test, for detection of *Helicobacter pylori* and resistance to clarithromycin in paraffin-embedded biopsy sections. J Clin Microbiol 2005;43:3494–6.

45. Cerqueira L, Fernandes RM, Ferreira RM, et al. PNA-FISH as a new diagnostic method for the determination of clarithromycin resistance of Helicobacter pylori. BMC Microbiol 2011;11:101.
46. Cerqueira L, Fernandes RM, Ferreira RM, et al. Validation of a fluorescence in situ hybridization method using peptide nucleic acid probes for detection of Helicobacter pylori clarithromycin resistance in gastric biopsy specimens. J Clin Microbiol 2013;51:1887–93.
47. Fontenete S, Guimaraes N, Leite M, et al. Hybridization-based detection of Helicobacter pylori at human body temperature using advanced locked nucleic acid (LNA) probes. PLoS One 2013;8:e81230.
48. Xing JZ, Clarke C, Zhu L, et al. Development of a microelectronic chip array for high-throughput genotyping of Helicobacter species and screening for antimicrobial resistance. J Biomol Screen 2005;10:235–45.
49. Lapierre MA, O'Keefe M, Taft BJ, et al. Electrocatalytic detection of pathogenic DNA sequences and antibiotic resistance markers. Anal Chem 2003;75:6327–33.
50. De Francesco V, Zullo A, Ierardi E, et al. Phenotypic and genotypic Helicobacter pylori clarithromycin resistance and therapeutic outcome: benefits and limits. J Antimicrob Chemother 2010;65:327–32.
51. Monno R, Giorgio F, Carmine P, et al. Helicobacter pylori clarithromycin resistance detected by Etest and TaqMan real-time polymerase chain reaction: a comparative study. APMIS 2012;120:712–7.
52. Liou JM, Chang CY, Sheng WH, et al. Genotypic resistance in Helicobacter pylori strains correlates with susceptibility test and treatment outcomes after levofloxacin- and clarithromycin-based therapies. Antimicrob Agents Chemother 2011;55:1123–9.
53. Francavilla R, Lionetti E, Castellaneta S, et al. Clarithromycin-resistant genotypes and eradication of Helicobacter pylori. J Pediatr 2010;157:228–32.
54. Lee JH, Shin JH, Roe IH, et al. Impact of clarithromycin resistance on eradication of Helicobacter pylori in infected adults. Antimicrob Agents Chemother 2005;49:1600–3.
55. Moore RA, Beckthold B, Wong S, et al. Nucleotide sequence of the gyrA gene and characterization of ciprofloxacin-resistant mutants of Helicobacter pylori. Antimicrob Agents Chemother 1995;39:107–11.
56. Tankovic J, Lascols C, Sculo Q, et al. Single and double mutations in gyrA but not in gyrB are associated with low- and high-level fluoroquinolone resistance in Helicobacter pylori. Antimicrob Agents Chemother 2003;47:3942–4.
57. Glocker E, Kist M. Rapid detection of point mutations in the gyrA gene of Helicobacter pylori conferring resistance to ciprofloxacin by a fluorescence resonance energy transfer-based real-time PCR approach. J Clin Microbiol 2004;42:2241–6.
58. Bogaerts P, Berhin C, Nizet H, et al. Prevalence and mechanisms of resistance to fluoroquinolones in Helicobacter pylori strains from patients living in Belgium. Helicobacter 2006;11:441–5.
59. Cattoir V, Nectoux J, Lascols C, et al. Update on fluoroquinolone resistance in Helicobacter pylori: new mutations leading to resistance and first description of a gyrA polymorphism associated with hypersusceptibility. Int J Antimicrob Agents 2007;29:389–96.
60. Kese D, Gubina M, Kogoj R, et al. Detection of point mutations in the gyrA gene of Helicobacter pylori isolates in Slovenia. Hepatogastroenterology 2009;56:925–9.

61. Wang LH, Cheng H, Hu FL, et al. Distribution of *gyr*A mutations in fluoroquinolone-resistant *Helicobacter pylori* strains. World J Gastroenterol 2010;16:2272–7.
62. Garcia M, Raymond J, Garnier M, et al. Distribution of spontaneous gyrA mutations in 97 fluoroquinolone-resistant *Helicobacter pylori* isolates collected in France. Antimicrob Agents Chemother 2012;56:550–1.
63. Rimbara E, Noguchi N, Kawai T, et al. Fluoroquinolone resistance in *Helicobacter pylori*: role of mutations at position 87 and 91 of GyrA on the level of resistance and identification of a resistance conferring mutation in GyrB. Helicobacter 2012;17:36–42.
64. Ontsira Ngoyi EN, Atipo Ibara BI, Moyen R, et al. Molecular detection of *Helicobacter pylori* and its antimicrobial resistance in Brazzaville, Congo. Helicobacter 2015. [Epub ahead of print].
65. Nishizawa T, Suzuki H, Umezawa A, et al. Rapid detection of point mutations conferring resistance to fluoroquinolone in *gyr*A of *Helicobacter pylori* by allele-specific PCR. J Clin Microbiol 2007;45:303–5.
66. Gerrits MM, Berning M, Van Vliet AH, et al. Effects of 16S rRNA gene mutations on tetracycline resistance in *Helicobacter pylori*. Antimicrob Agents Chemother 2003;47:2984–6.
67. Trieber CA, Taylor DE. Mutations in the 16S rRNA genes of *Helicobacter pylori* mediate resistance to tetracycline. J Bacteriol 2002;184:2131–40.
68. Dailidiene D, Bertoli MT, Miciuleviciene J, et al. Emergence of tetracycline resistance in *Helicobacter pylori*: multiple mutational changes in 16S ribosomal DNA and other genetic loci. Antimicrob Agents Chemother 2002;46:3940–6.
69. Nonaka L, Connell SR, Taylor DE. 16S rRNA mutations that confer tetracycline resistance in *Helicobacter pylori* decrease drug binding in *Escherichia coli* ribosomes. J Bacteriol 2005;187:3708–12.
70. Wu JY, Kim JJ, Reddy R, et al. Tetracycline-resistant clinical *Helicobacter pylori* isolates with and without mutations in 16S rRNA-encoding genes. Antimicrob Agents Chemother 2005;49:578–83.
71. Glocker E, Berning M, Gerrits MM, et al. Real-time PCR screening for 16S rRNA mutations associated with resistance to tetracycline in *Helicobacter pylori*. Antimicrob Agents Chemother 2005;49:3166–70.
72. Lawson AJ, Elviss NC, Owen RJ. Real-time PCR detection and frequency of 16S rDNA mutations associated with resistance and reduced susceptibility to tetracycline in *Helicobacter pylori* from England and Wales. J Antimicrob Chemother 2005;56:282–6.
73. Ribeiro ML, Gerrits MM, Benvengo YH, et al. Detection of high-level tetracycline resistance in clinical isolates of *Helicobacter pylori* using PCR-RFLP. FEMS Immunol Med Microbiol 2004;40:57–61.
74. Toledo H, Lopez-Solis R. Tetracycline resistance in Chilean clinical isolates of *Helicobacter pylori*. J Antimicrob Chemother 2010;65:470–3.
75. Heep M, Beck D, Bayerdorffer E, et al. Rifampin and rifabutin resistance mechanism in *Helicobacter pylori*. Antimicrob Agents Chemother 1999;43:1497–9.
76. Qureshi NN, Morikis D, Schiller NL. Contribution of specific amino acid changes in penicillin binding protein 1 to amoxicillin resistance in clinical *Helicobacter pylori* isolates. Antimicrob Agents Chemother 2011;55:101–9.
77. Hoffman PS, Goodwin A, Johnsen J, et al. Metabolic activities of metronidazole-sensitive and -resistant strains of *Helicobacter pylori*: repression of pyruvate oxidoreductase and expression of isocitrate lyase activity correlate with resistance. J Bacteriol 1996;178:4822–9.

78. Wang G, Wilson TJ, Jiang Q, et al. Spontaneous mutations that confer antibiotic resistance in *Helicobacter pylori*. Antimicrob Agents Chemother 2001;45:727–33.
79. Marais A, Bilardi C, Cantet F, et al. Characterization of the genes *rdx*A and *frx*A involved in metronidazole resistance in *Helicobacter pylori*. Res Microbiol 2003; 154:137–44.
80. Mendz GL, Megraud F. Is the molecular basis of metronidazole resistance in microaerophilic organisms understood? Trends Microbiol 2002;10:370–5.
81. van Amsterdam K, Bart A, van der Ende A. A *Helicobacter pylori* TolC efflux pump confers resistance to metronidazole. Antimicrob Agents Chemother 2005;49: 1477–82.
82. Miendje Deyi VY, Burette A, Bentatou Z, et al. Practical use of GenoType(R) HelicoDR, a molecular test for *Helicobacter pylori* detection and susceptibility testing. Diagn Microbiol Infect Dis 2011;70:557–60.
83. Tanih NF, Ndip RN. Molecular detection of antibiotic resistance in South African isolates of *Helicobacter pylori*. Gastroenterol Res Pract 2013;2013:259457.

When Is Endoscopic Follow-up Appropriate After *Helicobacter pylori* Eradication Therapy?

Ernst J. Kuipers, MD, PhD

KEYWORDS

- *Helicobacter pylori* • Eradication • Endoscopy • Follow-up • Biopsy • Peptic ulcer
- Atrophic gastritis • MALT lymphoma

KEY POINTS

- The roles of *Helicobacter pylori* and eradication therapy have been firmly established in a range of gastroduodenal disorders.
- Confirmation of successful *H pylori* eradication is needed in patients with persistent or recurrent symptoms as well as in those with complicated peptic ulcer.
- Further endoscopic surveillance after *H pylori* eradication is needed in patients with advanced premalignant gastric lesions, previous early gastric cancer, and gastric mucosa associated lymphoid tissue lymphoma and in carriers of a hereditary cancer syndrome with gastric cancer risk.

INTRODUCTION

The introduction of acid suppressants and the recognition of *Helicobacter pylori* as a pathogen revolutionized gastroenterology practice. It meant that chronic, debilitating conditions, such as peptic ulcer disease, could be treated with a course of antibiotics. Patients were relieved from the stigma of suffering from a psychosomatic disease and from long treatments and hospital admissions, often ending in surgery. A younger generation of physicians may easily underestimate this impact. The author and colleagues previously estimated it for the Netherlands alone, a small country with 17 million inhabitants. The improvement in peptic ulcer treatment led to a yearly gain of 46,000 quality-adjusted life-years and annual savings of at least €1.8 billion.[1] These major changes

Competing interests: none.
Department of Gastroenterology and Hepatology, Erasmus MC University Medical Center, s-Gravendijkwal 230, 3015 CE, Rotterdam, The Netherlands
E-mail address: e.j.kuipers@erasmusmc.nl

Gastroenterol Clin N Am 44 (2015) 597–608
http://dx.doi.org/10.1016/j.gtc.2015.05.006
0889-8553/15/$ – see front matter © 2015 Elsevier Inc. All rights reserved.

have not removed the necessity for endoscopic follow-up for a proportion of patients with *H pylori*–associated conditions. They need follow-up to monitor the underlying disease and/or to confirm successful bacterial eradication when persistent colonization puts patients at significant risk for disease recurrence or progression. This article focuses on the need for endoscopic follow-up after *H pylori* eradication therapy (**Table 1**).

Table 1
Need for follow-up after *H pylori* eradication therapy

Disease Category	Condition	Endoscopic Follow-up After *H pylori* Eradication Therapy	Purpose of Follow-up
Dyspepsia	Uninvestigated dyspepsia	Only in case persistent/ recurrent symptoms	Establish diagnosis, reassess *H pylori* status
	Functional dyspepsia	Only in case persistent/ recurrent symptoms and lack of noninvasive *H pylori* test	Reassess *H pylori* status
Peptic ulcer	Duodenal ulcer, uncomplicated	Only in case persistent/ recurrent symptoms and lack of noninvasive *H pylori* test	Reassess *H pylori* status
	Gastric ulcer, uncomplicated, unsuspected, negative histology, and evident cause	Only in case persistent/ recurrent symptoms and lack of noninvasive *H pylori* test	Reassess *H pylori* status
	Gastric ulcer, possibly malignant, negative baseline histology	Repeat gastroscopy with biopsy sampling	Reconfirm benign cause, reassess *H pylori* status
	Gastric or duodenal ulcer, complicated	Only if noninvasive *H pylori* test not available	Reassess *H pylori* status
Premalignant lesions	OLGIM stage III & IV	Surveillance gastroscopy with biopsy sampling	Monitor disease progression, reassess *H pylori* status
	Dysplasia	Surveillance gastroscopy with biopsy sampling	Monitor disease progression, reassess *H pylori* status
Gastric malignancy	Early gastric cancer, after endoscopic treatment	Surveillance gastroscopy with biopsy sampling	Monitor disease recurrence, reassess *H pylori* status
	MALT lymphoma	Surveillance gastroscopy with biopsy sampling	Monitor disease remission, reassess *H pylori* status
	Familial gastric cancer	Only if noninvasive *H pylori* test not available	Reassess *H pylori* status
	Hereditary cancer syndrome	Surveillance gastroscopy with biopsy sampling	Monitor disease occurrence, reassess *H pylori* status

Abbreviations: MALT, mucosa-associated lymphoid tissue; OLGIM, Operative Link on Gastric Intestinal Metaplasia Assessment.

HELICOBACTER PYLORI ERADICATION

The first antimicrobial therapy for intragastric flagellated bacilli was introduced more than 100 years ago.[2] This treatment in particular consisted of high doses of bismuth, often for prolonged periods. Soon after the first culture of H pylori, attempts were made to eradicate this bacterium. For that purpose, bismuth therapy was combined with other antimicrobials.[3,4] Since those first successful attempts, the success rates of eradication therapy plateaued. Other drugs, such as proton pump inhibitors and a range of antimicrobials, were introduced in various combinations. Many combinations of a proton pump inhibitor with 1 to 3 antimicrobials as well as 3 to 4 antimicrobials including bismuth were applied over the years. These drugs were all given together or in sequential combinations. Many of these combinations first yielded promising eradication results. Unfortunately, further studies and use in daily clinical practice without exception showed limitations.[5] These limitations were among others caused by the rapid increase of antimicrobial resistance in H pylori. More complex regimens, such as the combination of 4 drugs, prolonged treatment, and sequential regimens often also decrease adherence, among others, because of side effects. This factor explains that, in many daily clinical practice settings, 15% to 40% of eradication attempts fail. This failure rate explains the need to assess the outcome of eradication treatment in some patients. Most of these patients do not need endoscopic follow-up. Their H pylori status can, thus, be reassessed noninvasively. Urea breath tests, fecal antigen tests, and conventional serology serve this purpose. Serology is, in most settings, not convenient because it needs a long time interval between treatment and reassessment. Urea breath tests are excellent for this purpose. They are highly accurate; patient burden is minimal; and costs are low. However, they are not always available. In practices where none of these noninvasive options are available, renewed endoscopy may be required to reassess H pylori status. This situation is preferentially avoided, both because of the patient burden and costs. Against this background, endoscopic follow-up after H pylori eradication pertains to the following situation.

UNINVESTIGATED AND NONULCER DYSPEPSIA

H pylori colonization and dyspepsia are both common phenomena, which explains the considerable overlap between the two (ie, a considerable proportion of patients with dyspeptic symptoms are H pylori positive). The causal relation between the two is, however, limited. The effect of H pylori eradication on nonulcer dyspepsia is, thus, also small. More than 15 prospective randomized controlled trials compared the effect of H pylori eradication with placebo in patients with nonulcer dyspepsia. On average, the number needed to treat to cure one patient with dyspepsia was 14.[6] It often took 6 to 12 months for symptoms to improve.

This finding implies that patients who receive H pylori eradication therapy for nonulcer dyspepsia first need adequate explanation that the effect on symptoms is not guaranteed and may take months. If a patient reports after 6 to 12 months of follow-up with persistent or recurrent symptoms, H pylori status may be reassessed. This reassessment will preferably be done by a noninvasive test. Endoscopy needs to be considered if noninvasive tests are not available.

A related category consists of patients who have received H pylori eradication after noninvasive testing only, without endoscopy. This category of uninvestigated dyspepsia includes patients with nonulcer dyspepsia as well as patients with other conditions, such as peptic ulcer. Patients with uninvestigated dyspepsia who report with persistent or recurrent symptoms after H pylori eradication are eligible for endoscopy. This eligibility allows reassessing *H pylori* status as well as evaluating the presence of specific disease, such as peptic ulcer.

PEPTIC ULCER

H pylori and nonsteroidal antiinflammatory drugs (NSAIDs) in most settings cause more than 90% of peptic ulcers. The remainder is caused by a range of other causes, including other microorganisms, other drugs,[7] and cancer. *H pylori* and NSAIDs interact in the etiology of ulcers; the risk for peptic ulcer is higher in an *H pylori*–positive NSAID user than in patients with either factor alone.[8] It is estimated that the lifetime risk for the development of peptic ulcer in the presence of *H pylori* lies in the order of 20%.[9] Once an individual develops an *H pylori*–associated peptic ulcer, he or she is at a more than 50% risk of recurrent ulcer disease within the next 24 months. This risk explains that peptic ulcer used to be a chronic, recurrent disease. Acid-suppressive maintenance therapy reduces the recurrence rate but does not prevent recurrent peptic ulcer. *H pylori* eradication leads to an almost complete cure of chronic recurrent ulcer disease. For that reason, *H pylori* eradication is the mainstay of treatment of peptic ulcers associated with *H pylori* colonization.[10] Eradication treatment is similarly important in *H pylori*-positive patients with peptic ulcer and simultaneous of aspirin or NSAIDs. Ulcer recurrence rates after eradication treatment are very low. Ulcers can reoccur in patients with recrudescent or renewed infection or patients taking ulcerogenic drugs, in particular NSAIDs or aspirin. Against this background, patients with uncomplicated duodenal disease do not require endoscopic follow-up or routine reassessment of their *H pylori* status after eradication treatment. In case of recurrent or persistent symptoms, the effect of eradication treatment needs to be assessed at least 4 weeks after treatment. This reassessment is preferentially done noninvasively, for instance, by means of urea breath testing. This approach does not pertain to all peptic ulcers. Two exceptions are gastric ulcer disease and complicated peptic ulcer.

Gastric ulcer disease can be caused by an underlying malignancy. This underlying malignancy includes adenocarcinoma, lymphoma, other primary gastric malignancies, as well as metastatic disease. This factor implies that assessment for the underlying cause not only requires assessment of *H pylori* status and drug use but also requires biopsy sampling from the ulcer rim itself. If this demonstrates an underlying malignancy, management first fully aims at cancer treatment. *H pylori* eradication only has a role during follow-up in those patients in whom (part of) the stomach is preserved (see later discussion). In patients with a gastric ulcer without histologic signs of malignancy, *H pylori* eradication is again the first treatment. However, because a single round of biopsy sampling may miss cancer, a follow-up endoscopy 1 month after the end of eradication treatment may be considered. This practice allows both to assess the effect of eradication treatment and to obtain additional ulcer histology to further exclude cancer. The yield of such surveillance is limited. Most studies date from the era of fiberoptic endoscopy or the early times of video endoscopy. They suggested a 2% to 5% cancer miss rate with initial endoscopy.[11] With these old roots, the practice of endoscopic surveillance for gastric ulcer is, nevertheless, still quite widely practiced. In a US survey among 6113 patients with gastric ulcers, 25% underwent surveillance endoscopy.[12] Current image-enhanced endoscopy techniques, such as narrow-band imaging, allow detailed assessment of the ulcer surroundings and targeted biopsies of visible lesions. This assessment likely enhances the yield of biopsy sampling and, thus, reduces the risk that any underlying malignancy is overseen. With this modern equipment, endoscopists may well consider to refrain from endoscopic surveillance in patients with negative histology and regular/benign-appearing ulcer with evident cause (in particular H pylori or NSAID use). Patients with initial negative histology, but irregular ulcer, no defined cause, and/or persistent symptoms should be considered for surveillance endoscopy with repeat biopsy sampling.[13]

A second group of patients with peptic ulcers for whom endoscopic follow-up is recommended after H pylori eradication consists of those with complicated peptic ulcer. The most common complication is ulcer hemorrhage, followed by perforation and gastric outlet stenosis. Peptic ulcer bleeding is a severe complication associated with significant morbidity and mortality.[14] Endoscopic therapy forms the mainstay of diagnosis and treatment. This therapy can be done by injection therapy, coagulation, or clipping. Although epinephrine injection may initially stop the bleed, it is insufficient as monotherapy for the treatment of bleeding peptic ulcer.[15] It should, therefore, be combined with other modalities. Patients who show, during endoscopy, active bleeding or stigmata of recent hemorrhage, in particular a visible vessel, should, after adequate endoscopic treatment, receive high-dose intravenous proton pump inhibitors.[15] After the acute phase, patients need to be assessed for the presence of H pylori and, if positive, receive eradication treatment. In a systematic review of 7 studies with 578 patients with bleeding peptic ulcer, rebleeding occurred in 3% after H pylori eradication versus 20% after acid-suppressive therapy alone.[16] The same approach pertains to patients with a perforated ulcer, for whom the initial treatment usually consists of surgical closure of the perforation. In a randomized trial comparing H pylori eradication versus 4 weeks omeprazole treatment of perforated peptic ulcer, recurrent ulcer occurred in 5% after eradication treatment versus 38% after omeprazole.[17] For patients with gastric outlet stenosis, the initial treatment may consist of balloon dilation, or sometimes surgery, followed by H pylori eradication if H pylori positive.[18] Because the risk of renewed complicated ulcer disease in any of these patients groups (bleeding, perforation, stenosis) is considerable, it is mandatory to assess H pylori status after eradication treatment. These patients will usually be kept on proton pump inhibitor therapy until confirmation of successful H pylori eradication. This therapy may affect the accuracy of urea breath testing, particularly the increase in the rate of false negatives. For that reason, follow-up of patients with previous complicated peptic ulcer is primarily done by endoscopy with renewed biopsy sampling from antrum and corpus to reassess H pylori status. Once H pylori eradication has been confirmed, further acid-suppressive therapy can be stopped because the risk of recurrent ulcer in the absence of H pylori and the risk for reinfection are both very low. However, if a patient with a history or complicated peptic ulcer has a strong need for NSAID/aspirin use without alternative options, gastroprotection by means of acid suppressive therapy is again needed.

PREMALIGNANT GASTRIC LESIONS AND EARLY GASTRIC CANCER

Intestinal-type adenocarcinoma is the predominant sporadic gastric cancer. The pathway toward this malignancy is characterized by chronic gastritis, leading to gland loss or atrophic gastritis, and replacement of specialized glands by intestinal metaplasia. Atrophy and metaplasia can eventually lead to dysplasia and invasive cancer.

This cascade is strongly determined by H pylori as the predominant cause of chronic active gastritis. Virtually all patients who are H pylori positive have chronic active gastritis. The level of inflammation tends to be stable throughout further life with H pylori and correlates with the risk for progression to peptic ulcer and gastric cancer.[19] The pattern and severity of gastritis depend on both host and bacterial characteristics, including bacterial cytotoxin-associated gene A (cagA) status and host acid output. Patients colonized with a cagA-positive, cytotoxin-producing strain tend to have more severe inflammation. Patients with normal to increased acid output have an antral-predominant gastritis, whereas patients with decreased acid output tend to have a corpus-predominant pan-gastritis. In all cases, chronic gastritis predisposes to gland loss. In a series of 107 subjects followed for an average 11.5 years, approximately half of the subjects who were H pylori positive eventually developed signs of gland loss compared with only a minority of subjects who were H pylori negative.[19] In the latter group, those with atrophic gastritis already tended to have widespread atrophy and metaplasia at baseline. Thus, they presumably reflected patients in whom H pylori had spontaneously disappeared as a result of a more hostile niche caused by the development of atrophy and metaplasia.

Once these conditions occur, the risk for further progression to invasive cancer significantly increases. In a prospective study of approximately 98,000 subjects with premalignant gastric lesions, the rate of progression to gastric cancer over a decade was approximately 1% in subjects with atrophic gastritis, 4% in those with atrophy and intestinal metaplasia, increasing to more than 30% in those with high-grade dysplasia at baseline.[20] These findings and other observations supported the notion that the risk of invasive cancer in these patient categories is higher than in some other conditions, such as Barrett esophagus and the situation after colonoscopy removal of sporadic adenomatous colorectal polyps. In contrast to these other conditions, international guidelines for the management of patients with premalignant gastric lesions were lacking.

This lack of guidelines was the reason for the recent development of the Management of precancerous conditions and lesions in the stomach (MAPS) guidelines, endorsed by the European Societies of Gastrointestinal Endoscopy and Pathology.[21] These guidelines recommend adequate endoscopic imaging of the gastric lining with routine biopsy sampling of the antrum and corpus and further sampling of any visible mucosal lesion. This practice should be followed by H pylori eradication treatment of all patients with evidence of persistent H pylori colonization.

This intervention has been shown to have a significant preventive effect on gastric cancer. A systematic review analyzed 6 randomized controlled trials comparing H pylori eradication with placebo for prevention of gastric cancer.[22] Subjects were then followed for 2 years or longer. Gastric cancer occurred in 1.6% of subjects after eradication versus 2.4% of controls (relative risk 0.66; 95% confidence interval 0.46–0.95).[22] Bacterial eradication, however, did not benefit those with intestinal metaplasia at baseline.[23] A similar lack of a preventive effect was observed in patients with gastric dysplasia.[24] This finding implies that H pylori eradication should be followed in these patients by further endoscopic surveillance, in particular of patients at the highest risk of gastric cancer. For that purpose, the MAPS guidelines recommended to use the Operative Link for Gastritis Assessment (OLGA) or the Operative Link on Gastric Intestinal Metaplasia Assessment (OLGIM) staging systems.[21] These systems cross-tabulate atrophy (OLGA) or intestinal metaplasia (OLGIM) of antrum and corpus, leading to 4 stages (OLGA/OLGIM I/II/III/IV).[25,26] Patients with moderate to severe atrophy/metaplasia of antrum and corpus (OLGA/OLGIM III and IV) are considered at the highest risk for progression to cancer. It is recommended to offer these patients endoscopic surveillance at 3-year intervals.[21]

In Japan, a comparable approach makes use of serologic screening. Serum pepsinogen I and II levels, their ratio, and H pylori serology define 4 categories (A/B/C/D). Groups A and B have normal pepsinogens and are respectively seronegative and seropositive for H pylori. Groups C and D have low pepsinogens (defined as a pepsinogen I <70 ng/mL and a pepsinogen (Pg) I/II ratio <3.0) and are respectively seropositive and seronegative for H pylori. A prospective study of 6983 subjects followed for an average 4.7 years in a health screening project showed that the risk for gastric cancer was significantly higher for stage C and D subjects than A and B subjects. Group D had the highest risk, with some 4.5% of subjects developing gastric cancer within 7 years.[27] Japanese patients are now eligible for H pylori eradication as part of a national prevention program (Sugano K, Tack J, Kuipers EJ, et al. Kyoto global consensus report on Helicobacter pylori gastritis. Gut. Submitted for publication.). Patients in groups C and D are eligible for additional endoscopic investigation and surveillance when histology confirms advanced atrophic gastritis.

Patients with early gastric cancer are primarily treated with endoscopic resection. Several studies have shown that additional H pylori eradication reduces the risk for metachronous gastric cancer. A first nonrandomized study treated 132 patients who were H pylori positive with early gastric cancer by endoscopic resection.[28] Sixty-five patients received additional H pylori eradication. After 3 years, 6 (9%) of the patients who were persistently H pylori positive had developed metachronous gastric cancer compared with nil of the patients treated with eradication therapy. A randomized study confirmed these results. It randomized 272 patients who were H pylori positive after endoscopic resection of early gastric cancer to additional eradication treatment or no further treatment.[29] After 3 years, 24 metachronous cancers had been diagnosed in the noneradication arm versus 9 in the eradication arm. Based on these findings, H pylori eradication is strongly recommended after endoscopic resection of early gastric cancer or a dysplastic lesion. Given the risk for local recurrence as well as metachronous lesions, such a measure should be followed by endoscopic surveillance.[21] This surveillance also allows to check the H pylori status after eradication treatment and prescribe second-line treatment in case of eradication failure.

HEREDITARY RISK FOR GASTRIC CANCER

In some cases, eradication therapy is given for preventive purposes only. This therapy in particular pertains to pateints with a first-degree family history of gastric cancer. These patients are at an increased risk for gastric cancer.[30] Several studies have shown that first-degree cancer relatives have a higher prevalence of H pylori as well as premalignant gastric lesions.[31] The Maastricht guidelines, therefore, recommend considering H pylori eradication in first-degree relatives of gastric cancer.[10] There are no prospective studies available to show the preventive effect of this strategy in these patients. Against this background, it is fair to assume that gastric cancer in these families is related to H pylori and follows similar pathways as in sporadic gastric cancer. For that purpose, endoscopy is indicated at least once to assess both H pylori status and the condition of the gastric lining. In most cases, this endoscopy will be the first approach, before eradication treatment of patients who are H pylori positive. Endoscopic follow-up is then afterward only indicated in case of signs of atrophic gastritis with or without intestinal metaplasia (see later discussion).

A combined approach of H pylori test and treat and endoscopic surveillance is recommended for carriers of a hereditary cancer syndrome with the risk for gastroduodenal cancer. This approach in particular pertains to carriers of the Lynch syndrome, familial adenomatous polyposis, and Peutz-Jeghers syndrome. It has long been recognized that gastric cancer forms part of the Lynch syndrome. In fact, in the first description of a family affected by the syndrome, gastric cancer was the predominant malignancy.[32] Over the past decades, gastric cancer incidence in families with Lynch syndrome declined. In a Dutch nationwide study, the author and colleagues previously showed a decrease of gastric cancer in patients with Lynch syndrome and a decrease in the lifetime risk for gastric cancer among patients with

Lynch syndrome to a lifetime risk of 5% in women and 8% in men.[33] The author thinks that this effect in particular relates to changes in the prevalence of H pylori. Other factors may contribute, such as the average age at infection and improvement of diet and other risk factors. The notion in the past was that gastric cancer was strongly clustered in some families with Lynch syndrome. The nationwide study by the author and colleagues, however, proved this untrue. The median number of gastric cancer cases in affected families was one. Eighty-five percent of the families in which gastric cancer occurred had only one affected family member.[33] It is assumed that timely H pylori eradication may reduce the risk for gastric cancer. Solid data to support this assumption are lacking. Nevertheless, an H pylori test-and-treat policy is recommended for Lynch syndrome carriers. This policy is accompanied by the recommendation to further endoscopic surveillance with targeted gastric biopsy sampling in Lynch syndrome carriers from 30 to 35 years of age onwards.[34] A similar approach is advocated for familial adenomatous polyposis[35] and patients with Peutz-Jeghers.[36] Both categories are more at risk for duodenal cancer, but gastric cancer also pertains to these syndromes. Endoscopic follow-up after H pylori eradication in particular aims at surveillance and early treatment of neoplastic conditions. This follow-up also allows checking the outcome of H pylori eradication treatment.

MUCOSA-ASSOCIATED LYMPHOID TISSUE LYMPHOMA

Gastric mucosa-associated lymphoid tissue (MALT) lymphoma is a rare condition (**Fig. 1**). In a nationwide survey using the Dutch national histology database PALGA, the author and colleagues previously identified 1419 patients with gastric MALToma over a 16-year period.[37] This finding was compatible with an annual incidence of 4.1 per 1 million inhabitants. The disease is strongly associated with chronic H pylori colonization of the stomach. A systematic review reported a 79% prevalence of H pylori among 1844 patients with MALToma in different series worldwide.[38] The investigators concluded that the prevalence per individual study depended on the methods of assessment. Studies that had used at least 2 methods per patient for assessment of H

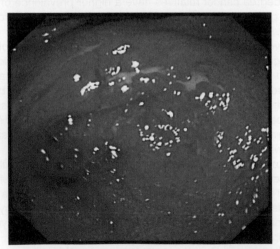

Fig. 1. Superficial, irregular ulceration of the gastric antrum caused by mucosa-associated lymphoid tissue lymphoma in a patient who is H pylori positive. Primary treatment consists of H pylori eradication with further endoscopic surveillance. This treatment allows assessment of bacterial eradication and, with further follow-up, lymphoma regression.

pylori status reported an average 85% *H pylori* prevalence in patients with MALToma. *H pylori* eradication benefits most of these patients and may over the course of several months to 2 years lead to complete and persistent regression of the lymphoma. A systematic review of 32 studies with 1408 patients reported that *H pylori* eradication led to complete MALToma remission in 77% of patients.[39] A later, large original study with 420 patients confirmed these findings.[40] Based on these observations, international guidelines recommend *H pylori* eradication as the first-line treatment of MALToma confined to the stomach.[10,41,42] These guidelines recommend to check *H pylori* status 1 month after eradication treatment by urea breath test. Endoscopic surveillance is needed to evaluate the effect of eradication treatment on the lymphoma. This surveillance is usually done at 3-month intervals during the first year, at 6-month intervals during the second year, and then annually until 5 years after eradication treatment. Further treatment is only given in case of persistent or recurrent lymphoma. The endoscopic surveillance also allows confirming that patients have no persistent or recurrent *H pylori* infection.

SUMMARY

The role of *H pylori* has been firmly established in a range of gastroduodenal disorders. *H pylori* colonization virtually always leads to immediate chronic active gastritis; the condition is remarkably stable throughout further life with *H pylori*. Although most patients with *H pylori* do not have any specific symptoms, there is a weak correlation with dyspeptic symptoms. In a subset of colonized patients, the persistent mucosal inflammation leads to complications, in particular peptic ulcer, atrophic gastritis, gastric cancer, and gastric MALT lymphoma. *H pylori* eradication may benefit patients with uninvestigated dyspepsia as well as those with functional dyspepsia. It is the therapy of choice for patients with *H pylori*–associated peptic ulcer. It is recommended for patients with premalignant gastric lesions and those with a familial risk of gastric cancer. Finally, it is the mainstay of treatment of patients with gastric MALT lymphoma. The effect of *H pylori* eradication treatment can be assessed by a variety of noninvasive methods, of which urea breath testing is in most settings the easiest and most reliable method. Further endoscopic follow-up is needed in patients with uninvestigated dyspepsia who do not respond to *H pylori* eradication. Patients with complicated peptic ulcer need thorough confirmation of successful *H pylori* eradication. Given the importance of adequate assessment and the fact that their use of acid suppressants interferes with urea breath testing, *H pylori* status is usually checked by repeat endoscopy. Finally, for several categories of patients, *H pylori* eradication alone is insufficient to completely prevent disease progression or recurrence. These categories include patients with premalignant gastric lesions (atrophy, metaplasia, and dysplasia), patients treated for early gastric cancer, and patients with gastric MALT lymphoma. These patients require adequate endoscopic surveillance, for which the interval depends on the baseline condition. This endoscopic surveillance also allows checking *H pylori* status.

REFERENCES

1. den Hoed CM, Isendoorn K, Klinkhamer W, et al. The societal gain of medical development and innovation in gastroenterology. United European Gastroenterol J 2013;1(5):335–45.
2. Pel PK. De ziekten van de maag ('Diseases of the stomach'). Amsterdam: De Erven Bohn; 1899.

3. Marshall BJ, Armstrong JA, Francis GJ, et al. Antibacterial action of bismuth in relation to Campylobacter pyloridis colonization and gastritis. Digestion 1987; 37(Suppl 2):16–30.

4. Rauws EA, Tytgat GN. Cure of duodenal ulcer associated with eradication of Helicobacter pylori. Lancet 1990;335(8700):1233–5.

5. Graham DY, Fischbach L. Helicobacter pylori treatment in the era of increasing antibiotic resistance. Gut 2010;59(8):1143–53.

6. Moayyedi P, Soo S, Deeks J, et al. Eradication of Helicobacter pylori for non-ulcer dyspepsia. Cochrane Database Syst Rev 2006;(2):CD002096.

7. Masclee GM, Valkhoff VE, Coloma PM, et al. Risk of upper gastrointestinal bleeding from different drug combinations. Gastroenterology 2014;147(4): 784–92.e9 [quiz: e13–4].

8. Huang JQ, Sridhar S, Hunt RH. Role of Helicobacter pylori infection and non-steroidal anti-inflammatory drugs in peptic-ulcer disease: a meta-analysis. Lancet 2002;359(9300):14–22.

9. Kuipers EJ, Thijs JC, Festen HP. The prevalence of Helicobacter pylori in peptic ulcer disease. Aliment Pharmacol Ther 1995;9(Suppl 2):59–69.

10. Malfertheiner P, Megraud F, O'Morain CA, et al. Management of Helicobacter pylori infection–the Maastricht IV/Florence Consensus Report. Gut 2012;61(5): 646–64.

11. Bustamante M, Devesa F, Borghol A, et al. Accuracy of the initial endoscopic diagnosis in the discrimination of gastric ulcers: is endoscopic follow-up study always needed? J Clin Gastroenterol 2002;35(1):25–8.

12. Saini SD, Eisen G, Mattek N, et al. Utilization of upper endoscopy for surveillance of gastric ulcers in the United States. Am J Gastroenterol 2008;103(8): 1920–5.

13. ASGE Standards of Practice Committee, Banerjee S, Cash BD, et al. The role of endoscopy in the management of patients with peptic ulcer disease. Gastrointest Endosc 2010;71(4):663–8.

14. Lau JY, Barkun A, Fan DM, et al. Challenges in the management of acute peptic ulcer bleeding. Lancet 2013;381(9882):2033–43.

15. Barkun AN, Bardou M, Kuipers EJ, et al. International consensus recommendations on the management of patients with nonvariceal upper gastrointestinal bleeding. Ann Intern Med 2010;152(2):101–13.

16. Gisbert JP, Khorrami S, Carballo F, et al. H. pylori eradication therapy vs. antisecretory non-eradication therapy (with or without long-term maintenance antisecretory therapy) for the prevention of recurrent bleeding from peptic ulcer. Cochrane Database Syst Rev 2004;(2):CD004062.

17. Ng EK, Lam YH, Sung JJ, et al. Eradication of Helicobacter pylori prevents recurrence of ulcer after simple closure of duodenal ulcer perforation: randomized controlled trial. Ann Surg 2000;231(2):153–8.

18. Cherian PT, Cherian S, Singh P. Long-term follow-up of patients with gastric outlet obstruction related to peptic ulcer disease treated with endoscopic balloon dilatation and drug therapy. Gastrointest Endosc 2007;66(3):491–7.

19. Kuipers EJ, Uyterlinde AM, Pena AS, et al. Long-term sequelae of Helicobacter pylori gastritis. Lancet 1995;345(8964):1525–8.

20. de Vries AC, van Grieken NC, Looman CW, et al. Gastric cancer risk in patients with premalignant gastric lesions: a nationwide cohort study in the Netherlands. Gastroenterology 2008;134(4):945–52.

21. Dinis-Ribeiro M, Areia M, de Vries AC, et al. Management of precancerous conditions and lesions in the stomach (MAPS): guideline from the European Society

of Gastrointestinal Endoscopy (ESGE), European Helicobacter Study Group (EHSG), European Society of Pathology (ESP), and the Sociedade Portuguesa de Endoscopia Digestiva (SPED). Endoscopy 2012;44(1):74–94.

22. Ford AC, Forman D, Hunt RH, et al. Helicobacter pylori eradication therapy to prevent gastric cancer in healthy asymptomatic infected individuals: systematic review and meta- analysis of randomised controlled trials. BMJ 2014;348:g3174.

23. Chen HN, Wang Z, Li X, et al. Helicobacter pylori eradication cannot reduce the risk of gastric cancer in patients with intestinal metaplasia and dysplasia: evidence from a meta-analysis. Gastric Cancer 2015. [Epub ahead of print].

24. Mera R, Fontham ET, Bravo LE, et al. Long term follow up of patients treated for Helicobacter pylori infection. Gut 2005;54(11):1536–40.

25. Rugge M, Genta RM, Group O. Staging gastritis: an international proposal. Gastroenterology 2005;129(5):1807–8.

26. Capelle LG, de Vries AC, Haringsma J, et al. The staging of gastritis with the OLGA system by using intestinal metaplasia as an accurate alternative for atrophic gastritis. Gastrointest Endosc 2010;71(7):1150–8.

27. Watabe H, Mitsushima T, Yamaji Y, et al. Predicting the development of gastric cancer from combining Helicobacter pylori antibodies and serum pepsinogen status: a prospective endoscopic cohort study. Gut 2005;54(6):764–8.

28. Uemura N, Mukai T, Okamoto S, et al. Effect of Helicobacter pylori eradication on subsequent development of cancer after endoscopic resection of early gastric cancer. Cancer Epidemiol Biomarkers Prev 1997;6(8):639–42.

29. Fukase K, Kato M, Kikuchi S, et al. Effect of eradication of Helicobacter pylori on incidence of metachronous gastric carcinoma after endoscopic resection of early gastric cancer: an open-label, randomised controlled trial. Lancet 2008; 372(9636):392–7.

30. Yaghoobi M, Bijarchi R, Narod SA. Family history and the risk of gastric cancer. Br J Cancer 2010;102(2):237–42.

31. Rokkas T, Sechopoulos P, Pistiolas D, et al. Helicobacter pylori infection and gastric histology in first-degree relatives of gastric cancer patients: a meta-analysis. Eur J Gastroenterol Hepatol 2010;22(9):1128–33.

32. Whartin AS. Heredity with reference to carcinoma: as shown by the study of the cases examined in the pathological laboratory of the University of Michigan, 1895-1913. Arch Intern Med 1913;12:546–55.

33. Capelle LG, Van Grieken NC, Lingsma HF, et al. Risk and epidemiological time trends of gastric cancer in Lynch syndrome carriers in the Netherlands. Gastroenterology 2010;138(2):487–92.

34. Vasen HF, Blanco I, Aktan-Collan K, et al. Revised guidelines for the clinical management of Lynch syndrome (HNPCC): recommendations by a group of European experts. Gut 2013;62(6):812–23.

35. Vasen HF, Moslein G, Alonso A, et al. Guidelines for the clinical management of familial adenomatous polyposis (FAP). Gut 2008;57(5):704–13.

36. van Lier MG, Wagner A, Mathus-Vliegen EM, et al. High cancer risk in Peutz-Jeghers syndrome: a systematic review and surveillance recommendations. Am J Gastroenterol 2010;105(6):1258–64 [author reply: 1265].

37. Capelle LG, de Vries AC, Looman CW, et al. Gastric MALT lymphoma: epidemiology and high adenocarcinoma risk in a nation-wide study. Eur J Cancer 2008; 44(16):2470–6.

38. Asenjo LM, Gisbert JP. Prevalence of Helicobacter pylori infection in gastric MALT lymphoma: a systematic review. Rev Esp Enferm Dig 2007;99(7):398–404 [in Spanish].

39. Zullo A, Hassan C, Cristofari F, et al. Effects of Helicobacter pylori eradication on early stage gastric mucosa-associated lymphoid tissue lymphoma. Clin Gastroenterol Hepatol 2010;8(2):105–10.

40. Nakamura S, Sugiyama T, Matsumoto T, et al. Long-term clinical outcome of gastric MALT lymphoma after eradication of Helicobacter pylori: a multicentre cohort follow-up study of 420 patients in Japan. Gut 2012;61(4):507–13.

41. Ruskone-Fourmestraux A, Fischbach W, Aleman BM, et al. EGILS consensus report. Gastric extranodal marginal zone B-cell lymphoma of MALT. Gut 2011; 60(6):747–58.

42. Dreyling M, Thieblemont C, Gallamini A, et al. ESMO Consensus conferences: guidelines on malignant lymphoma. Part 2: marginal zone lymphoma, mantle cell lymphoma, peripheral T-cell lymphoma. Ann Oncol 2013;24(4):857–77.

Gastric Cancer Risk in Patients with *Helicobacter pylori* Infection and Following Its Eradication

CrossMark

Massimo Rugge, MD

KEYWORDS

- *H pylori* • Gastric cancer risk • Gastric cancer prevention • Pepsinogens
- OLGA staging • Atrophic gastritis

KEY POINTS

- *Helicobacter pylori* is a first-class carcinogen; the eradication of the infection is a primary cancer-prevention strategy.
- In gastric mucosa, *H pylori* infection results in both (1) inflammation (ie, gastritis) and (2) structural modifications of the native anatomy/function (ie, precancerous lesions: atrophy/metaplasia, intraepithelial neoplasia [synonym dysplasia]).
- Anatomic changes are assessable by endoscopy/biopsy. Pepsinogen serology mirrors gastric mucosa atrophy with a high negative predictive value.
- Following *H pylori* eradication, the rate of reversion of the histology lesions decreases along with their increasing severity.
- Successful eradication invariably results in eliminating the *H pylori*–associated mucosal inflammation (ie, the inflammatory component of the mucosal damage).
- Mucosal atrophy and intestinal metaplasia may (at least partially) be reversed by *H pylori* eradication (the higher the gastritis stage, the lower/slower the reversion rate).
- Contradictory information is available on the benefit achievable by eradicating patients with advanced precancerous lesions (ie, intraepithelial neoplasia); beneficial effects have been reported only in association with low-grade lesions.
- In patients (endoscopically/surgically) treated for early gastric cancer, *H pylori* eradication delays/lowers the risk of metachronous cancers.
- The choice of eradicating is independent from both the severity of the mucosal damage and the (expected) rate of its reversibility; the mucosal status at eradication time only affects the timing/strategy of posteradication interventions (follow-up, ablation, surgical therapy).

This work was partly supported by a grant of the Italian Association for Cancer Research (AIRC Regional Grant 2008 No. 6421).

Potential competing interests: In 2010, the author was an unpaid consultant for Biohit HealthCare; at present, he has no competing interests to declare.

Surgical Pathology & Cytopathology Unit, Department of Medicine - DIMED, University of Padova, Via Aristide Gabelli, 61, Padova 35121, Italy

E-mail address: massimo.rugge@unipd.it

Gastroenterol Clin N Am 44 (2015) 609–624
http://dx.doi.org/10.1016/j.gtc.2015.05.009
0889-8553/15/$ – see front matter © 2015 Elsevier Inc. All rights reserved.

INTRODUCTION

The so-called epidemic or intestinal-type gastric cancer (GC) is the most frequent gastric neoplasia, and the fact that its (race-independent) incidence is declining throughout all developed countries supports the hypothesis that environmental factors play a major role in its cause. A second clinico-biological variant of GC is hereditary (ie, syndromic), and it is associated with specific mutational profiles; the epidemiologic impact of this variant is negligible.[1]

Irrespective of its morphologic/epidemiologic variants, GC is associated with a poor prognosis, with a 5-year overall survival rate lower than 30%.

The onset of intestinal-type GC is definitively associated with age (older than 50 years), which is consistent with the most accepted theory concerning the long natural history of GC. Chronic gastritis (mostly caused by H pylori infection) may represent the earliest phase of gastric oncogenesis. After several decades, long-standing inflammation extensively modifies the native gastric mucosa, creating a microenvironment prone to cancer development. This "cancerization field" consists of 2 main types of lesions: (1) inflammation of the gastric mucosa and (2) gastric mucosal atrophy characterized by both an absolute loss of resident glandular units and/or a metaplastic transformation (eg, intestinalization) of native glandular structures.[2] The metaplastic epithelium may further undergo dedifferentiation, acquiring most of the biological characteristics of neoplastic cells but still lacking invasion capability (intraepithelial neoplasia [IEN], formerly defined as dysplasia).[3] By acquiring stromal invasion capability, IEN ultimately progresses to invasive cancer.

GC's natural history, known as Correa oncogenic cascade, provides a biological rationale behind the multidisciplinary approach for primary and secondary prevention strategies.[4]

HELICOBACTER PYLORI INFECTION IS THE MOST IMPORTANT DETERMINANT OF GASTRIC CANCER RISK

As with most neoplastic diseases, GC is a multifactorial neoplasia. In most cases, environmental factors are the main cancer-promoting agents, but even in non-syndromic (ie, sporadic) cancers, host-related factors are involved in cancer promotion.

Among all possible environmental factors, H pylori is consistently recognized as the leading etiologic agent of GC.[5] In 1994, H pylori was recognized as a type I carcinogen; it is currently considered the most common etiologic agent linked to infection-related cancers, which represent 5.5% of the global cancer burden.[6] **Fig. 1** outlines the most relevant etio-pathogenetic factors involved in sporadic GCs.

Globally, about 3.5 billion people have the H pylori infection, and solid evidence supports a fecal-oral and/or gastric-oral transmission pattern that takes place early in life.[7] The rates of H pylori infection vary considerably by geographic area, with a generally higher prevalence in developing countries.[8] A large percentage of those who are infected develop non–self-limiting gastric inflammation; approximately 10% develop peptic (duodenal or gastric) ulcers; 3% develop gastric adenocarcinoma, with less than 0.5% developing mucosa-associated lymphoid tissue lymphoma.

The variable outcome of the infection probably depends on the infection's bacterial properties, on environmental cofactors, as well as on host-related immune response modulation.[9] All these variables must be taken into consideration when GC risk following H pylori eradication is being assessed.[10]

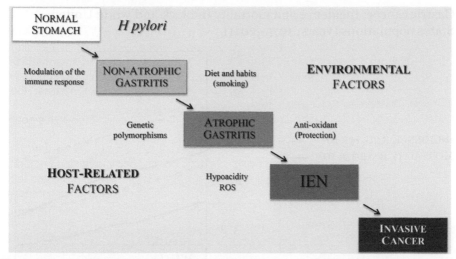

Fig. 1. Main phenotypic changes occurring in gastric oncogenetic cascade; some of the main environmental and host-related factors involved in the etiopathogenesis are also shown (ROS, reactive oxygen species [synonym: dysplasia]).

GASTRIC CANCER RISK: EPIDEMIOLOGIC TRENDS

In highly developed countries, survival curves of patients with GC have consistently demonstrated a continuous decline in cancer-related mortality (**Fig. 2**). This trend is, however, only partially explained by the advent of more efficient therapies; more realistically it seems to be the consequence of a declining cancer burden. In this epidemiologic setting, both GC and *H pylori* infection show the same declining incidence pattern. These two consistent patterns constitute a solid rationale for assuming that eradication of *H pylori* is an appropriate strategy for the primary prevention of GC.

Vaccinations constitute the ideal primary prevention against any infectious disease, but no vaccines are as yet available to prevent *H pylori* infection.[10] Although primary intervention strategies basically rely on efforts to eradicate the bacteria, the best approach to eradication therapy has been, and continues to be, under debate (also in view of the emergence of antibiotic-resistant *H pylori* strains).[11–16]

GASTRIC CANCER RISK: THE ASSESSMENT

GC risk can be assessed using both noninvasive and invasive methods.

Noninvasive approaches include assessment of demographic variables (age, sex, and ethnicity), subjective symptoms (clinical history and current symptoms), and laboratory findings (serology).

Invasive procedures include endoscopy and histology evaluation, which are 2 faces of the same coin: both are expensive and require a high level of technical expertise and a well-organized health care system.

Demographics

Nonsyndromic malignancies are associated with an age-related increased risk. With regard to GC, patients' age also reflects the time between when the person was

Gastric cancer: Incidence and mortality in black and white United
States populations (years: 1975–2011)

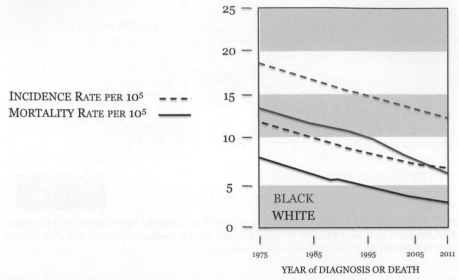

Fig. 2. Cancer of the stomach (both sexes) in black and white populations; Incidence and US
death rates (http://surveillance.cancer.gov/joinpoint/).

infected and the onset of the organic lesions (ie, extensive mucosal atrophy) in which
intestinal-type GC most frequently develops.

In all ethnic groups, solid epidemiologic data link GC to the male sex.[17] As it has
been supported by reports confirming significant differences in GC incidence in
various ethnic groups living in the same country, ethnicity per se seems to be a
risk factor. Age-adjusted incidence rates of GC were found to vary between 29.3
per 100,00 and 3.4 per 100,000, respectively, in Chinese and Malaysian males,
both living in Singapore. Even larger, significant differences were found between
Korean and Filipino populations living in Los Angeles (35.5 vs 6.8, respectively).[17]
The available studies on the effect of ethnicity, however, mostly disregard the differences in the incidence of H pylori infection (Chinese vs Malays), the virulence of the
infecting strains, and the diet (eg, Korans and Filipino populations in Los Angeles).
The relationships between GC risk and dietary constituents (salt and nitrites as
causal agents and fruits and vegetables as protective ones), lifestyle, and, more in
general, socioeconomic status need to be further addressed and more exactly
quantified.[17]

Noninvasive Methods

The noninvasive assessment of GC risk basically relies on the well-established
assumption that the risk of cancer parallels the incidence of atrophic gastritis; the
latter can be reliably assessed by functionally testing the status of the gastric mucosa
with serum pepsinogens, currently considered the best indicators of gastric atrophy.[18]
Pepsinogens (pepsinogen I [PgI] and pepsinogen II [PgII], in particular) are aspartic
proteinases produced by gastric epithelia and secreted into the gastric lumen, where
they are transformed into pepsin. PgI is produced in the chief cells of the oxyntic

mucosa, whereas PgII is produced in both corpus and antral stomach mucosa.[19] Any decrease in the oxyntic gland population (ie, corpus atrophy) leads to a reduction in the serum levels of PgI resulting in a lower PgI/PgII ratio. Pepsinogen testing was implemented long before *H pylori* was discovered and was rediscovered as a marker of GC risk (but not of GC itself).

In a large cohort of 22,000 Finnish subjects, the sensitivity and specificity for PgI/PgII value for the detection of atrophic gastritis were 83% and 93%, respectively.[20] According to a recent study by K. Miki,[21] a PgI/PgII ratio less than 3.0 should be considered a reliable indicator of gastric atrophy and, ultimately, of increased cancer risk; similar results were more recently outlined with regard to a Japanese population by Iijima and coworkers.[22] In addition, according to a long-term Italian follow-up study, a PgI/PgII ratio less than 3.0 was found to be significantly correlated with both the severity and the topography of atrophy, as assessed by gastritis staging.[23] According to that same study, the pepsinogen ratio at the patients' enrollment significantly predicted their cancer risk, as assessed at the end of the 12-year follow-up. A meta-analysis on the sensitivity and specificity of PgI and PgII values as screening tests for advanced precancerous lesions (ie, dysplasia) were associated with a PgI/PgII ratio less than 3, with a negative predictive value (NPV) greater than 95%.[24]

More recently, H. Tu and coworkers[25] reported on a cohort of 2039 Chinese subjects in whom the PgI/PgII ratio was tested as a predictor of progression of gastric precancerous lesions.[25] In that study population, the odds ratio (OR) for patients whose PgI/PgII ratio decreased 50% or more with respect to those in whom it increased 50% or more was 1.40 (confidence interval [CI] 1.08–1.81); among patients in whom both the PgII and anti–*H pylori* immunoglobulin G levels were increased 50% or more with respect to patients whose values decreased 50% or more, the OR was 3.18 (CI 2.05–4.93).[25]

According to available evidence, serum pepsinogen values should never be regarded as cancer biomarkers but should be considered functional indicators of extensive mucosa atrophy and, therefore, as markers of a cancer-prone gastric microenvironment. The predictive value of pepsinogen testing is limited in patients harboring antrum-restricted atrophy, which explains those (unusual) cases in which normal PgI values are associated with overt gastric carcinoma.[26] Moreover, as wisely observed by A. Shiotani and colleagues,[27] the reliability of pepsinogen testing "clearly depends on the cut-off of serum pepsinogen levels as well as the definition used to identify atrophy."[27]

A panel of serologic tests (GastroPanel; Biohit HealthCare) including serum pepsinogens (PgI and PgII), gastrin 17 (G-17), and anti–*H pylori* antibodies has recently been proposed as a tool for the serologic screening (serologic biopsy) of dyspeptic patients. The rationale behind including anti-Helicobacter pylori (Hp) serology is clearly based on its contribution to the morphogenesis of the gastric atrophy. G-17 (a subfraction of total gastrin consisting of 17 amino-acids) is, instead, synthesized/secreted exclusively by gastric antral G cells; serum G-17 is expected to be significantly reduced in the event of severe antral atrophy.[27] G-17, instead, increases significantly in hypochlorhydric patients because of severe atrophy affecting the gastric corpus mucosa. An increased serum G-17 level can, as a result, be confidently assumed to be a marker of autoimmune (corpus-restricted) atrophic gastritis. G-17 is, unfortunately, unstable in serum and requires stabilization with highly standardized procedures for sampling and processing.[28,29] In populations with a low prevalence of atrophic gastritis, the NPV of the serologic panel in identifying atrophic gastritis is as high as 97% (95% CI = 95%–99%).[20,28] More recently, a multicenter study testing the accuracy of the GastroPanel in assessing atrophic gastritis demonstrated an acceptable NPV

(NPV = 92%; 95% CI = 86%–98%) but failed to identify 5 out of the 10 atrophic patients (sensitivity = 50%) included in the cohort of the 85 subjects studied.[30]

The most recent (and actually not the last) step in pepsinogens' validation as markers of atrophic gastritis was made at the Kyoto Global Consensus Conference (Kyoto, February 2014) where the experts involved unequivocally agreed on the following statement: "Serological tests (pepsinogen I and II and anti-*H pylori* antibody) are useful for identifying patients at increased risk for gastric cancer (Grade of Recommendation: Strong; Evidence Level: High)."[31]

Invasive Methods

Invasive procedures for assessing GC risk are basically 2: (1) endoscopy associated to a standard biopsy protocol and (2) histology.

Endoscopy and biopsy protocols

Significant technical progress has been achieved in endoscopic approaches. Conventional endoscopy is currently considered inadequate to assess both early and advanced precancerous lesions that are assessable with high diagnostic accuracy by last-generation, image-enhanced endoscopy (chromo-endoscopy, narrow-band imaging).[32–34]

Irrespective of the endoscopic instruments that are available, gastric biopsy sampling constitutes an essential step in the assessment of organic gastric diseases. The rationale behind how and where biopsy samples should be obtained is based both on normal gastric anatomy/function and the biology of gastric diseases. According to D.Y. Graham, in fact: "taking biopsies should not be an afterthought; obtaining biopsy samples is part of a logical process aimed to provide informative clinico-biologic, diagnostic, therapeutic, and prognostic information." (Graham DY, personal communication, 2007)

The gastric mucosa includes 2 structural/functional compartments: (1) the distal mucosecreting and (2) the proximal oxyntic: this biological heterogeneity results in different patterns of gastric inflammatory diseases. As a consequence, histologic assessment of gastritis requires separate analyses of an adequate number of biopsy specimens obtained from each of the 2 mucosal compartments. At least 5 biopsies (3 from the antrum [including the incisura angularis] and 2 from the gastric body) should be available to assess both the cause and the severity of inflammatory/atrophic disease, including their risk of malignancy.[35,36]

In the *H pylori* gastritis model, several studies support the hypothesis that atrophic/metaplastic lesions are initially located in the region of the incisura angularis. These observations support the recommendation that incisura angularis biopsy samples be obtained both at the initial assessment of precancerous lesions and while monitoring their (possible) regression after eradication; it can be assumed, in fact, that atrophic/metaplastic lesions regress following the opposite topographic sequence characterizing their development. Consistent with that view, atrophy at the incisura angularis could be considered a histologic timer of gastric disease.[37–40]

Histology

Histologically confirmed extensive gastric atrophy is consistently associated with an increased risk of GC. Any strategy addressing GC secondary prevention should then specifically focus on the histologic diagnosis of early (ie, atrophy/intestinal metaplasia) and advanced (ie, IEN) precancerous lesions.[41–43]

Gastric atrophy is defined as the "loss of appropriate glands."[35,44] This definition includes 2 phenotypes of atrophic transformation: (1) the shrinkage or complete disappearance of glandular units that are replaced by fibrosis of the lamina propria (ie, a reduced glandular mass with no modification of the native glandular phenotype) and/ or (2) the replacement of the native glands by metaplastic ones featuring a new commitment (so-called metaplastic atrophy caused by intestinal metaplasia [IM] and/or pseudopyloric metaplasia). Metaplastic atrophy does not necessarily imply a numerical reduction in the glandular units, but the metaplastic replacement of the native glands ultimately results in a decrease in the population of glandular structures appropriate to the compartment concerned.

In 1991, an international consensus document (the Revised Sydney System) set out to standardize the histologic assessment of gastric inflammatory diseases and provided a detailed list of elementary lesions (inflammation, atrophy, intestinal metaplasia) included in the spectrum of gastric mucosa inflammatory diseases.[36] A scoring system was also proposed for each of these lesions (graded variables).

The descriptive philosophy behind the Sydney System has recently been replaced by new approaches to gastritis histology reporting that aim to enable a clearer stratification of gastritis-associated GC risk.[45–47] These new diagnostic formats suggest histologically reporting gastritis in terms of stage: by scoring atrophy/IM microscopically in both oxyntic and antral/angular biopsy samples, the staging frame (stages 0–IV) ranks gastritis according to GC risk.[45–47] The staging format was unexpectedly omitted from the recent guidelines addressing the management of gastric precancerous conditions/lesions.[28] Although those guidelines recognize the prognostic reliability of the staging approach, they base their working recommendations entirely on the topographic spread of atrophy/metaplasia, without taking into consideration the (more significant) prognostic value linked to gastritis staging.[28] Two staging systems have been proposed for GC risk estimation: Operative Link on Gastritis Assessment (OLGA) and Operative Link on Gastric Intestinal Assessment.[46,47] Both of these distinguish gastritis into 5 stages (stage 0 to stage 4), indicating a progressively increasing risk of GC.[46,47]

The OLGA staging system was put forward in 2005 by an International group of pathologists and gastroenterologists.[35,45,46] According to the OLGA proposal, the gastritis stage is obtained by combining the atrophy scores as assessed in both antral and oxyntic biopsy samples.[35] With regard to the dyspeptic patient population, gastritis staging significantly discriminates different classes of cancer risk (low risk: stages 0, I, and II vs high risk: stages III and IV).[23,43] Moreover, a significant correlation has also been demonstrated between the severity of the organic lesions (OLGA stage) and gastric mucosa functional parameters, in particular, with serum pepsinogens.[23]

GASTRIC CANCER RISK IN ERADICATED PATIENTS

The best primary prevention strategy against *H pylori* infection (and its neoplastic consequences) would be vaccination to prevent *H pylori* infection; no vaccines are, however, currently available. As a consequence, if and how the GC risk can be lowered by eradicating the established infection have become clinically important questions. In this scenario, the main issues to be addressed can be summarized as following:

- *H pylori* eradication as a primary prevention of GC
- How to assess cancer risk after *H pylori* eradication
- How to quantify GC risk after *H pylori* eradication
- *H pylori* eradication to prevent metachronous GC

Helicobacter pylori Eradication as a Primary Prevention of Gastric Cancer

In November 2006, the Bangkok Gastric Cancer Consensus Conference recommended *H pylori* screening and treatment to prevent GC for asymptomatic patients belonging to high-risk populations (GC incidence >20 per 100,000 per year).[48] Rather than screening for the infection in asymptomatic patients, the Maastricht IV Consensus Conference recommended that *H pylori* eradication should be used as GC prevention only in selected populations including (1) first-degree relatives of family members with GC; (2) persons at high risk of gastritis; (3) patients with chronic gastric acid inhibition for longer than 1 year; and (4) heavy smokers and individuals with other environmental risk factors like high exposure to dust, coal, quartz, cement.[11]

In the natural history of GC, the gastritis-associated cancer risk increases with the time that has elapsed from when the *H pylori* infection was established. In GC prevention, the benefit that can be achieved by eradicating *H pylori* is a function of the organic lesions (ie, the level of cancer risk) at the time the therapy is carried out. Theoretically then, the less advanced the gastric disease, the greater will be the beneficial effect of eradication.[27] This hypothesis is not contradicted by the possible occurrence of GC in already eradicated patients: in fact, when eradication therapy is obtained in patients who have already developed advanced precancerous lesions, the progression to cancer may become independent from the *H pylori* status.[49,50] The high prevalence of progression to cancer of the high-grade IEN (ie, high-grade dysplasia) consistently qualifies this lesion as a point of no return; less defined information is available concerning the progression/reversibility of low-grade IEN lesions.[49,50]

As in other models of environmental carcinogenesis, it is plausible that in formerly exposed patients, the risk of cancer decreases (more or less slowly) when the (main) etiologic agent has been removed; conversely, cancer risk is expected to increase continuously in those who are currently exposed. A validated example is that provided by the carcinogenetic cascade of smoking-related lung cancers, in which mortality rates differ according to the smoking status (**Fig. 3**).[51,52] The lung cancer mortality rate in current smokers has been estimated to be approximately twice as high with respect to that in never smokers at 40 years of age; after 30 years of abstinence, the mortality rate of former-smokers returns to that of never-smokers.[51,52]

With regard to *H pylori* infection, age is a surrogate marker of the severity of the gastric lesions (ie, the stage of the organic disease); the benefit of eradication consequently differs depending on the patients' age.[27] When (as in the gastric setting) the environmental carcinogen is a transmissible agent, its elimination may result in 2 beneficial effects: (1) it removes the dangerous effect of the carcinogen in the single patient and (2) it dries the source of transmission in the population that is exposed to the bacteria.

Unfortunately, no long-term follow-up studies are as yet available; in particular, there is little information regarding 2 important variables: (1) the effect of age on eradication and (2) the status of the gastric mucosa at the time of eradication. Based on other oncogenetic models, the expected benefits could be hypothesized, as outlined in **Fig. 4**.

How to Assess/Quantify Cancer Risk After Helicobacter pylori Eradication

How to assess and to quantify the variation in cancer risk following eradication therapy are issues that continue to be debated. Assessment methods, however, basically do not differ from those usually applied in the assessment of cancer risk among patients infected with *H pylori*; both invasive and noninvasive types of testing have already been discussed earlier.

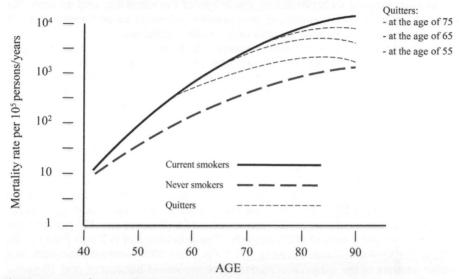

Fig. 3. Age-specific mortality rates according to the smoking status calculated based on the models selected for lung cancer. The mortality rate of former smokers, after 15 and 30 years since quitting, was estimated to decline to approximately 40% and 15%, respectively, of the mortality rate of continuous current smokers. After 30 years of abstinence, the mortality rate of former smokers would be similar to the mortality rate of never smokers. (*Adapted from* Katanoda K, Saika K, Yamamoto S, et al. Projected cancer mortality among Japanese males under different smoking prevalence scenarios: evidence for tobacco control goal setting. Jpn J Clin Oncol 2011;41:486; with permission.)

The variables that need to be taken into consideration to quantify the posteradication residual cancer risk are numerous. Patients should, in fact, be stratified according to different risk criteria, including the geographical-associated GC risk, the profile of the *H pylori* strain, the patients' comorbidities and sex/age, the severity of the gastric

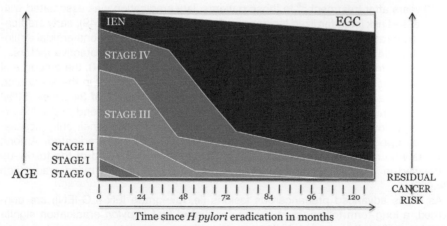

Fig. 4. Presumptive model of the beneficial effects achievable through *H pylori* eradication according to the OLGA stage or to the presence of IEN (synonym dysplasia) at the eradication time. EGC, early GC.

disease at the time of the therapeutic intervention, the procedures applied for disease assessment (invasive vs noninvasive), the length of the follow-up, and so forth. No studies have as yet been conducted (and possibly will never be performed) that will be able to include such a wide number of normalized variables.

The recent availability of molecular biological techniques may, theoretically, open new avenues. No molecular studies on large populations are as yet available; in fact, there is still no well-defined *H pylori*–related molecular deregulation that can be consistently considered a marker of cancer risk fluctuations. It is also important to remember that these methods require solid tissue samples, which per se represent an additional limitation. (Circulating) regulating microRNAs might represent an innovative diagnostic/therapeutic strategy.[53–55]

The study design that has most frequently been used is one that assesses the differences in cancer risk in infected versus eradicated populations.

To assess the effect of *H pylori* eradication in reducing GC risk, in 2009 Fuccio and colleagues[56] performed a meta-analysis of 7 randomized controlled trials that were conducted between 2000 and 2008. All the studies were carried out in geographic areas with a high incidence of GC (incidence rate >20 cases per 10^5 persons per year) and involved a total of 6695 subjects. The prevalence of GC was found to be 1.1% in the 3388 eradicated subjects and 1.7% in the 3307 untreated subjects. In a pooled analysis of the subjects considered, all monitored between 4 and 10 years, the relative risk for GC was 0.65 (95% CI: 0.43 to 0.98). Based on these results, the investigators concluded that *"Helicobacter pylori* eradication treatment seems to reduce gastric cancer risk."[56]

A longitudinal Japanese study was conducted on middle-aged men infected with *H pylori* (3656 *Hp* +ve patients) to evaluate the preventive effects of its eradication (obtained in 473 patients) on GC development (mean follow-up = 9.3 years; SD = 0.7).[57] A significant reduction (*P*<.05; log-rank test) in cancer incidence was observed after eradication in the Pg test-negative (PgI >70 ng/mL and PgI/PgII ratio >3.0) subjects. The results obtained support the hypothesis that GC risk in eradicated patients depends on the extension of atrophic gastritis before eradication and showed that eradication was beneficial in most of the pepsinogen-test-negative subjects.

A cohort of 80,000 Taiwanese patients with ulcers was eradicated early after symptom onset or within 1 year from the time the ulcer diagnosis was made and monitored for 10 years after treatment.[58] In those patients, late eradication was associated with an increased risk (standardized incidence ratio 1.36, 95% CI 1.24–1.49); early eradication (hazard ratio [HR] 0.77) and frequent assumption of aspirin or nonsteroidal antiinflammatory drugs (HR 0.65) were both found to be independent protective factors.

According to a long-term Italian follow-up study published in 2010, the outcome of gastritis (as assessed by OLGA staging) was significantly different in the eradicated versus noneradicated patients. The study also reported that 17 of 34 cases (50%) with persistent *H pylori* infection had a higher OLGA stage at the end of the follow-up (mean follow-up 12 years, range 12–17 years) with respect to their entry assessment, as opposed to 2 of 48 (4%) whose *H pylori* had been eradicated. Among patients who maintained the infection, the OLGA stage at the end of the follow-up decreased in 3 of 34 cases (9%) versus 8 of 48 (17%) after *H pylori* eradication (*P*<.005).[23]

As far as advanced precancerous lesions (ie, low-grade IEN [LG-IEN]) are concerned, a long-term follow-up study demonstrated that *H pylori* eradication significantly modified the natural history of the disease as it was associated to a reversibility of morphologic alterations already showing a neoplastic profile. A significantly lower risk of evolution to high-grade noninvasive neoplasia or to invasive GC was found to be associated with *H pylori* eradication when the pathologic outcome of LG-IEN in patients infected with *H pylori* (81 patients; follow-up: mean 43 months, range 12–160 months) was compared with that in eradicated ones (30 patients; follow-up: mean 37 months; range 12–119 months) (**Fig. 5**).[59,60] Although a sampling bias cannot be entirely excluded in any of the biopsy follow-up studies demonstrating a regression of precancerous lesions, both the biopsy protocols applied and/or the number of patients enrolled in these studies can be considered genuine proof of the reversibility of the lesions considered.[27,61]

In the GC setting, the most extreme preventive interventions involve patients already treated (mucosectomy or gastric resection) for a previous GC (ie, prevention of metachronous GC). Because of their previous cancer, these persons can be consistently considered at high risk; they constitute a unique model to evaluate the beneficial effects of eradication when it is carried out in such an extreme clinico-biological context.

In 2008, a Japanese study set out to assess the prevalence of metachronous GCs that developed after radical endoscopic mucosal resection of an early GC (EGC).[62] That multicenter trial randomized 544 patients with EGC into 2 groups (272 patients each) according to their *H pylori* status (eradicated vs noneradicated patients, the latter acting as controls). At the 3-year follow-up, the prevalence of metachronous GCs was reduced by one-third in the eradicated subjects (metachronous cancers OR = 0.35; 95% CI = 0.161–0.775; P = .009), thus demonstrating a significant beneficial effect of the prophylactic eradication after endoscopic resection. More recently, these results were only partially confirmed by a retrospective study involving 268 patients with *H pylori* +ve who underwent endoscopic resection of EGC. A total of 177 patients were successfully eradicated, whereas 91 maintained the infection. When the 5-year follow-up period was completed, the incidence in the eradicated group was significantly ($P<.007$) lower with respect to that observed in the infected group. During the overall follow-up period (1.1 to 11.1 years; median 3.0 years), metachronous GC developed in 14% of the infected versus 8.5% in the eradicated patients (P = .262, log-rank test).[63] A multivariate logistic regression analysis also demonstrated that severe mucosal atrophy at baseline and after a follow-up longer than 5 years was an independent risk factor for the development of metachronous GC.[62] Recently, a

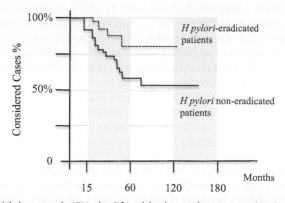

Fig. 5. Patients with low-grade IEN: the life table shows the progression into high-grade IEN or into invasive GC in *H pylori*–positive versus *H pylori*–eradicated patients ($P<.04$). After *H pylori* eradication, all patients had follow-up (endoscopy, with extensive biopsy sampling) longer than 12 months. (*Adapted from* Rugge M, Russo VM, Guido M. Review article: what have we learnt from gastric biopsy? Aliment Pharmacol Ther 2003;17:68; with permission.)

meta-analysis (involving 6237 patients in 13 studies) compared the prevalence of metachronous GC in H pylori–eradicated versus non-eradicated patients; the initial malignancy had been endoscopically treated in all the patients considered, but no information was available about the stage of the initial cancer. Both the pooled OR in the eradicated group (OR = 0.42; 95% CI = 0.32–0.56) and a subgroup analysis of 3 prospective trials (OR = 0.39; 95% CI = 0.20–0.75) consistently demonstrated a lower incidence of metachronous GC in the eradicated patients.[64] Taken together, these results confirm the beneficial effect of H pylori eradication but also show that the more advanced the gastric atrophy is, the more difficult it is to reverse the carcinogenetic cascade. Ablation of early neoplastic lesions does not, in fact, prevent the progression of other (coexistent) advanced precancerous lesions.[65] Late-onset of metachronous cancers, which have been documented by Yuji Maehata and coworkers,[63] would be consistent with both the carcinogenetic cascade theory and with experimental studies demonstrating that bacterial eradication delays the development of high-grade intra-epithelial lesions. In fact, one study confirmed that it took longer for metachronous cancers to develop in eradicated mice.[66]

The effect of H pylori eradication after surgical resection for GC has not yet been clearly elucidated. A tendency toward a decreasing prevalence of the H pylori infection in the gastric remnant has been documented and interpreted as a favorable consequence of an unfavorable microenvironment following gastric resection (biliary enterogastric reflux).[67] Spontaneous clearance of H pylori infection has also been reported within a year of gastric surgery.[68] A randomized clinical trial conducted by S.J. Cho and colleagues[69] demonstrated that both atrophy (P = .0046), and IM (P = .0284) were significantly less prevalent in the H pylori–eradicated than in the H pylori–persistent patients 36 months after subtotal gastrectomy. These observations might offer indirect evidence supporting the advisability of eradication therapy in patients who have undergone gastrectomy.

SUMMARY

As H pylori is a first-class carcinogen, it is more than plausible that eradication of the infection would prove beneficial for the (primary) prevention of cancer.

The pre-eradication assessment of the severity of the gastric disease (using both noninvasive and invasive methods) may contribute to quantifying the clinical benefit that is achievable, but it should not affect the decision to eradicate (which should be considered mandatory in any patient with H pylori +ve). Eradication before gastric atrophy sets in offers the best chance for the greatest reduction in risk, but the beneficial effects of treatment still persist even in advanced age and in advanced disease.

Solid evidence supports the view that the more severe the gastric disease is at the time of eradication, the less reversible already established mucosal lesions will be. The reversibility of inflammatory lesions is supported by undeniable evidence; the regression of mucosal atrophy/metaplasia has also been confirmed by several recent histologic studies.

Already established (advanced) organic lesions may progress to cancer even in eradicated patients; as a consequence, the mucosal lesions as assessed at the time of eradication should serve as a reference point for scheduling posteradication follow-up examinations (secondary prevention strategy).

The advisability of eradication has been debated with regard to those patients in whom the gastric disease is so advanced that the horse has already bolted. This is, probably, a false problem: the severity the organic lesions should influence tailored secondary preventive strategies (or the endoscopic or surgical therapy for invasive cancer) but is irrelevant to the decision to eradicate or not to eradicate. Even in patients with EGC, eradication seems to at least delay cancer recurrence (if not to prevent metachronous cancer); the cost-benefit balance in this restricted number of patients is, again, in favor of eradication therapy.

REFERENCES

1. Cancer Genome Atlas Research Network. Comprehensive molecular characterization of gastric adenocarcinoma. Nature 2014;513:202–9.
2. Rugge M, Capelle LG, Fassan M. Individual risk stratification of gastric cancer: evolving concepts and their impact on clinical practice. Best Pract Res Clin Gastroenterol 2014;28:1043–53.
3. Rugge M, Correa P, Dixon MF, et al. Gastric dysplasia: the Padova international classification. Am J Surg Pathol 2000;24:167–76.
4. Correa P. Gastric cancer: overview. Gastroenterol Clin North Am 2013;42:211–7.
5. Lochhead P, El-Omar EM. Helicobacter pylori infection and gastric cancer. Best Pract Res Clin Gastroenterol 2007;2:281–97.
6. Parkin DM, Bray F, Ferlay J, et al. Global cancer statistics, 2002. CA Cancer J Clin 2005;55:74–108.
7. Ernst PB, Gold BD. The disease spectrum of Helicobacter pylori: the immunopathogenesis of gastroduodenal ulcer and gastric cancer. Annu Rev Microbiol 2000;54:615–40.
8. Malaty HM. Epidemiology of Helicobacter pylori infection. Best Pract Res Clin Gastroenterol 2007;21:205–14.
9. Wroblewski LE, Peek RM Jr, Wilson KT. Helicobacter pylori and gastric cancer: factors that modulate disease risk. Clin Microbiol Rev 2010;23:713–39.
10. Zhang S, Desrosiers J, Aponte-Pieras JR, et al. Human immune responses to H. pylori HLA class II epitopes identified by immunoinformatic methods. PLoS One 2014;9:e94974.
11. Malfertheiner P, Megraud F, O'Morain CA, et al, European Helicobacter Study Group. Management of Helicobacter pylori infection–the Maastricht IV/Florence Consensus Report. Gut 2012;61:646–64.
12. Graham DY. Helicobacter pylori update: gastric cancer, reliable therapy, and possible benefits. Gastroenterology 2015;148(4):719–31.e3.
13. Kimko H, Thyssen A, Mould DR, et al. Helicobacter pylori treatment in children: defining a dose for rabeprazole as a part of a triple therapy regimen. J Clin Pharmacol 2015;55(5):592–600.
14. Zhu R, Chen K, Zheng YY, et al. Meta-analysis of the efficacy of probiotics in Helicobacter pylori eradication therapy. World J Gastroenterol 2014;20:18013–21.
15. Sakakibara M, Ando T, Ishiguro K, et al. Usefulness of Helicobacter pylori eradication for precancerous lesions of the gastric remnant. Gastroenterol Hepatol 2014;4:60–4.
16. Yoon H, Kim N. Diagnosis and management of high risk group for gastric cancer. Gut Liver 2015;9:5–17.
17. Kelley JR, Duggan JM. Gastric cancer epidemiology and risk factors. J Clin Epidemiol 2003;56:1–9.
18. Sipponen P, Graham DY. Importance of atrophic gastritis in diagnostics and prevention of gastric cancer: application of plasma biomarkers. Scand J Gastroenterol 2007;42:2–10.
19. Di Mario F, Cavallaro LG. Non-invasive tests in gastric diseases. Dig Liver Dis 2008;40:523–30.

20. Väänänen H, Vauhkonen M, Helske T, et al. Non-endoscopic diagnosis of atrophic gastritis with a blood test. Correlation between gastric histology and serum levels of gastrin-17 and pepsinogen I: a multicentre study. Gastroenterol Hepatol 2003;15:885–91.
21. Miki K. Gastric cancer screening using the serum pepsinogen test method. Gastric Cancer 2006;9:245–53.
22. Iijima K, Abe Y, Kikuchi R, et al. Serum biomarker tests are useful in delineating between patients with gastric atrophy and normal, healthy stomach. World J Gastroenterol 2009;15:853–9.
23. Rugge M, de Boni M, Pennelli G, et al. Gastritis OLGA-staging and gastric cancer risk: a twelve-year clinico-pathological follow-up study. Aliment Pharmacol Ther 2010;31:1104–11.
24. Dinis-Ribeiro M, da Costa-Pereira A, Lopes C, et al. Validity of serum pepsinogen I/II ratio for the diagnosis of gastric epithelial dysplasia and intestinal metaplasia during the follow-up of patients at risk for intestinal-type gastric adenocarcinoma. Neoplasia 2004;6:449–56.
25. Tu H, Sun L, Dong X, et al. Temporal changes in serum biomarkers and risk for progression of gastric precancerous lesions: a longitudinal study. Int J Cancer 2015;136:425–34.
26. Correa P. Serum pepsinogens in gastric cancer screening. Dig Dis Sci 2010;55: 2123–5.
27. Shiotani A, Cen P, Graham DY. Eradication of gastric cancer is now both possible and practical. Semin Cancer Biol 2013;23:492–501.
28. Dinis-Ribeiro M, Areia M, de Vries AC, et al. Management of precancerous conditions and lesions in the stomach (MAPS): guideline from the European Society of Gastrointestinal Endoscopy (ESGE), European Helicobacter Study Group (EHSG), European Society of Pathology (ESP), and the Sociedade Portuguesa de Endoscopia Digestiva (SPED). Endoscopy 2012;44:74–94.
29. Leja M, Kupcinskas L, Funka K, et al. Value of gastrin-17 in detecting antral atrophy. Adv Med Sci 2011;56:145–50.
30. McNicholl AG, Forné M, Barrio J, et al. Accuracy of GastroPanel for the diagnosis of atrophic gastritis. Eur J Gastroenterol Hepatol 2014;26(9):941–8.
31. Sugano K, Tack J, Kuipers EJ, et al. Kyoto Global Consensus Report on Helicobacter pylori gastritis. Gut, in press.
32. Gonen C, Simsek I, Sarioglu S, et al. Comparison of high resolution magnifying endoscopy and standard videoendoscopy for the diagnosis of Helicobacter pylori gastritis in routine clinical practice: a prospective study. Helicobacter 2009;14:12–21.
33. Uedo N, Ishihara R, Iishi H, et al. Endoscopy. A new method of diagnosing gastric intestinal metaplasia: narrow-band imaging with magnifying endoscopy. Endoscopy 2006;38:819–24.
34. Okubo M, Tahara T, Shibata T, et al. Usefulness of magnifying narrow-band imaging endoscopy in the Helicobacter pylori-related chronic gastritis. Digestion 2011;83:161–6.
35. Rugge M, Pennelli G, Pilozzi E, et al. Gastritis: the histology report. Dig Liver Dis 2011;43:S373–84.
36. Dixon MF, Genta RM, Yardley JH, et al. Classification and grading of gastritis. The updated Sydney System. International Workshop on the Histopathology of Gastritis, Houston 1994. Am J Surg Pathol 1996;20:1161–81.
37. Kimura K. Chronological transition of the fundic-pyloric border determined by stepwise biopsy of the lesser and greater curvatures of the stomach. Gastroenterology 1972;63:584–92.

38. El-Zimaity HM, Graham DY. Evaluation of gastric mucosal biopsy site and number for identification of Helicobacter pylori intestinal metaplasia: role of the Sydney System. Hum Pathol 1999;30:72–7.
39. Rugge M, Cassaro M, Pennelli G, et al. Atrophic gastritis: pathology and endoscopy in the reversibility assessment. Gut 2003;52:1387–8.
40. Isajevs S, Liepniece-Karele I, Janciauskas D, et al. The effect of incisura angularis biopsy sampling on the assessment of gastritis stage. Eur J Gastroenterol Hepatol 2014;26:510–3.
41. Pizzi M, Saraggi D, Fassan M, et al. Secondary prevention of epidemic gastric cancer in the model of Helicobacter pylori-associated gastritis. Dig Dis 2014; 32:265–74.
42. Rugge M, Fassan M, Graham DY. Clinical guidelines: secondary prevention of gastric cancer. Nat Rev Gastroenterol Hepatol 2012;9:128–9.
43. Rugge M, Capelle LG, Cappellesso R, et al. Precancerous lesions in the stomach: from biology to clinical patient management. Best Pract Res Clin Gastroenterol 2013;27:205–13.
44. Rugge M, Correa P, Dixon MF, et al. Gastric mucosal atrophy: interobserver consistency using new criteria for classification and grading. Aliment Pharmacol Ther 2002;16(7):1249–59.
45. Rugge M, Genta RM, OLGA Group. Staging gastritis: an international proposal. Gastroenterology 2005;129:1807–8.
46. Rugge M, Genta RM. Staging and grading of chronic gastritis. Hum Pathol 2005; 36:228–33.
47. Capelle LG, de Vries AC, Haringsma J, et al. The staging of gastritis with the OLGA system by using intestinal metaplasia as an accurate alternative for atrophic gastritis. Gastrointest Endosc 2010;71:1150–8.
48. Talley NJ, Fock KM, Moayyedi P. Gastric Cancer Consensus conference recommends Helicobacter pylori screening and treatment asymptomatic persons from high-risk populations to prevent gastric cancer. Am J Gastroenterol 2008;103:510–4.
49. de Vries AC, Kuipers EJ, Rauws EA. Helicobacter pylori eradication and gastric cancer: when is the horse out of the barn? Am J Gastroenterol 2009;104:1342–5.
50. Rugge M, de Boni M, Pennelli G, et al. OLGA can guard the barn. Am J Gastroenterol 2009;104:3101–2.
51. Katanoda K, Saika K, Yamamoto S, et al. Projected cancer mortality among Japanese males under different smoking prevalence scenarios evidence for tobacco control goal setting. Jpn J Clin Oncol 2011;41:483–9.
52. Bach PB, Kattan MW, Thornquist MD, et al. Variations in lung cancer risk among smokers. Natl Cancer Inst 2003;95:470–8.
53. Fassan M, Volinia S, Palatini J, et al. MicroRNA expression profiling in human Barrett's carcinogenesis. Int J Cancer 2011;129:1661–70.
54. Zabaleta J. MicroRNA: a bridge from H. pylori infection to gastritis and gastric cancer development. Front Genet 2012;3:294.
55. Wang R, Wen H, Xu Y, et al. Circulating microRNAs as a novel class of diagnostic biomarkers in gastrointestinal tumors detection: meta-analysis based on 42 articles. PLoS One 2014;9:e113401.
56. Fuccio L, Zagari RM, Eusebi LH, et al. Meta-analysis: can Helicobacter pylori eradication treatment reduce the risk for gastric cancer? Ann Intern Med 2009; 151:121–8.
57. Yanaoka K, Oka M, Ohata H, et al. Eradication of Helicobacter pylori prevents cancer development in subjects with mild gastric atrophy identified by serum pepsinogen levels. Int J Cancer 2009;125:2697–703.

58. Wu CY, Kuo KN, Wu MS, et al. Early Helicobacter pylori eradication decreases risk of gastric cancer in patients with peptic ulcer disease. Gastroenterology 2009;137:1641–8.

59. Rugge M, Russo VM, Guido M. Review article: what have we learnt from gastric biopsy? Aliment Pharmacol Ther 2003;17:68–74.

60. Rugge M, Cassaro M, Di Mario F, et al. Interdisciplinary Group on Gastric Epithelial Dysplasia (IGGED). The long term outcome of gastric non-invasive neoplasia. Gut 2003;52:1111–6.

61. Hojo M, Miwa H, Ohkusa T, et al. Alteration of histological gastritis after cure of Helicobacter pylori infection. Aliment Pharmacol Ther 2002;16:1923–32.

62. Fukase K, Kato M, Kikuchi S, et al. Effect of eradication of Helicobacter pylori on incidence of metachronous gastric carcinoma after endoscopic resection of early gastric cancer: an open-label, randomised controlled trial. Lancet 2008;372: 392–7.

63. Maehata Y, Nakamura S, Fujisawa K, et al. Long-term effect of Helicobacter pylori eradication on the development of metachronous gastric cancer after endoscopic resection of early gastric cancer. Gastrointest Endosc 2012;75:39–46.

64. Yoon SB, Park JM, Lim CH, et al. Effect of *Helicobacter pylori* eradication on metachronous gastric cancer after endoscopic resection of gastric tumors: a meta-analysis. Helicobacter 2014;19:243–8.

65. Graham DY, Uemura N. Natural history of gastric cancer after Helicobacter pylori eradication in Japan: after endoscopic resection, after treatment of the general population, and naturally. Helicobacter 2006;11:139–43.

66. Lee CW, Rickman B, Rogers AB, et al. *Helicobacter pylori* eradication prevents progression of gastric cancer in hypergastrinemic INS-GAS mice. Cancer Res 2008;68:3540–8.

67. Lin YS, Chen MJ, Shih SC, et al. Management of Helicobacter pylori infection after gastric surgery. World J Gastroenterol 2014;20:5274–82.

68. Suh S, Nah JC, Uhm MS, et al. Changes in prevalence of Helicobacter pylori infection after subtotal gastrectomy. Hepatogastroenterology 2012;59:646–8.

69. Cho SJ, Choi IJ, Kook MC, et al. Randomised clinical trial: the effects of Helicobacter pylori eradication on glandular atrophy and intestinal metaplasia after subtotal gastrectomy for gastric cancer. Aliment Pharmacol Ther 2013;38:477.

Molecular Pathogenesis of *Helicobacter pylori*-Related Gastric Cancer

Takahiro Shimizu, MD, PhD, Hiroyuki Marusawa, MD, PhD,
Norihiko Watanabe, MD, PhD, Tsutomu Chiba, MD, PhD*

KEYWORDS

- Gastric cancer • *Helicobacter pylori* • Inflammation • Genetics • Epigenetics

KEY POINTS

- *Helicobacter pylori*-related gastric carcinogenesis is associated with interactions between bacterial virulence factors and host inflammatory responses.
- Comprehensive analyses of gastric cancer genomes provide us with clues to identifying the molecular pathogenesis of gastric carcinogenesis as well as therapeutic targets.
- The expression of activation-induced cytidine deaminase (AID) in gastric epithelium induced by *H pylori* infection and resultant inflammation have a crucial role in the induction of genetic alterations during *H pylori*-related gastric carcinogenesis.

INTRODUCTION

Gastric cancer is the third leading cause of cancer-related death worldwide.[1] *Helicobacter pylori* infection is the most common causative factor of gastric cancer among various factors including host genetic and environmental factors.[2,3] Since its discovery in 1984 by Marshall and Warren,[4] many epidemiologic studies have investigated the relationship between *H pylori* and gastric cancer.[5,6] Also, many investigators have revealed complex interactions between the virulence factors of *H pylori*, resultant chronic inflammation, and gastric carcinogenesis.[7–9] Recently, advances in sequence technology revealed the whole picture of human gastric cancer genome.[10–12] These results can contribute to uncovering the molecular mechanisms of gastric

Author Contributions: Each of the authors has been involved equally and has read and approved the final manuscript. Each meets the criteria for authorship established by the International Committee of Medical Journal Editors and verifies the validity of the results reported. Potential Conflicts: The authors have no conflicts of interest.
Department of Gastroenterology and Hepatology, Graduate School of Medicine, Kyoto University, 54 Kawara-cho, Shogoin, Sakyo-ku, Kyoto 606-8507, Japan
* Corresponding author.
E-mail address: chiba@kuhp.kyoto-u.ac.jp

Gastroenterol Clin N Am 44 (2015) 625–638
http://dx.doi.org/10.1016/j.gtc.2015.05.011
0889-8553/15/$ – see front matter © 2015 Elsevier Inc. All rights reserved.

gastro.theclinics.com

carcinogenesis and also to the targeted therapy for gastric cancer. This review focuses on the recent developments in the molecular mechanisms of H pylori-related gastric carcinogenesis.

CLASSIFICATIONS AND CHARACTERIZATIONS OF GASTRIC CANCER

Gastric cancer is histologically heterogeneous and classified by various histologic classification systems. The commonly used classifications are those of Lauren[13] and the World Health Organization.[14] The former classification is composed of 2 subtypes, intestinal type and diffuse type, and the latter classification has 4 subtypes, papillary, tubular, mucinous, and poorly cohesive. Intestinal-type gastric cancer shows cohesive groups of tumor cells with a glandular architecture. These types of cancers typically generate from H pylori-infected gastric mucosa with chronic gastritis, atrophy, and metaplastic changes. While intestinal metaplasia has been focused as a precursor to gastric cancer, recently, spasmolytic-polypeptide-expressing metaplasia (SPEM) has also been highlighted as another metaplastic lesion. SPEM is generated through the transdifferentiation of chief cells after parietal cell loss due to H pylori infection and gives rise to intestinal metaplasia in the presence of inflammation.[15,16] SPEM is thought to be the initial preneoplastic metaplasia predisposing to gastric cancer, although further analysis is needed. Diffuse-type gastric cancer, by contrast, is composed of scattered poorly cohesive cells with poor cellular differentiation. This type emerges in H pylori-infected mucosa with or without atrophic and metaplastic changes as well as the mucosa unrelated with H pylori infection.

On the other hand, recent innovative technologies enable us to classify gastric cancers based on tumor molecular biology. Several reports revealed that gastric cancer is genomically heterogeneous and is classified into several types by comprehensive molecular evaluation, contributing to understanding not only the molecular pathogenesis of gastric carcinogenesis but also the targets for personalized therapy.[10–12] The Cancer Genome Atlas research network proposes that gastric cancer is divided into 4 subtypes: tumors that test positive for Epstein-Barr virus (EBV), tumors with microsatellite instability (MSI), tumors with chromosomal instability (CIN), and genomically stable (GS) tumors.[10] EBV-positive cancers display PIK3CA mutations, extreme DNA hypermethylation, and amplification of JAK2, PD-L1, and PD-L2. MSI tumors have epigenetic silencing of MLH1, one of DNA mismatch repair genes, in the context of a CpG island methylator phenotype.[11] MSI can lead to subsequent genetic changes, including small insertions and deletions, in hundreds to thousands of genes. It has been reported that the frequency of MSI was higher in intestinal-type gastric cancer, old-aged women, and distal gastric cancer, and these tumors are usually diagnosed at the earlier stage.[17] Interestingly, early gastric cancer genomes with MSI showed a comparable level of mutations to advanced MSI gastric cancer in terms of the number, sequence composition, and functional consequences of mutations.[18] These results suggest that the genetic or epigenetic alterations characterized as MSI may already be achieved in early gastric cancer genomes. CIN tumors account for 50% of gastric cancers, and most of them are histologically of the intestinal type. These types of cancers typically have TP53 mutations and marked aneuploidy and focal amplification, including receptor tyrosine kinases, VEGFA, and cell cycle mediators (CCNE1, CCND1, and CDK6). These genomic amplifications are possible targets for therapeutic inhibitors. Intriguingly, TP53 mutations are frequently seen in noncancerous gastritis mucosa with H pylori infection[19] and various chromosomal aberrations are present in gastric adenoma.[20] These findings suggest that TP53 mutations and various chromosomal alterations are early events during H pylori-related gastric carcinogenesis with atrophy-metaplasia-dysplasia sequence. GS tumors that lack the specific features are predominantly the diffuse histologic subtype, and half of them harbor mutations or fusion in *CDH1* or RHO family genes.[21,22]

In addition, Lei and colleagues[12] classified gastric tumors into 3 subtypes by gene expression profile. Proliferative-type tumors have CIN, *TP53* mutations, and DNA hypomethylation, consistent with CIN-type tumors. Tumors of mesenchymal type contain cells with features of cancer stem cells, suggesting that this type of cancer may generate from stem cell regions in gastric mucosa. Furthermore, metabolic-type tumors are likely to express genes characterized in SPEM, a particular kind of metaplasia in the stomach, which has been proposed as an intermediate step during gastric carcinogenesis. This fact suggests that these tumors may generate from metaplastic regions in *H pylori*-related gastritis.

Taken together, the combination of histologic and genetic analyses is essential for understanding the process of gastric cancer development. Although each cancer has a very different profile, these analyses provide several processes from early genetic events to progressive *H pylori*-related gastric carcinogenesis (**Fig. 1**). In addition to these approaches for uncovering gastric carcinogenesis, molecular mechanisms of how *H pylori* infection induce emergence of cancer cells are also important.

HELICOBACTER PYLORI VIRULENCE FACTORS ON GASTRIC EPITHELIUM DURING GASTRIC CARCINOGENESIS
Roles of CagA in Gastric Carcinogenesis

Among various virulence factors of *H pylori* that may be involved in gastric carcinogenesis, the *cag* pathogenicity island (cytotoxin-associated gene [cag] PAI) is a well-characterized molecule.[23] Several genes within this island encode the CagA protein and the type IV secretion system (T4SS) that delivers bacterial agents into gastric epithelial cells.[24] A large amount of clinical data showed that the *cagA*-positive strains are considered to be more potent in gastric cancer development than *cagA*-negative strains, although *cagA*-negative strains also cause gastric cancer.[25,26] Importantly, the oncogenic potential of CagA was directly demonstrated by the observation that transgenic mice systemically expressing CagA protein spontaneously developed gastrointestinal carcinomas and hematopoietic malignancies.[27] CagA is translocated into the cytoplasm of gastric epithelial cells by the T4SS during bacterial attachment.[24] Once translocated into host cytoplasm, CagA may bind to the inner surface of the cell membrane, be tyrosine-phosphorylated at Glu-Pro-Ile-Tyr-Ala (EPIYA) motif by Src family kinases and Abl kinases, and then interact with a variety of human proteins to lower the threshold for neoplastic transformation.[28] Phosphorylated CagA can specifically bind to the SH2-domain-containing protein tyrosine phosphatase (SHP2) and activate this molecule, leading to the activation of the Ras-Erk pathway.[29,30] CagA-mediated SHP2 signaling also dephosphorylates focal adhesion kinase, a kinase regulating cell shape and motility, and then inhibits its kinase activity, causing impaired focal adhesions that are associated with an elongated cell shape known as the hummingbird phenotype and elevated cell motility.[31] On the other hand, nonphosphorylated CagA also exerts effects within the cells that contribute to carcinogenesis. CagA inhibits PAR1 activity by binding this protein kinase, leading to the disruption of tight junctions and loss of cell polarity.[32] CagA also interacts with E-cadherin via PAR1, leading to activation of β-catenin.[33] In addition to PAR1, nonphosphorylated CagA can associate with the c-Met receptor tyrosine kinase, the phospholipase C-γ, and the adaptor protein Grb2.[34,35] Taken together, CagA contributes to gastric carcinogenesis via the interaction with multiple signaling pathways.

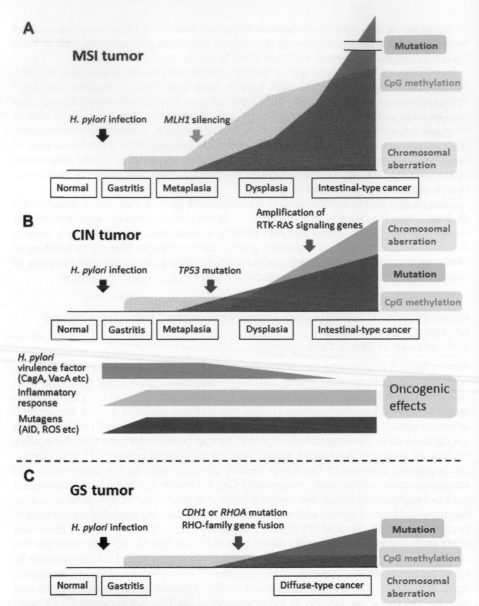

Fig. 1. Schematic summary of molecular pathogenesis of *H pylori*-related gastric cancer. (*A*) Molecular events of MSI tumors. MSI tumors have CpG island methylator phenotype characteristics and epigenetic silencing of *MLH1*, leading to increasing number of mutations. (*B*) Molecular events of CIN tumors. CIN tumors have *TP53* mutations and various chromosomal aberrations, including RTK-RAS signaling genes. Both MSI tumors and CIN tumors are typically intestinal-type tumors and are generated through atrophic gastritis-metaplasia-dysplasia sequence. While *H pylori* virulence factors exert oncogenic effects on gastric mucosa during *H pylori* infection, inflammatory responses and the resultant overexpression of mutagens, including AID and reactive oxygen species, continue to play oncogenic roles on the gastric mucosa even if *H pylori* is eradicated. (*C*) Molecular events of GS tumors. GS tumors are predominantly diffuse-type tumors and have *CDH1* or *RHOA* mutations or RHO family gene fusions.

Recently, it has been reported that CagA interacts with tumor suppressors, including RUNX3 and p53. Interaction of CagA with RUNX3 induces the ubiquitination and degradation of RUNX3 that impairs its ability as a tumor-suppressive transcriptional factor.[36] CagA also interacts with the apoptosis-stimulating protein p53 (ASPP2) and prevents ASPP2 from inducing apoptosis through activation of p53.[37] Together, CagA can act directly with tumor suppressors, contributing to malignant transformation of gastric epithelial cells.

CagA is also considered to mediate cell reprogramming. It has reported that CagA can deregulate Wnt signaling and then induce Wnt target genes, including CDX1, an intestinal-specific transcriptional factor.[33] Interestingly, ectopically expressed CDX1 transactivates stemness-associated reprogramming factors SALL4 and KLF5 that can convert gastric epithelial cells into tissue stemlike progenitor cells, which then transdifferentiated into intestinal epithelial cells.[38] Considering from the aspect of cancer stem cell theory, these results also suggest that cells dedifferentiated by CagA may become cells of origin of gastric cancer as cancer stem-cell-like cells.

Roles of Vacuolating Cytotoxin A in Gastric Carcinogenesis

The vacuolating cytotoxin A (VacA) is a toxin secreted by *H pylori* that is associated with increased disease risk. VacA has a variety of effects on epithelial cells, including vacuolation characterized by a collection of large vesicles as well as induction of apoptosis and suppression of T-cell responses, which results in the longevity of infection.[39] VacA and CagA counterregulate the effects of each other on the host cells, contributing to effective mechanisms to promote persistent colonization of *H pylori*.[40] One mechanism is that VacA induces autophagy-dependent degradation of CagA by triggering reactive oxygen species (ROS) via the binding of VacA m1 to low-density lipoprotein receptor-related protein-1 on host cells.[41] Interestingly, CagA can escape from the ROS-induced autophagy in cells expressing a variant 9 form of CD44 (CD44v9), one of the gastric cancer stem cell markers because CD44v9 increases the level of intracellular glutathione that neutralizes ROS. Therefore, CagA is thought to be able to remain longer in gastric cancer stem cells, perhaps contributing to initiation and progression of gastric cancer. Taken together, *H pylori* can avoid the induction of excess cellular damage and maintain long-term persistence in host cells as well as increase oncogenic functions in cancer stem cell population even if *H pylori* is eradicated.

Role of Peptidoglycan in Gastric Carcinogenesis

In addition to CagA, components of *H pylori* peptidoglycan are also delivered into host cells through T4SS and trigger several signaling pathways related with carcinogenesis. Peptidoglycan is recognized by NOD1, an intracellular pathogen recognition molecule, and then leads to activation of nuclear factor (NF)-κB-dependent proinflammatory responses, such as secretion of interleukin (IL)-8, β-defensin2, and PI3K-AKT signaling, lowering the threshold for malignant transformation by decreasing apoptosis and increasing proliferation and cell migration.[42,43]

HELICOBACTER PYLORI-INDUCED INFLAMMATORY RESPONSES DURING GASTRIC CARCINOGENESIS

Inflammation has been well recognized as the key risk factor for many types of cancers.[44–46] *Helicabacter pylori* infection causes inflammation of the gastric mucosa with inflammatory cell infiltration, including T cells and activated mononuclear cells. *Helicobacter pylori*-induced gastritis is characterized by the enhanced production of a variety of proinflammatory cytokines, such as IL-1β, tumor necrosis factor (TNF)-α, IL-6, IL-8, IL-11, and others, in the gastric mucosa, and these cytokines are thought to play important roles in cancer development.[47] Among them, IL-1β has been focused as the factor that links gastric inflammation and gastric cancer. Polymorphisms in the IL-1β gene are linked with the increase of IL-1β production and risk of gastric cancer related with H pylori infection.[48] IL-1β is upregulated by H pylori infection and induces NF-κB activation in both inflammatory and epithelial cells and hepatocyte growth factor.[49]

In addition to IL-1β, TNF-α may increase the risk for gastric cancer. TNF-α polymorphisms that increase TNF-α production are associated with an increased risk of gastric cancer and its precursors.[50] TNF-α produced by macrophages promotes Wnt/β-catenin signaling in gastric epithelial cells through inhibition of GSK3β.[51] Also, the activation of TNF-α/TNFR1 signaling in the tumor microenvironment promotes gastric tumor development through induction of Noxo1 and Gna14, which contribute to maintaining the tumor cells in an undifferentiated state.[52] Importantly, IL-1β and TNF-α enhance NF-κB activation, a key transcription factor mediating inflammation and cancer development. NF-κB activation promotes growth, suppresses apoptosis of epithelial cells, and stimulates the production of growth factors and cytokines such as epidermal growth factor and IL-6, enhances cyclooxygenase (COX)-2 induction, and increases ROS production.[53,54] The induced COX2 has various functions, including enhancement of cell growth and angiogenesis.

IL-6 levels are also increased in the H pylori-induced gastritis mucosa. IL-6 activates signal transducer and activator of transcription 3 and thereby enhances cell growth and stimulates growth factor production, including RegIα.[55,56]

Thus, these mediators of inflammation form a complex of regulatory networks and seem to work in concert to enhance cancer development.

GENETIC AND EPIGENETIC ALTERATIONS DURING GASTRIC CARCINOGENESIS
Mechanisms of Induction of Genetic Alterations

Comprehensive cancer genome analyses reveal not only a snapshot of current cancer status but also a footprint of its carcinogenesis process. Recent studies show that the mutation signature that accumulates in tumor tissues provides the clue to identifying the cause of genetic alterations during tumor development.[57] Nucleotide alterations that accumulated in gastric cancer genomes were enriched with C:G>T:A transition, followed by C:G>A:T transversion.[10,19,58,59] C:G>T:A transition mutations typically represent involvement of deamination process, although exogenous mutagens, such as UV light can also induce these mutations. C:G>A:T transversion mutations are considered to be caused by ROS and tobacco. Furthermore, most gastric cancers have chromosomal aberrations.

Deamination
The mechanisms that induce deamination are of 2 types, spontaneous deamination and activation of endogenous deaminase by the apolipoprotein B mRNA editing enzyme, catalytic polypeptide-like (APOBEC) family. Spontaneous deamination is the most frequent cause of spontaneously generated mutations, that is, deamination of 5-methylcytosine in CpG sequences, resulting in C:G>T:A transitions.[60] This mutation signature is correlated with age and seen in almost all cancers of various tissues. Among these cancer types, gastrointestinal cancers, including gastric cancer, particularly have C:G>T:A mutations in the context of CpG.[57,61] These results indicate that some factors that can promote methylation or deamination are involved in the elevated rate of these mutations in gastric cancer in addition to spontaneous methylation.

On the other hand, the APOBEC family members are cytidine deaminases that are capable of inducing nucleotide alterations by converting cytidine to uracil coupled to repair systems and DNA replication machineries.[62] Among the APOBEC family members, AID can induce genetic alterations in human DNA sequences and plays a key role in generating immune diversity through induction of both somatic hypermutation and class-switch recombination in immunoglobulin genes.[63,64] APOBEC3A and 3B also have the capacity to induce genetic alterations in human DNA.[65,66] Although their normal functions are unknown, APOBEC3A and 3B are thought to elicit mutations in several cancer types, such as breast cancer and lung cancer.[61] Similar to AID, these enzymes can deaminate C on target nucleotides to produce U, generating a U:G mismatch. The generated U:G mismatches can usually be repaired to C:G by the high-fidelity repair system. If the mismatch is not repaired before DNA replication, DNA polymerase will insert an A nucleotide opposite the U nucleotide, resulting in a C:G>T:A transition. Alternatively, recognition of a U:G mismatch by uracil DNA glycosylase or mismatch repair protein, such as MSH2 and MSH6, induces various patterns of nucleotide alterations.[67] In contrast, nicks in the near sites of both strand sequences are generated by the repair process of generated U:G mismatches, resulting in DNA double-strand breaks followed by chromosomal aberrations.[68]

While APOBEC3A and 3B favor C residues flanked by 5'-T, AID exhibits a strong preference for deaminating C residues flanked by a 5'-purine (G or A).[69,70] In whole exome sequencing analyses of gastric cancer, the C:G>T:A mutations in gastric cancer genomes predominantly accumulated in the context of GpCpX or ApCpX (C is the mutated base and X is any base) as well as CpG.[19,71] In particular, these mutational signatures are more frequent in MSI gastric cancer, consistent with the mechanism that defect of mismatch repair genes enhances the characteristics of AID-mediated cytidine deamination. Furthermore, the predominant pattern of mutations in *H pylori*-infected gastritis is also C:G>T:A in GpCpX motifs. These results suggest that AID is deeply involved in the induction of somatic mutations during *H pylori*-related gastric carcinogenesis.

Under physiologic conditions, AID expression is limited to activated B cells for inducing somatic hypermutation and class-switch recombination in immunoglobulin genes. By contrast, AID protein is aberrantly expressed in a substantial proportion of *H pylori*-associated human gastric epithelium and gastric cancer tissues, although no AID expression is observed in normal gastric mucosa.[72,73] In particular, mononuclear cell infiltration and intestinal metaplasia correlate with AID expression.[74] After eradication of *H pylori*, AID expression is significantly decreased but is still higher than that in *H pylori*-negative gastric mucosa. Intriguingly, infection with *cag*PAI-positive *H pylori* ectopically induces a high expression of AID in human gastric epithelial cell lines, whereas *cag*PAI-negative *H pylori* has no effect on AID expression.[73] Also, inflammatory cytokines, such as TNF-α, increase the expression of endogenous AID protein in gastric epithelial cells through the NF-κB pathway. Furthermore, aberrant AID expression in gastric epithelial cells induced by these stimuli causes several somatic mutations in tumor-related genes, including the tumor suppressor *TP53* gene. Consistent with this result, *TP53* mutations are frequently seen in chronic gastritis mucosa with *H pylori* infection.[19] These findings suggest that AID is a key molecule for the induction of somatic mutations during *H pylori*-related gastric carcinogenesis.

Oxidative stress

Generation of ROS and reactive nitrogen species (RNS) in human stomach are considered potential genotoxic factors in gastric mucosa.[75] *Helicobacter pylori* stimulates the production of ROS and RNS by inflammatory cells and gastric epithelial cells.[76]

These agents bind with nucleic acids, resulting in generation of altered nucleotides. These modified nucleic acids could induce putative DNA damage, including single- or double-strand breaks, DNA intrastrand adducts, and DNA protein cross-links.[77] In addition, ROS alters the mismatch repair function and allows mutations to accumulate in microsatellite sequences. One of the common products of free radical attack on DNA, 8-hydroxydeoxyguanine, is considered to be a biomarker of oxidative stress. The typical mutation pattern induced by this product represents C:G>A:T transversions.

Helicobacter pylori CagA also upregulates spermine oxidase (SMO) in gastric epithelial cells. SMO metabolizes the polyamine spermine into spermidine and generates H_2O_2. While H_2O_2 causes apoptosis and DNA damage, a subpopulation of DNA damaged cells are resistant to apoptosis, resulting in increased risk for gastric cancer.[78]

Chromosomal instability

Apart from nucleotide alterations, chromosomal aberrations are the other hallmark of gastric cancer. While it is considered that hypomethylation can induce chromosome breakage events,[79] one notable thing is that CIN-type cancers frequently have TP53 mutations in many cancer types, including gastric cancer.[80] This observation suggests that dysfunction of p53 may induce chromosomal aberration.[81] The fact that TP53 mutation is present in chronic gastritis mucosa with H pylori infection indicates that early mutations in TP53 gene may be involved in CIN during gastric carcinogenesis.[19] On the other hand, AID expression in gastric epithelial cells can cause chromosomal aberrations at various chromosomal loci as well as mutations.[82] In human cases, the relative copy numbers of CDKN2A/CDKN2B are reduced in a subset of gastric cancer tissues compared with the surrounding noncancerous gastric mucosa. In addition, oral infection of wild-type mice with H pylori reduces the copy number of the Cdkn2b-Cdkn2a locus, whereas no such changes are observed in the gastric mucosa of H pylori-infected AID-deficient mice. These findings suggest that aberrant AID expression in gastric epithelial cells with H pylori infection induces chromosomal aberrations as well as mutations.

Mechanisms of Induction of Epigenetic Alterations

In cancer cells, the presence of regional hypermethylation and global hypomethylation has been shown.[83] Regional hypermethylation refers to aberrant DNA methylation of specific promoter CpG islands physiologically kept unmethylated.[84] Recent comprehensive genome analyses revealed that many tumor suppressor genes that have promoter CpG islands, such as MLH1, MGMT, and CDKN2A, can be inactivated permanently in gastric cancer by aberrant DNA methylation as driver genes.[11,85] Also, increasing DNA methylation of non-CpG islands is suggested to be involved in induction of mutation during gastric carcinogenesis.[10] Interestingly, methylation levels of passenger genes in gastric mucosa with H pylori infection correlate with gastric cancer risk.[86] This accumulation of aberrant DNA methylation in noncancerous tissues with chronic inflammation is considered to form an epigenetic field for cancerization.[87] Along with the accumulation of genetic alterations, an epigenetic field defect is considered to be deeply related with gastric carcinogenesis. By contrast, gastric cancer as well as gastric mucosa with H pylori infection display global hypomethylation.[88] Global hypomethylation has shown to be causally involved in carcinogenesis by inducing genomic instability.[79]

The mechanisms by which H pylori infection induces DNA methylation remain unknown. Several mechanisms are proposed to explain aberrant promoter methylation in carcinogenesis, such as overexpression of DNA methyltransferases and reduction of DNA demethylation activity.[89] Expression levels of several inflammatory-related genes, such as CXCL2, IL-1β, NOS2, and TNF-α, were seen to be parallel with methylation levels in gastric mucosa of Mongolian Gerbils with *H pylori* infection.[90] Suppression of inflammation by the immunosuppressive drug cyclosporine A in *H pylori*-infected Mongolian Gerbils blocks induction of aberrant DNA methylation in gastric mucosa, although the number of *H pylori* was not changed. Furthermore, a polymorphism of the IL-1β promoter was associated with the presence of the CpG island methylation phenotype in gastric cancers.[91] These findings indicate that chronic inflammation, rather than *H pylori* itself, is important for induction of aberrant DNA methylation. Interestingly, Niwa and colleagues[92] revealed that a demethylating agent, 5-aza-2'-deoxycytidine can decrease *H pylori*-induced gastric cancers in Mongolian Gerbils. Removal of induced DNA methylation and/or suppression of DNA methylation induction could become a target for prevention of chronic inflammation-associated cancers.

Mechanisms of Induction of microRNA Alterations

Micro RNAs (miRNAs) are short noncoding RNAs that can regulate the expression of many target genes posttranscriptionally and are related with various cellular functions. Gastric cancer cells have dysregulation of expression of many miRNAs involved in cell cycle progression, inhibition of apoptosis, cell invasion, and so on, thus contributing to carcinogenesis.[93] The alteration of miRNA expression in epithelial cells can occur through various mechanisms such as NF-κB activation and cytokine stimulation following *H pylori* infection. For example, CagA has been shown to attenuate let-7 expression by histone and DNA methylation and then lead to the activation of the Ras pathway in gastric epithelial cells.[94] Recently, epigenetic silencing of miR-210 has been shown to increase the proliferation of gastric epithelium during *H pylori* infection, contributing to gastric cancer development.[95] However, mechanisms of how *H pylori* infection induce epigenetic changes in these miRNAs remain unknown.

SUMMARY

Many investigators have revealed molecular mechanisms of gastric carcinogenesis related with *H pylori*. Recent comprehensive analyses of gastric cancers also provide us with clues to identifying the mechanisms. This review focuses on major genetic patterns of gastric cancers, but the mechanisms of some cancer types are still unknown.[57] In addition, some important mechanisms, such as the induction of epigenetic alterations, are also unresolved. To gain further understanding of molecular pathogenesis of *H pylori*-related gastric carcinogenesis, further investigations from the broad perspective, including molecular mechanisms, comprehensive analyses, and epidemiologic studies, are needed.

REFERENCES

1. Ferlay J, Soerjomataram I, Dikshit R, et al. Cancer incidence and mortality worldwide: sources, methods and major patterns in GLOBOCAN 2012. Int J Cancer 2015;136(5):E359–86.
2. Correa P. A human model of gastric carcinogenesis. Cancer Res 1988;48(13): 3554–60.
3. Blaser MJ, Musser JM, Berg DE. Bacterial polymorphisms *Helicobacter pylori* genetic diversity and risk of human disease. J Clin Invest 2001;107(7):767–73.

4. Marshall BJ, Warren JR. Unidentified curved bacilli in the stomach of patients with gastritis and peptic ulceration. Lancet 1984;1(8390):1311–5.
5. Uemura N, Okamoto S, Yamamoto S, et al. *Helicobacter pylori* infection and the development of gastric cancer. N Engl J Med 2001;345(11):784–9.
6. Chiba T, Marusawa H, Seno H, et al. Mechanism for gastric cancer development by *Helicobacter pylori* infection. J Gastroenterol Hepatol 2008;23(8 Pt 1): 1175–81.
7. Polk DB, Peek RM. *Helicobacter pylori*: gastric cancer and beyond. Nat Rev Cancer 2010;10(6):403–14.
8. Wroblewski LE, Peek RM. *Helicobacter pylori* in gastric carcinogenesis: mechanisms. Gastroenterol Clin North Am 2013;42(2):285–98.
9. Wang F, Meng W, Wang B, et al. *Helicobacter pylori*-induced gastric inflammation and gastric cancer. Cancer Lett 2014;345(2):196–202.
10. Bass AJ, Thorsson V, Shmulevich I, et al. Comprehensive molecular characterization of gastric adenocarcinoma. Nature 2014;513(7517):202–9.
11. Zouridis H, Deng N, Ivanova T, et al. Methylation subtypes and large-scale epigenetic alterations in gastric cancer. Sci Transl Med 2012;4(156):156ra140.
12. Lei Z, Tan IB, Das K, et al. Identification of molecular subtypes of gastric cancer with different responses to PI3-kinase inhibitors and 5-fluorouracil. Gastroenterology 2013;145(3):554–65.
13. Lauren P. The two histological main types of gastric carcinoma: diffuse and so-called intestinal-type carcinoma. An attempt at a histo-clinical classification. Acta Pathol Microbiol Scand 1965;64:31–49.
14. Bosman FT, Carneiro F, Hruban RH, et al. WHO classification of tumours of the digestive system 4th edition. Lyon (France): IARC; 2010.
15. Goldenring JR, Nam KT, Wang TC. Spasmolytic polypeptide-expressing metaplasia and intestinal metaplasia: time for reevaluation of metaplasias and the origins of gastric cancer. Gastroenterology 2010;138(7):2207–10, 2210.e1.
16. Nam KT, Lee H-J, Sousa JF, et al. Mature chief cells are cryptic progenitors for metaplasia in the stomach. Gastroenterology 2010;139(6):2028–37.e9.
17. Kim H, An JY, Noh SH, et al. High microsatellite instability predicts good prognosis in intestinal-type gastric cancers. J Gastroenterol Hepatol 2011;26(3): 585–92.
18. Kim T-M, Jung S-H, Kim MS, et al. The mutational burdens and evolutionary ages of early gastric cancers are comparable to those of advanced gastric cancers. J Pathol 2014;234(3):365–74.
19. Shimizu T, Marusawa H, Matsumoto Y, et al. Accumulation of Somatic Mutations in TP53 in Gastric Epithelium With *Helicobacter pylori* Infection. Gastroenterology 2014;147(2):407–17.e3.
20. Uchida M, Tsukamoto Y, Uchida T, et al. Genomic profiling of gastric carcinoma in situ and adenomas by array-based comparative genomic hybridization. J Pathol 2010;221(1):96–105.
21. Wang K, Yuen ST, Xu J, et al. Whole-genome sequencing and comprehensive molecular profiling identify new driver mutations in gastric cancer. Nat Genet 2014;46(6):573–82.
22. Kakiuchi M, Nishizawa T, Ueda H, et al. Recurrent gain-of-function mutations of RHOA in diffuse-type gastric carcinoma. Nat Genet 2014;46(6):583–7.
23. Hatakeyama M. *Helicobacter pylori* CagA and gastric cancer: a paradigm for hit-and-run carcinogenesis. Cell Host Microbe 2014;15(3):306–16.
24. Fischer W. Assembly and molecular mode of action of the *Helicobacter pylori* Cag type IV secretion apparatus. FEBS J 2011;278(8):1203–12.

25. Parsonnet J, Friedman GD, Orentreich N, et al. Risk for gastric cancer in people with CagA positive or CagA negative *Helicobacter pylori* infection. Gut 1997;40:297–301.
26. Blaser MJ, Perez-perez GI, Kleanthous H, et al. Infection with *Helicobacter pylori* strains possessing cagA is associated with an increased risk of developing adenocarcinoma of the Stomach1. Cancer Res 1995;55:2111–6.
27. Ohnishi N, Yuasa H, Tanaka S, et al. Transgenic expression of *Helicobacter pylori* CagA induces gastrointestinal and hematopoietic neoplasms in mouse. Proc Natl Acad Sci U S A 2008;105(3):1003–8.
28. Mueller D, Tegtmeyer N, Brandt S, et al. c-Src and c-Abl kinases control hierarchic phosphorylation and function of the CagA effector protein in Western and East Asian *Helicobacter pylori* strains. J Clin Invest 2012;122(4):1553–66.
29. Higashi H, Tsutsumi R, Muto S, et al. SHP-2 tyrosine phosphatase as an intracellular target of *Helicobacter pylori* CagA protein. Science 2002;295(5555):683–6.
30. Saito Y, Murata-Kamiya N, Hirayama T, et al. Conversion of *Helicobacter pylori* CagA from senescence inducer to oncogenic driver through polarity-dependent regulation of p21. J Exp Med 2010;207(10):2157–74.
31. Segal ED, Cha J, Lo J, et al. Altered states: involvement of phosphorylated CagA in the induction of host cellular growth changes by *Helicobacter pylori*. Proc Natl Acad Sci 1999;96(25):14559–64.
32. Saadat I, Higashi H, Obuse C, et al. *Helicobacter pylori* CagA targets PAR1/MARK kinase to disrupt epithelial cell polarity. Nature 2007;447(7142):330–3.
33. Murata-Kamiya N, Kurashima Y, Teishikata Y, et al. *Helicobacter pylori* CagA interacts with E-cadherin and deregulates the beta-catenin signal that promotes intestinal transdifferentiation in gastric epithelial cells. Oncogene 2007;26(32):4617–26.
34. Mimuro H, Suzuki T, Tanaka J, et al. Grb2 is a key mediator of *Helicobacter pylori* CagA protein activities. Mol Cell 2002;10(4):745–55.
35. Churin Y, Al-Ghoul L, Kepp O, et al. *Helicobacter pylori* CagA protein targets the c-Met receptor and enhances the motogenic response. J Cell Biol 2003;161(2):249–55.
36. Tsang YH, Lamb A, Romero-Gallo J, et al. *Helicobacter pylori* CagA targets gastric tumor suppressor RUNX3 for proteasome-mediated degradation. Oncogene 2010;29(41):5643–50.
37. Buti L, Spooner E, Van der Veen AG, et al. *Helicobacter pylori* cytotoxin-associated gene A (CagA) subverts the apoptosis-stimulating protein of p53 (ASPP2) tumor suppressor pathway of the host. Proc Natl Acad Sci U S A 2011;108(22):9238–43.
38. Fujii Y, Yoshihashi K, Suzuki H, et al. CDX1 confers intestinal phenotype on gastric epithelial cells via induction of stemness-associated reprogramming factors SALL4 and KLF5. Proc Natl Acad Sci U S A 2012;109:20584–9.
39. Cover TL, Blanke SR. *Helicobacter pylori* VacA, a paradigm for toxin multifunctionality. Nat Rev Microbiol 2005;3(4):320–32.
40. Oldani A, Cormont M, Hofman V, et al. *Helicobacter pylori* counteracts the apoptotic action of its VacA toxin by injecting the CagA protein into gastric epithelial cells. PLoS Pathog 2009;5(10):e1000603.
41. Tsugawa H, Suzuki H, Saya H, et al. Reactive oxygen species-induced autophagic degradation of *Helicobacter pylori* CagA is specifically suppressed in cancer stem-like cells. Cell Host Microbe 2012;12(6):764–77.
42. Viala J, Chaput C, Boneca IG, et al. Nod1 responds to peptidoglycan delivered by the *Helicobacter pylori* cag pathogenicity island. Nat Immunol 2004;5(11):1166–74.

43. Watanabe T, Asano N, Fichtner-feigl S, et al. NOD1 contributes to mouse host defense against *Helicobacter pylori* via induction of type I IFN and activation of the ISGF3 signaling pathway. J Clin Invest 2010;120(5):1645–62.
44. Grivennikov SI, Greten FR, Karin M. Immunity, inflammation, and cancer. Cell 2010;140(6):883–99.
45. Chiba T, Marusawa H, Ushijima T. Inflammation-associated cancer development in digestive organs: mechanisms and roles for genetic and epigenetic modulation. Gastroenterology 2012;143(3):550–63.
46. Shimizu T, Marusawa H, Endo Y, et al. Inflammation-mediated genomic instability: roles of activation-induced cytidine deaminase in carcinogenesis. Cancer Sci 2012;103(7):1201–6.
47. Lamb A, Chen LF. Role of the *Helicobacter pylori*-induced inflammatory response in the development of gastric cancer. J Cell Biochem 2013;114(3):491–7.
48. El-Omar EM, Carrington M, Chow WH, et al. Interleukin-1 polymorphisms associated with increased risk of gastric cancer. Nature 2000;404(6776):398–402.
49. Noach LA, Bosma NB, Jansen J, et al. Mucosal tumor necrosis factor-alpha, interleukin-1 beta, and interleukin-8 production in patients with *Helicobacter pylori* infection. Scand J Gastroenterol 1994;29(5):425–9.
50. El-Omar EM, Rabkin CS, Gammon MD, et al. Increased risk of noncardia gastric cancer associated with proinflammatory cytokine gene polymorphisms. Gastroenterology 2003;124(5):1193–201.
51. Oguma K, Oshima H, Aoki M, et al. Activated macrophages promote Wnt signalling through tumour necrosis factor-alpha in gastric tumour cells. EMBO J 2008; 27(12).1671–81.
52. Oshima H, Ishikawa T, Yoshida GJ, et al. TNF-α/TNFR1 signaling promotes gastric tumorigenesis through induction of Noxo1 and Gna14 in tumor cells. Oncogene 2013;33(29):3820–9.
53. Pikarsky E, Porat RM, Stein I, et al. NF-kappaB functions as a tumour promoter in inflammation-associated cancer. Nature 2004;431(7007):461–6.
54. Maeda S, Akanuma M, Mitsuno Y, et al. Distinct mechanism of *Helicobacter pylori*-mediated NF-kappa B activation between gastric cancer cells and monocytic cells. J Biol Chem 2001;276(48):44856–64.
55. Sekikawa A, Fukui H, Fujii S, et al. REG Ialpha protein may function as a trophic and/or anti-apoptotic factor in the development of gastric cancer. Gastroenterology 2005;128(3):642–53.
56. Sekikawa A, Fukui H, Fujii S, et al. REG Ialpha protein mediates an anti-apoptotic effect of STAT3 signaling in gastric cancer cells. Carcinogenesis 2008;29(1):76–83.
57. Alexandrov LB, Nik-Zainal S, Wedge DC, et al. Signatures of mutational processes in human cancer. Nature 2013;500(7463):415–21.
58. Wang K, Kan J, Yuen ST, et al. Exome sequencing identifies frequent mutation of ARID1A in molecular subtypes of gastric cancer. Nat Genet 2011;43(12): 1219–23.
59. Zang ZJ, Cutcutache I, Poon SL, et al. Exome sequencing of gastric adenocarcinoma identifies recurrent somatic mutations in cell adhesion and chromatin remodeling genes. Nat Genet 2012;44(5):570–4.
60. Pfeifer GP. Mutagenesis at methylated CpG sequences. Curr Top Microbiol Immunol 2006;301:259–81.
61. Burns MB, Temiz NA, Harris RS. Evidence for APOBEC3B mutagenesis in multiple human cancers. Nat Genet 2013;45(9):977–83.
62. Cascalho M. Advantages and disadvantages of cytidine deamination. J Immunol 2004;172(11):6513–8.

63. Muramatsu M, Kinoshita K, Fagarasan S, et al. Class switch recombination and hypermutation require activation-induced cytidine deaminase (AID), a potential RNA editing enzyme. Cell 2000;102(5):553–63.
64. Honjo T, Kinoshita K, Muramatsu M. Molecular mechanism of class switch recombination: linkage with somatic hypermutation. Annu Rev Immunol 2002;20:165–96.
65. Shinohara M, Io K, Shindo K, et al. APOBEC3B can impair genomic stability by inducing base substitutions in genomic DNA in human cells. Sci Rep 2012;2:806.
66. Burns MB, Lackey L, Carpenter MA, et al. APOBEC3B is an enzymatic source of mutation in breast cancer. Nature 2013;494(7437):366–70.
67. Liu M, Schatz DG. Balancing AID and DNA repair during somatic hypermutation. Trends Immunol 2009;30(4):173–81.
68. Revy P, Muto T, Levy Y, et al. Activation-induced cytidine deaminase (AID) deficiency causes the autosomal recessive form of the Hyper-IgM syndrome (HIGM2). Cell 2000;102(5):565–75.
69. Schmitz K-M, Petersen-Mahrt SK. AIDing the immune system-DIAbolic in cancer. Semin Immunol 2012;24(4):241–5.
70. Beale RCL, Petersen-Mahrt SK, Watt IN, et al. Comparison of the differential context-dependence of DNA deamination by APOBEC enzymes: correlation with mutation spectra in vivo. J Mol Biol 2004;337(3):585–96.
71. Nagarajan N, Bertrand D, Hillmer AM, et al. Whole-genome reconstruction and mutational signatures in gastric cancer. Genome Biol 2012;13(12):R115.
72. Marusawa H, Chiba T. *Helicobacter pylori*-induced activation-induced cytidine deaminase expression and carcinogenesis. Curr Opin Immunol 2010;22(4): 442–7.
73. Matsumoto Y, Marusawa H, Kinoshita K, et al. *Helicobacter pylori* infection triggers aberrant expression of activation-induced cytidine deaminase in gastric epithelium. Nat Med 2007;13(4):470–6.
74. Nagata N, Akiyama J, Marusawa H, et al. Enhanced expression of activation-induced cytidine deaminase in human gastric mucosa infected by *Helicobacter pylori* and its decrease following eradication. J Gastroenterol 2014;49(3):427–35.
75. Hussain SP, Harris CC. Inflammation and cancer: an ancient link with novel potentials. Int J Cancer 2007;121(11):2373–80.
76. Handa O, Naito Y, Yoshikawa T. Redox biology and gastric carcinogenesis: the role of *Helicobacter pylori*. Redox Rep 2011;16(1):1–7.
77. Federico A, Morgillo F, Tuccillo C, et al. Chronic inflammation and oxidative stress in human carcinogenesis. Int J Cancer 2007;121(11):2381–6.
78. Chaturvedi R, Asim M, Romero-Gallo J, et al. Spermine oxidase mediates the gastric cancer risk associated with *Helicobacter pylori* CagA. Gastroenterology 2011;141(5):1696–708.e1–2.
79. Chen RZ, Pettersson U, Beard C, et al. DNA hypomethylation leads to elevated mutation rates. Nature 1998;395(6697):89–93.
80. Ciriello G, Miller ML, Aksoy BA, et al. Emerging landscape of oncogenic signatures across human cancers. Nat Genet 2013;45(10):1127–33.
81. Weiss MB, Vitolo MI, Mohseni M, et al. Deletion of p53 in human mammary epithelial cells causes chromosomal instability and altered therapeutic response. Oncogene 2010;29(33):4715–24.
82. Matsumoto Y, Marusawa H, Kinoshita K, et al. Up-regulation of activation-induced cytidine deaminase causes genetic aberrations at the CDKN2b-CDKN2a in gastric cancer. Gastroenterology 2010;139(6):1984–94.
83. Feinberg AP, Tycko B. The history of cancer epigenetics. Nat Rev Cancer 2004; 4(2):143–53.

84. Yamashita S, Hosoya K, Gyobu K, et al. Development of a novel output value for quantitative assessment in methylated DNA immunoprecipitation-CpG island microarray analysis. DNA Res 2009;16(5):275–86.
85. Sepulveda AR, Yao Y, Yan W, et al. CpG methylation and reduced expression of O6-methylguanine DNA methyltransferase is associated with Helicobacter pylori infection. Gastroenterology 2010;138(5):1836–44.
86. Maekita T, Nakazawa K, Mihara M, et al. High levels of aberrant DNA methylation in Helicobacter pylori-infected gastric mucosae and its possible association with gastric cancer risk. Clin Cancer Res 2006;12(3 Pt 1):989–95.
87. Ushijima T. Epigenetic field for cancerization. J Biochem Mol Biol 2007;40(2): 142–50.
88. Bae JM, Shin S-H, Kwon H-J, et al. ALU and LINE-1 hypomethylations in multistep gastric carcinogenesis and their prognostic implications. Int J Cancer 2012; 131(6):1323–31.
89. Zhao C, Bu X. Promoter methylation of tumor-related genes in gastric carcinogenesis. Histol Histopathol 2012;27(10):1271–82.
90. Niwa T, Tsukamoto T, Toyoda T, et al. Inflammatory processes triggered by Helicobacter pylori infection cause aberrant DNA methylation in gastric epithelial cells. Cancer Res 2010;70(4):1430–40.
91. Yoo EJ, Park SY, Cho NY, et al. Influence of IL1B polymorphism on CpG island hypermethylation in Helicobacter pylori-infected gastric cancer. Virchows Arch 2010;456(6):647–52.
92. Niwa T, Toyoda T, Tsukamoto T, et al. Prevention of Helicobacter pylori-induced gastric cancers in gerbils by a DNA demethylating agent. Cancer Prev Res (Phila) 2013;6(4):263–70.
93. Link A, Kupcinskas J, Wex T, et al. Macro-role of microRNA in gastric cancer. Dig Dis 2012;30(3):255–67.
94. Hayashi Y, Tsujii M, Wang J, et al. CagA mediates epigenetic regulation to attenuate let-7 expression in Helicobacter pylori-related carcinogenesis. Gut 2013; 62(11):1536–46.
95. Kiga K, Mimuro H, Suzuki M, et al. Epigenetic silencing of miR-210 increases the proliferation of gastric epithelium during chronic Helicobacter pylori infection. Nat Commun 2014;5:4497.

Helicobacter pylori Eradication to Eliminate Gastric Cancer: The Japanese Strategy

CrossMark

Masahiro Asaka, MD, PhD[a],*, Katsuhiro Mabe, MD, PhD[a],
Rumiko Matsushima, MD[b], Momoko Tsuda, MD[b]

KEYWORDS

- Gastric cancer • *Helicobacter pylori* • Elimination of gastric cancer
- Eradication of *Helicobacter pylori*

KEY POINTS

- *Helicobacter pylori* eradication therapy for chronic gastritis achieved world-first coverage by the Japanese national health insurance scheme in 2013, making a dramatic decrease of gastric cancer–related deaths more realistic.
- Combining *H pylori* eradication therapy with endoscopic surveillance can prevent the development of gastric cancer. Even if gastric cancer develops, most patients are likely to be diagnosed while it is at an early stage, possibly resulting in a large decrease of gastric cancer deaths.
- Success with the elimination of gastric cancer in Japan could lead other countries with a high incidence of gastric cancer (China, Korea, and Latin American countries) to consider a similar strategy, suggesting the potential for elimination of gastric cancer around the world.

INTRODUCTION

After the discovery of *Helicobacter pylori* in 1983,[1] the causal relationship between this bacterium and gastritis and/or gastric cancer has been steadily elucidated. In 1994, *H pylori* was classified as a definite carcinogen by the International Agency for Research on Cancer of the World Health Organization.[2] Subsequently, many clinical studies were conducted in various countries to determine whether eradication of *H pylori* could contribute to the prevention of gastric cancer. However, the very low incidence of gastric cancer among the subjects meant that sufficient data for statistical analysis

Conflict of Interest: M. Asaka and K. Mabe belongs to the donation-funded department by Eizai Co LTD at Hokkaido University Graduate School of Medicine.
[a] Cancer Preventive Medicine, Hokkaido University Graduate School of Medicine, Kita 12, Nishi 7, Kita-ku, Sapporo 060-0812, Japan; [b] Department of Gastroenterology, Hokkaido University Graduate School of Medicine, Kita 12, Nishi 7, Kita-ku, Sapporo 060-0812, Japan
* Corresponding author.
E-mail address: maasaka@med.hokudai.ac.jp

Gastroenterol Clin N Am 44 (2015) 639–648
http://dx.doi.org/10.1016/j.gtc.2015.05.010
0889-8553/15/$ – see front matter © 2015 Elsevier Inc. All rights reserved.

gastro.theclinics.com

were not obtained. In 2008, a randomized multicenter clinical study conducted in Japan revealed that eradication of *H pylori* reduced the incidence of secondary gastric cancer by approximately two-thirds after endoscopic mucosal resection of early gastric cancer,[3] suggesting the usefulness of *H pylori* eradication for prevention of gastric cancer. However, this study also showed that *H pylori* eradication did not completely eliminate gastric cancer. Therefore, to eliminate gastric cancer, periodic surveillance would be required after *H pylori* eradication. Thus, to achieve the elimination of gastric cancer in Japan, the important issue is how to combine primary prevention through *H pylori* eradication with secondary prevention through surveillance. Fortunately, the Ministry of Health, Labor and Welfare of Japan (MHLW) approved national health insurance coverage for eradication therapy in patients with gastritis caused by *H pylori* infection (chronic active gastritis) on February 21, 2013, for the first time in the world.[4]

PREVIOUS PREVENTIVE MEASURES FOR GASTRIC CANCER IN JAPAN

In Japan, the prevention of cancer, including gastric cancer, has primarily focused on secondary measures for early detection of cancer, rather than on primary prevention aimed at elimination of the causes. Indirect barium contrast imaging has been used as the screening method for gastric cancer, but despite the long interest and emphasis, the screening rate was only 9.6% in 2010.[5] Screening for gastric cancer based on barium contrast imaging also does not have a high sensitivity for detecting early cancer[6] and is associated with considerable exposure to radiation. Furthermore, targeting all people age 40 or older for screening is a major problem, as people younger than 50 account for only approximately 3% of all patients with gastric cancer in Japan.[7] Moreover, patients who are *H pylori*–negative with minimal or no atrophy of the gastric mucosa are very unlikely to develop gastric cancer,[8–10] such that these patients are unlikely to benefit from annual barium contrast screening and are still exposed to the adverse effects of radiation.

The most serious disadvantage with Japan's attempts to prevent gastric cancer was the inability to implement primary prevention, which is understandable, as the cause of gastric cancer had not been identified in the 1970s when programs of screening for this cancer were begun. However, we now know that more than 95% of gastric cancers are due to *H pylori* infection in Japan and Korea.[9,10] As a general rule for cancers caused by infections, such as liver cell cancer and cervical carcinoma, primary prevention based on preventing the infection or early eradication before significant damage is done is preferred over screening. Primary preventive measures for gastric cancer have yet to be started in Japan, and Japan has relied on barium contrast screening for 30 years. The aging of the population has increased the population at risk and thus the number of patients dying of gastric cancer has remained unchanged at approximately 50,000 per year.[11] The lack of a reduction in the total number of deaths despite the decline in age-standardized mortality rates provided important evidence to the Japanese government that current programs were not effective in the prevention of gastric cancer deaths.

CURRENT STATUS AND CHARACTERISTICS OF SCREENING FOR GASTRIC CANCER IN JAPAN

Approximately 60% of patients with gastric cancer worldwide are found in only 3 East Asian countries (Japan, China, and Korea), and the disease seems to be endemic to this area.[12] Gastric cancer was the most common cause of cancer death in Japan until it was replaced by lung cancer in 1995.[13] Thanks to concerted efforts by clinical and fundamental researchers, the concept of early gastric cancer was proposed in Japan in 1963. At that time, early gastric cancer was defined as a lesion with infiltration of tumor cells limited to the mucosa or submucosa, irrespective of lymph node metastasis.[14,15]

The prognosis of early gastric cancer is far better than that of advanced cancer, with a 5-year survival rate exceeding 90%.[16] Therefore, many studies in Japan have focused on how to effectively diagnose early gastric cancer. As a result, early cancer now accounts for nearly 60% of all gastric cancers detected in Japan. This has not been reported in any other country and suggests high diagnostic capability for early cancer in the country. The efforts made so far have led to an overall 5-year survival rate of more than 60% for patients with gastric cancer in Japan.[17] In other countries, including the United States and Europe, the 5-year survival rate of patients with gastric cancer is reported to be only 10% to 25% (**Fig. 1**).[18–20] This is not because treatment of gastric cancer is superior in Japan to that in other countries, but because the detection rate of early cancer is much lower outside Japan. In the United States and Europe, intramucosal carcinoma is not even considered to be cancer, and is classified as dysplasia. Thus, researchers in the United States and Europe have speculated that the diagnosis and treatment of precancerous lesions as early gastric cancer improves the prognosis in Japan compared with other countries. There is undoubtedly a difference of diagnostic criteria between Japan and the United States/Europe. Although Japanese pathologists make a diagnosis of gastric cancer based on the presence of atypical nuclei in gastric mucosal cells and atypical glandular or ductal structures, pathologists in the United States and Europe will diagnose gastric dysplasia instead of gastric cancer when atypical glandular and ductal structures do not extend beyond the muscularis mucosa.[21] This difference in the diagnostic criteria for gastric cancer between Japan and the United States/Europe is an issue that seems to be difficult to resolve.[22] However, based on the findings that 30% to 60% of lesions diagnosed as dysplasia show progression to gastric cancer within a few years,[23–25] and that examination of larger biopsy specimens leads to diagnosis of more lesions as cancer,[26] high-grade dysplasia should be classified as intramucosal gastric cancer and be treated aggressively to improve the prognosis of gastric cancer.

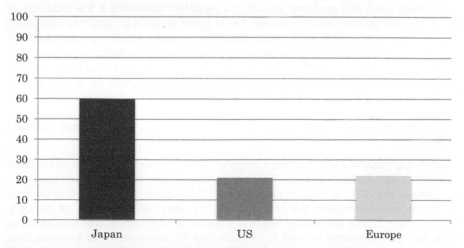

Fig. 1. Five-year survival rates (%) of gastric cancer in various countries.

THE EFFECT OF *HELICOBACTER PYLORI* ERADICATION FOR GASTRIC CANCER PREVENTION

After it became clear that *H pylori* infection is an important risk factor for gastric cancer, the issue of whether *H pylori* eradication therapy can decrease the incidence of gastric cancer has attracted increasing attention. Intervention studies to assess the preventive effect of *H pylori* eradication on gastric cancer have been conducted in healthy individuals worldwide. However, the incidence of gastric cancer is very low in Western countries and the study populations enrolled in those countries were not large enough to detect a significant effect of eradication therapy, resulting in the discontinuation of most studies.

You and colleagues[27] reported a study of 3365 Chinese patients who were randomized to an *H pylori* eradication group, a garlic group, or a vitamin group, and then were followed for 7.3 years in 2006. They found no difference of gastric cancer among the 3 groups. However, longer follow-up for 15 years subsequently revealed a significant reduction of gastric cancer in the *H pylori* eradication group (odds ratio 0.61; $P = .032$).[28] Because the incidence of progression from *H pylori*–positive atrophic gastritis to gastric cancer is very low, it has been suggested that it would be difficult to demonstrate a significant difference unless the sample size is increased or the observation period is longer. Gail and colleagues[29] recently reported that *H pylori* eradication at later times also has a benefit in that it stops the progression of damage and the age-related increase in cancer incidence.

We conducted a clinical trial with a small sample size and short follow-up period that involved patients who had undergone endoscopic mucosal resection for early gastric cancer, a population in which gastric cancer is very likely to develop. To investigate the ectopic recurrence of gastric cancer, 544 patients who had received endoscopic treatment for early gastric cancer were randomly allocated to *H pylori* eradication or noneradication groups and were followed for 3 years by annual endoscopic examination. Metachronous recurrence was detected in 9 and 24 subjects from the eradication group and the noneradication group, respectively, and there was a significantly lower relapse rate in the eradication group ($P<.01$ according to intention-to-treat analysis).[3] *H pylori* eradication therapy reduced the incidence of differentiated gastric cancer by at least two-thirds irrespective of whether the patients had atrophic gastritis, intestinal metaplasia, or early gastric cancer. Data obtained up to 8 to 10 years after completion of this study were also analyzed, revealing a persistent difference in the incidence of metachronous gastric cancer between the *H pylori* eradication and noneradication groups (Kato M, Kikuchi S, Asaka M. Long-term preventive effect of *H pylori* eradication on the incidence of metachronous gastric cancer after endoscopic resection of primary early gastric cancer. BMJ. Submitted for publication). Thus, our findings indicate that the preventive effect of *H pylori* eradication therapy on gastric cancer persists for a long time.

HEALTH INSURANCE COVERAGE FOR *HELICOBACTER PYLORI* ERADICATION THERAPY IN JAPAN

Cancers are classified into 2 broad categories: lifestyle-related and infection-related cancers. In the United States and Europe, cancers related to infection account for a low percentage (10% or less) of all cancers.[30,31] In Japan, however, it has become clear that infection-related cancers account for approximately 25% of cancers, including liver cancer caused by hepatitis viruses, cervical cancer due to papillomavirus, and gastric cancer related to *H pylori* (**Fig. 2**). Because it has become clear that most gastric cancer is due to *H pylori* infection rather than lifestyle factors, it is

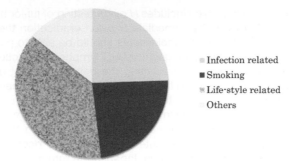

Fig. 2. Cause of cancer in Japan.

time for major revision of the preventive strategies for gastric cancer. When it is suspected that a cancer is caused by infection, proactive preventive measures are likely to lead to a dramatic decrease in the incidence of that cancer, resulting in a significant decrease of cancer mortality. In Japan, preventive measures for liver cancer have been focused on hepatitis virus infection since 2002, leading to a reduction of mortality.[32,33] However, the annual number of deaths from gastric cancer has remained at approximately 50,000 for the past few decades,[34] suggesting that the current preventive measures are inadequate. Even though there is a difference in the causative agent between liver cancer (viruses) and gastric cancer (a bacterium), preventive measures for gastric cancer should not be completely different from those for liver cancer. Thus, the fundamental measures for preventing gastric cancer should be shifted from conventional secondary prevention based on barium X-ray screening to primary prevention focused on H pylori eradication therapy.

In 2009, the Japanese Society for Helicobacter Research published a guideline in which it is recommended that all H pylori–infected people receive bacterial eradication therapy.[35] In response to this, the MHLW approved the extension of national health insurance coverage to H pylori eradication therapy for 3 indications (ie, patients with gastric mucosa-associated lymphoid tissue [MALT] lymphoma, patients who have undergone endoscopic surgery for early gastric cancer, and patients with idiopathic thrombocytopenic purpura [ITP]), in addition to patients with gastroduodenal ulcer. This was the first time in the world that insurance coverage has been provided for H pylori eradication therapy for indications other than gastroduodenal ulcer and represents an innovative approach. Regarding the potential expansion of health insurance coverage for eradication therapy to include patients with chronic gastritis, the Japanese Society of Gastroenterology, the Japan Gastroenterological Endoscopy Society, and the Japanese Society for Helicobacter Research submitted a joint petition to the minister of the MHLW. This public knowledge–based application led to the inclusion of H pylori eradication therapy for patients with chronic gastritis on February 21, 2013. The MHLW notification states that eradication therapy is covered by the national health insurance scheme when a patient with endoscopically diagnosed chronic gastritis is positive for H pylori.

STRATEGY FOR THE ELIMINATION OF GASTRIC CANCER IN JAPAN

The strategy for adolescents should be different from that for elderly persons to eliminate gastric cancer in Japan. This is because bacterial eradication in adolescents achieves nearly 100% prevention of gastric cancer, but the incidence of this cancer increases with advancing age.[36] We recommend a screen-and-treat approach as the strategy for adolescents, which includes *H pylori* testing of junior high school and high school students, followed by immediate *H pylori* eradication therapy for those with a positive result. Eradication in adolescents should be able to prevent *H pylori*–related diseases, such as peptic ulcer, gastric MALT lymphoma, functional dyspepsia, gastric polyps, and ITP, as well as preventing the development of nearly 100% of gastric cancers (**Fig. 3**). It is estimated that approximately 5% of all teenagers in Japan are positive for *H pylori*,[37] suggesting that the cost of this approach would not be so high. Some local governments in Japan have already scheduled free *H pylori* testing for junior high school students. We are expecting a screen-and-treat approach as the strategy for adolescents will contribute to the dramatic decrease of *H pylori*–related diseases, such as gastric cancer, in Japan in the future.

The recent expansion of health insurance coverage allows individuals with symptoms such as gastric heaviness to present to hospital for the diagnosis and treatment of *H pylori*–associated gastritis. To obtain health insurance coverage, endoscopy must be performed first for the diagnosis of gastritis, and most patients seem to have chronic gastritis by the time they undergo endoscopy. We expect that many patients with gastric cancer will be discovered during this endoscopic examination. This project thus includes a form of endoscopic screening supported by medical insurance. All patients in whom gastritis is diagnosed are supposed to receive *H pylori* eradication therapy. In patients with obvious atrophic gastritis, periodic endoscopic follow-up is recommended every 1 or 2 years, even after eradication therapy, whereas patients with no or mild atrophy and those who are negative for *H pylori* infection can be followed by optional screening instead of strategic screening (**Fig. 4**).[38]

Although it is not clear to what extent the use of eradication therapy in patients with *H pylori*–induced gastritis will inhibit the development of gastric cancer, a good model may be peptic ulcer, for which *H pylori* eradication therapy was first covered by the Japanese national health scheme in 2000. Since then, the incidence of peptic ulcer has decreased dramatically by approximately 60% over 10 years (**Fig. 5**). In addition, the medical costs of treating ulcers have decreased by 47% during that period.[38] Although it is unclear whether the results obtained with gastric cancer will be comparable to those for peptic ulcer, *H pylori* eradication therapy (etiologic treatment) for *H pylori*–associated gastritis will lead to a long-term decrease of gastric cancer. Such treatment will inhibit the development of peptic ulcer and gastric polyps as well as gastric cancer, suggesting a greater reduction of medical costs than that achieved by providing insurance coverage for *H pylori* eradication therapy in patients with peptic ulcer.

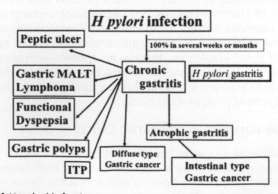

Fig. 3. Progress of *H pylori* infection.

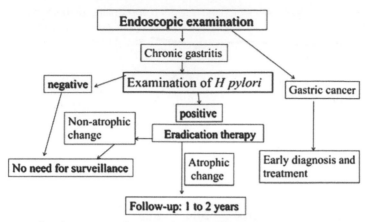

Fig. 4. Strategy for elimination of gastric cancer deaths in Japan.

There are 2 potential outcomes of the gastric cancer elimination project suggested here with regard to gastric cancer–related deaths in Japan. One is a definite decrease in the incidence of gastric cancer resulting from the widespread use of *H pylori* eradication therapy (a direct effect of this therapy). The other is a decrease in the number of deaths resulting from an increase in the diagnosis of early gastric cancer owing to mandatory endoscopy at the time of presentation for chronic gastritis. The target would be to eventually increase the proportion of early gastric cancer from the current 60% to approximately 90%, which would make it possible to increase the 5-year survival rate for patients with gastric cancer in Japan to approximately 90%. Because the baby boomer generation represents a huge population turning 65 and entering the cancer-prone years, the number of deaths from gastric cancer is likely to increase

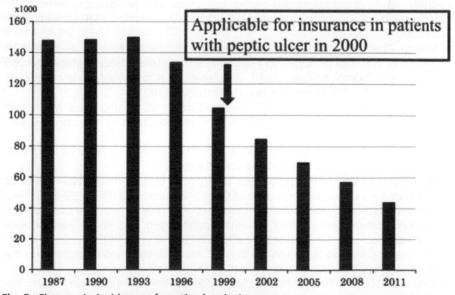

Fig. 5. Changes in incidence of peptic ulcer in Japan.

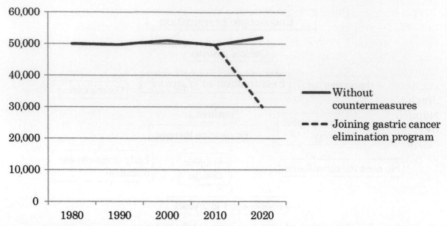

Fig. 6. Anticipated gastric cancer deaths in Japan, with or without countermeasures.

in 2020 without any countermeasures. In contrast, if the gastric cancer elimination project is successful, and approximately 50% of persons with *H pylori* infection receive eradication therapy, the number of deaths from gastric cancer will decrease to approximately 30,000 in 2020 **(Fig. 6)**.[39]

REFERENCES

1. Warren JR, Marshall BJ. Unidentified curved bacilli on gastric epithelium in active chronic gastritis. Lancet 1983;1:1273–5.
2. International agency for research on cancer. World Health Organization: schistosomes, liver flukes and *Helicobacter pylori*. IARC Monogr Eval Carcinog Risks Hum 1994;61:177–241.
3. Fukase K, Kato M, Kikuchi S, et al. Effect of eradication of *Helicobacter pylori* on incidence of metachronous gastric carcinoma after endoscopic resection of early gastric cancer: an open-label, randomised controlled trial. Lancet 2008; 372:392–7.
4. Takeda Pharmaceutical Company. *Helicobacter pylori* gastritis approved as additional indication in Japan for *Helicobacter pylori* eradication by triple therapy with proton pump inhibitor. 2013. Available at: http://www.takeda.com/news/2013/20130221_5659.html. Accessed February 21, 2013.
5. Health promotion and community health report in 2010. Japanese Ministry of Health, Labour and Welfare. Statistical Surveys conducted by Ministry of Health, Labour and Welfare. 2010. p. 15.
6. Hamashima C, Shibuya D, Yamazaki H, et al. The Japanese guidelines for gastric cancer screening. Jpn J Clin Oncol 2008;38:259–67.
7. Trends in age-specific incidence rate, The Editorial Board of the Cancer Statistics in Japan. Foundation for Promotion of Cancer Research. 2011. p. 29–36.
8. Inoue K, Fujisawa T, Haruma K. Assessment of degree of health of the stomach by concomitant measurement of serum pepsinogen and serum *Helicobacter pylori* antibodies. Int J Biol Markers 2010;25:207–12.
9. Uemura N, Okamoto S, Yamamoto S, et al. *Helicobacter pylori* infection and the development of gastric cancer. N Engl J Med 2001;345:784–9.
10. Yoon H, Kim N, Lee HS, et al. *Helicobacter pylori*-negative gastric cancer in South Korea: incidence and clinicopathologic characteristics. Helicobacter 2011;16:382–8.

11. Trends in site-specific crude mortality rate 1965–2010, The Editorial Board of the Cancer Statistics in Japan. Foundation for Promotion of Cancer Research. 2011. p. 26.
12. Ferlay J, Shin HR, Bray F, et al. Estimates of worldwide burden of cancer in 2008: GLOBOCAN 2008. Int J Cancer 2010;127:2893–917.
13. Marugame T, Matsuda T, Kamo K, et al. Cancer incidence and incidence rates in Japan in 2001 based on the data from 10 population-based cancer registries. Jpn J Clin Oncol 2007;37:884–91.
14. Nagayo T, Ito M, Yokoyama H, et al. Early phases of human gastric cancer: morphological study. Gann 1965;56:101–20.
15. Nakamura K, Sugano H, Takagi K. Carcinoma of the stomach in incipient phase: its histogenesis and histological appearances. Gann 1968;59:251–8.
16. Kaneko E, Nakamura T, Umeda N, et al. Outcome of gastric carcinoma detected by gastric mass survey in Japan. Gut 1977;18:626–30.
17. Survival rate in the member hospitals of the association of clinical cancer centers diagnosed in 2000–2004, The Editorial Board of the Cancer Statistics in Japan. Foundation for Promotion of Cancer Research. 2012. p. 76–7.
18. Noguchi Y, Yoshikawa T, Tsuburaya A, et al. Is gastric carcinoma different between Japan and the United States? Cancer 2000;89:2237–46.
19. Hundahl SA, Phillips JL, Menck HR. The National Cancer data base report on poor survival of U.S. gastric carcinoma patients with gastrectomy. Cancer 2000;88:921–32.
20. Comparison of 5-year survival rates between Japan and Western countries. The Editorial Board of the Cancer Statistics in Japan. Foundation for Promotion of Cancer Research. 2006. p. 59.
21. Schlemper RJ, Itabashi M, Kato Y, et al. Difference in diagnostic criteria for gastric carcinoma between Japanese and Western pathologists. Lancet 1997; 349:1725–9.
22. Schlemper RJ, Riddell RH, Kato Y, et al. The Vienna classification of gastrointestinal epithelial neoplasia. Gut 2000;47:251–5.
23. Yamada H, Ikegami M, Shimoda T, et al. Long-term follow-up study of gastric adenoma/dysplasia. Endoscopy 2004;36:390–6.
24. Park SY, Jeon SW, Jung MK, et al. Long-term follow-up study of gastric intraepithelial neoplasias: progression from low-grade dysplasia to invasive carcinoma. Eur J Gastroenterol Hepatol 2008;20:966–70.
25. Dinis-Ribeiro M, Areia M, De Vries AC, et al. Management of precancerous conditions and lesions in the stomach (MAPS): guideline from the European Society of Gastrointestinal Endoscopy (ESGE), European Helicobacter Study Group (EHSG), European Society of Pathology(ESP), and the Sociedade Portuguesa de Endoscopia Digestiva (SPED). Endoscopy 2012;44:74–94.
26. Dixon MF. Gastrointestinal epithelial neoplasia: Vienna revised. Gut 2002;51:130–1.
27. You WC, Brown LM, Zhang L, et al. Randomized double-blind factorial trial of three treatments to reduce the prevalence of precancerous gastric lesions. J Natl Cancer Inst 2006;98:974–83.
28. Ma JL, Zhang L, Linda M, et al. Fifteen-year effects of *Helicobacter pylori*, garlic, and vitamin treatments on gastric cancer incidence and mortality. J Natl Cancer 2012;104:488–92.
29. Gail MH, You WC, Li WQ. Effects of *Helicobacter pylori* treatment on gastric cancer incidence and mortality in subgroups. Response. J Natl Cancer Inst 2014;106 [pii:dju348].
30. Harvard Report on Cancer Prevention. Volume 1: causes of human cancer. Cancer Causes Control 1996;7(Suppl 1):S3–59.

31. Olsen JH, Andersen A, Dreyer L, et al. Summary of avoidable cancers in the Nordic countries. APMIS Suppl 1997;76:141–6.
32. Tsukuma H, Tanaka H, Ajiki W, et al. Liver cancer and its prevention. Asian Pac J Cancer Prev 2005;6:244–50.
33. Makuuchi M, Kokudo N, Arii S, et al. Development of evidence-based clinical guidelines for the diagnosis and treatment of hepatocellular carcinoma in Japan. Hepatol Res 2008;38:37–51.
34. Trends in site-specific crude mortality rate 1965–2010. The Editorial Board of the Cancer Statistics in Japan. Foundation for Promotion of Cancer Research. Tokyo: 2011. p. 26.
35. Asaka M, Kato M, Takahashi S, et al. Guidelines for the management of Helicobacter pylori infection in Japan: 2009 revised edition. Helicobacter 2010; 15:1–20.
36. Asaka M. A new approach for elimination of gastric cancer in Japan. Int J Cancer 2013;132:1272–6.
37. Akamatsu T, Ichikawa S, Okudaira S, et al. Introduction of an examination and treatment for Helicobacter pylori infection in high school health screening. J Gastroenterol 2011;46:1353–60.
38. Asaka M, Kato M, Sakamoto N. Roadmap to eliminate gastric cancer with Helicobacter pylori eradication and consecutive surveillance in Japan. J Gastroenterol 2014;249:1–8.
39. Asaka M. Strategy to eliminate gastric cancer deaths in Japan. Helicobacter pylori eradication as a strategy for preventing gastric cancer. IARC Working Group Rep 2014;8:21–7.

Treatment Strategy for Gastric Mucosa-Associated Lymphoid Tissue Lymphoma

Shotaro Nakamura, MD, PhD*, Takayuki Matsumoto, MD, PhD

KEYWORDS

- Gastric lymphoma • MALT lymphoma • *Helicobacter pylori* • Radiotherapy
- Chemotherapy • Rituximab

KEY POINTS

- Infection with *H pylori* is found in 80% to 90% of gastric MALT lymphoma cases.
- First-line treatment of gastric MALT lymphomas should be *H pylori* eradication independent of the stage.
- *H pylori* eradication achieves complete remission in 60% to 90% of cases.
- Strategies for nonresponders to eradication, including "watch and wait," radiotherapy, chemotherapy, or rituximab immunotherapy, should be tailored.

INTRODUCTION

Extranodal marginal zone lymphoma of mucosa-associated lymphoid tissue (MALT lymphoma) is an indolent non-Hodgkin lymphoma composed of morphologically heterogeneous small B cells including marginal zone (centrocyte-like) cells, monocytoid cells, and scattered immunoblasts and centroblast-like cells.[1] MALT lymphoma occurs in various extranodal organs, and the stomach is the most common site; it comprises 7% to 9% of all B-cell lymphomas, 3% to 6% of all gastric malignant neoplasms, and 40% to 50% of primary gastric lymphomas.[1–4] In most patients with gastric MALT lymphoma, *Helicobacter pylori* plays a causative role in the development of the disease, and the eradication of *H pylori* leads to a complete remission of the lymphoma in 60% to 90% of cases.[5,6]

Here we review recent trends and the current knowledge regarding the diagnosis and treatment strategy for patients with gastric MALT lymphoma.

Disclosure Statement: The authors disclose no conflicts of interest.
Division of Gastroenterology, Department of Internal Medicine, School of Medicine, Iwate Medical University, Uchimaru 19-1, Morioka 020-8505, Japan
* Corresponding author.
E-mail address: shonaka@iwate-med.ac.jp

Gastroenterol Clin N Am 44 (2015) 649–660
http://dx.doi.org/10.1016/j.gtc.2015.05.012
0889-8553/15/$ – see front matter © 2015 Elsevier Inc. All rights reserved.

PATHOGENESIS
Helicobacter pylori

In 1991, Wotherspoon and colleagues[7] first reported a link of *H pylori* with gastric MALT lymphoma by histologic detection of the bacteria in most cases. This association was supported by subsequent epidemiologic and histopathologic studies.[8,9] Infection with *H pylori* is observed in 80% to 90% of patients with gastric MALT lymphoma,[6–11] and 60% to 80% of the cases respond to *H pylori* eradication therapy.[5,6] In such *H pylori*–dependent cases, the growth of lymphoma cells is largely driven by *H pylori*–generated immune responses including signaling from CD40 and CD86 through bystander T-cell help.[12–15] A proliferation-inducing ligand (APRIL), a tumor necrosis factor (TNF) superfamily member, produced by macrophages in the *H pylori*–infected gastric mucosa also plays an important role in promoting the survival and proliferation of neoplastic B cells.[16]

Genetic Aberrations

MALT lymphoma is genetically characterized by the replicable chromosomal translocations t(11;18) (q21;q21)/*API2-MALT1*, t(1;14) (p22;q32)/*BCL10-IGH*, t(14;18) (q32;q21)/*IGH-MALT1*, and t(3;14) (p13;q32)/*FOXP1-IGH*.[1,12,17] These translocations are considered to exert their oncogenic activities through constitutive activation of the nuclear factor kappa B (NF-κB) pathway, leading to expression of several genes for cell survival and proliferation.[12] Among these aberrations, t(11;18)/*API2-MALT1* is the most frequent translocation, which is detected in 15% to 24% of gastric MALT lymphoma cases. The translocation fuses the N-terminal region of the *API2* to the C-terminal region of the *MALT1* and generates a functional chimeric fusion, which gains the ability to activate the NF-κB pathway.[12,17] Clinically, t(11;18)/*API2-MALT1* is frequently associated with the absence of *H pylori* infection, and most the translocation-positive cases do not respond to *H pylori* eradication therapy.[6,10,17,18] Interestingly, t(11;18)-positive MALT lymphomas rarely transform to diffuse large B-cell lymphoma.[19]

The TNF-α–induced protein 3 gene (*TNFAIP3, A20*), which has been recently identified as the target of 6q23 deletion in MALT lymphomas, is an important negative regulator of NF-κB.[12,20,21] The mutation and/or deletion of *A20*, which leads to A20 inactivation, is observed frequently in MALT lymphoma of the ocular adnexa, salivary glands, thyroid, and liver. Such A20-mediated oncogenic activities in MALT lymphoma are considered to depend on the NF-κB activation triggered by TNF or other unidentified molecules.[12] By contrast, *A20* deletion was detected only in 2 of 29 (7%) cases of gastric MALT lymphomas.[21] Further investigations with larger numbers of patients are warranted to determine to what extent A20 inactivation contributes to the development of gastric MALT lymphoma.

DIAGNOSIS
Histopathology

The definite diagnosis of gastric MALT lymphoma should be based on the histopathologic criteria by the World Health Organization classification, using the tissue specimens appropriately obtained by biopsy or surgical resection.[1,22,23] Histologically, the small- to medium-sized neoplastic lymphoid cells (centrocyte-like cells) infiltrate around reactive follicles showing marginal zone growth pattern, which often infiltrate into gastric glands causing destruction of the epithelial cells (lymphoepithelial lesions).[1,22] Immunohistochemically, the tumor cells exhibit CD20$^+$, CD79a$^+$, CD5$^-$, CD10$^-$, CD23$^-$, CD43$^{+/-}$, and cyclin D1$^-$. When large neoplastic cells are present in solid or sheets, the diagnosis of an associated diffuse large B-cell lymphoma should be made.[1] Staining for Ki-67 may help the identification of diffuse large B-cell lymphoma. The diagnosis should be confirmed by an expert hematopathologist.[22,23]

The differential diagnosis of gastric MALT lymphoma includes the reactive inflammatory conditions, such as *H pylori*–related chronic gastritis.[1] Distinction from gastritis is based mainly on the presence of a dense infiltrate of monotonous B cells extending away from lymphoid follicles, the presence of cytologic atypia of lymphoid cells, Dutcher bodies, and characteristic lymphoepithelial lesions. Wotherspoon score is widely used for the confident histologic diagnosis of gastric MALT lymphoma on biopsy specimens (**Table 1**).[24] The consensus report of the European Gastro-Intestinal Lymphoma Study (EGILS) group recommends that a minimum of 10 biopsy samples should be taken from visible lesions and endoscopically normal-appearing mucosa.[22] The demonstration of immunoglobulin light chain (κ or λ) restriction by immunohistochemistry or in situ hybridization, and analyses for clonality of the rearranged immunoglobulin genes by polymerase chain reaction, may help a diagnosis of B-cell lymphoma.[1,22] Cytogenetic analyses using G-banding, reverse-transcription polymerase chain reaction, and/or fluorescence in situ hybridization for t(11;18)/*API2-MALT1* or other specific chromosomal translocations are useful for confirming the diagnosis of MALT lymphoma.[1,22,23]

Endoscopic Findings

Standard endoscopic or macroscopic classifications for gastric lymphomas have not been established to date. In Western countries, gastric B-cell lymphomas were endoscopically classified either as ulcerative (34%–69%), mass/polypoid (26%–35%), diffusely infiltrating (15%–40%), or other types.[25–27] In our previous study,[28] 197 consecutive Japanese cases of primary gastric B-cell lymphoma (MALT lymphomas

Table 1
Histologic scoring system for diagnosis of gastric MALT lymphoma (Wotherspoon score)

Grade	Description	Histologic Features
0	Normal	Scattered plasma cells in lamina propria; no lymphoid follicles.
1	Chronic active gastritis	Small clusters of lymphocytes in lamina propria; no lymphoid follicles; no lymphoepithelial lesions.
2	Chronic active gastritis with florid lymphoid follicle formation	Prominent lymphoid follicles with surrounding mantle zone and plasma cells; no lymphoepithelial lesions.
3	Suspicious lymphoid infiltrate in lamina propria, probably reactive	Lymphoid follicles surrounded by small lymphocytes that infiltrate diffusely in lamina propria and occasionally into epithelium.
4	Suspicious lymphoid infiltrate in lamina propria, probably lymphoma	Lymphoid follicles surrounded by centrocyte-like cells that infiltrate diffusely in lamina propria and into epithelium in small groups.
5	MALT lymphoma	Presence of dense diffuse infiltrate of centrocyte-like cells in lamina propria with prominent lymphoepithelial lesions.

Data from Wotherspoon AC, Doglioni C, Diss TC, et al. Regression of primary low-grade B-cell gastric lymphoma of mucosa-associated lymphoid tissue type after eradication of *Helicobacter pylori*. Lancet 1993;342:575–7.

and diffuse large B-cell lymphomas) were macroscopically classified as superficial-spreading (46%), mass-forming (41%), diffuse-infiltrating (6%), or other types (8%).[28] It should be noted that the most frequent macroscopic type in gastric MALT lymphomas is superficial-spreading type (**Fig. 1**). This type of lymphoma is occasionally misdiagnosed as depressed-type early gastric cancer. By contrast, gastric diffuse large B-cell lymphomas often present as mass-forming type lesions, mimicking advanced gastric cancers.[27,28] Recently, Zullo and colleagues[29] proposed another endoscopic classification of gastric MALT lymphoma, which includes ulcerative (52%), hypertrophic (24%), normal/hyperemic (13%), exophytic (10%), and petechial hemorrhage types (1%).

Clinical Staging

To determine the optimal management strategy for malignant lymphomas, appropriate clinical staging is essential. It is controversial as to which classification is the best system for staging of gastric MALT lymphoma. Generally, the Lugano International Conference (Blackledge) classification (I, II_1, II_2, IIE, or IV; **Table 2**) or Ann Arbor staging system with its modifications by Musschoff and Radaszkiewicz (I_1E, I_2E, II_1E, II_2E, IIIE, or IV) have been widely applied to patients with gastrointestinal lymphomas.[30] Recently, however, the EGILS consensus report and European Society of Medical Oncology guidelines also recommend to use the Paris staging system, a modification of the TNM system including the degree of the spread of lymphoma assessed by endoscopic ultrasound (see **Table 2**).[22,23,31] In addition to esophagogastroduodenoscopy, the following are recommended for the initial staging work-up: physical examination (including peripheral lymph nodes and Waldeyer ring), complete hematologic biochemical examinations (including lactate dehydrogenase and β_2-microblobulin), computerized tomography of abdomen and pelvis, and endoscopic ultrasound.[22] We consider that ileocolonoscopy, bone marrow aspiration or biopsy, fluorine-18 fluorodeoxyglucose PET, and endoscopic examinations of the small bowel (balloon-assisted endoscopy or capsule endoscopy) should also be considered.[32]

TREATMENTS
Helicobacter pylori Eradication

The first-line treatment of all gastric MALT lymphomas is *H pylori* eradication therapy independent of the stage.[22,23] In patients with stage I/II_1 disease, complete remission is achieved in 60% to 90% of cases only by *H pylori* eradication.[4–6] Histologic evaluation of posttreatment biopsies should be based on the Groupe d'Etude des

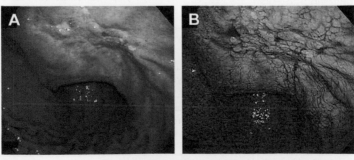

Fig. 1. Endoscopic images of superficial-spreading type gastric MALT lymphoma. (*A*, *B*) A superficially depressed lesion, mimicking early gastric cancer, with erosions and reddish granular mucosa can be seen on the lesser curvature of the lower corpus.

Table 2
Comparison of the Lugano and Paris staging systems for gastrointestinal lymphomas

	Lugano Staging System[30]	Paris Staging System[31]	Tumor Extension
Stage I	Tumor confined to the GI tract (single primary site or multiple, noncontiguous lesions)	T1m N0 M0 T1sm N0 M0 T2 N0 M0 T3 N0 M0	Mucosa Submucosa Muscularis propria Serosa
Stage II	Tumor extending into abdomen	—	—
II$_1$	Local nodal involvement	T1-3 N1 M0	Perigastric lymph nodes
II$_2$	Distant nodal involvement	T1-3 N2 M0	More distant regional nodes
Stage IIE	Penetration of serosa to involve adjacent organs or tissues	T4 N0-2 M0	Invasion of adjacent structures with or without abdominal lymph nodes
Stage IV	Disseminated extranodal involvement or concomitant supradiaphragmatic nodal involvement	T1-4 N3 M0 T1-4 N0-3 M1 T1-4 N0-3 M2 T1-4 N0-3 M0-2 BX T1-4 N0-3 M0-2 B0 T1-4 N0-3 M2 B1	Extra-abdominal lymph nodes And/or additional distant GI sites Or non-GI sites Bone marrow not assessed Bone marrow not involved Bone marrow involvement

Abbreviations: B, describes the bone marrow assessment; GI, gastrointestinal; M, describes distant dissemination; N, describes the regional lymph node involvement; T, describes the gastric wall infiltration.

Data from Zucca E, Copie-Bergman C, Ricardi U, et al. Gastric marginal zone lymphoma of MALT type: ESMO Clinical Practice Guidelines for diagnosis, treatment and follow-up. Ann Oncol 2013;24:vi144-8.

Lymphomes de l'Adulte grading system (**Table 3**),[22,23,33] because Wotherspoon score (see **Table 1**), recommended for initial diagnosis, is no longer considered adequate for response assessment during follow-up.[22] As for the regimen for *H pylori* eradication, proton pump inhibitor plus clarithromycin-based triple therapy composed of a double dose of a proton pump inhibitor plus clarithromycin and amoxicillin or metronidazole for 7 or 14 days has been recommended[22] but is now considered obsolete (discussed elsewhere in this issue in the article on practical aspects in choosing an *H pylori* therapy). Success of bacterial eradication should be confirmed by urea breath test or stool antigen test.[22,23] A first evaluation of lymphoma regression using endoscopy and biopsy should be performed 3 to 6 months after completion of successful treatment. Further follow-up should be performed every 4 to 6 months thereafter until complete remission (complete histologic response or probable minimal residual disease, see **Table 3**) is documented. Although complete remission is obtained usually within 6 to 12 months, it may be delayed up to 24 to 71 months in some cases.[5,22]

In a systematic review of the data from 32 published studies including 1408 patients with gastric MALT lymphoma, the complete remission rate after *H pylori* eradication was 78%.[5] Various predictive factors for resistance to *H pylori* eradication therapy have been reported, including absence of *H pylori* infection, advanced stage, proximal location in the stomach, endoscopic nonsuperficial type, deep tumor invasion in the gastric wall, and t(11;18)/*API2-MALT1* translocation.[5,6,17,18,22,34]

Table 3
GELA histologic grading system for posttreatment evaluation of gastric MALT lymphoma

Score	Lymphoid Infiltrate	LEL	Stromal Changes	Clinical Significance
Complete histologic response	Absent or scattered plasma cells and small lymphoid cells in the LP	Absent	Normal or empty LP and/or fibrosis	Complete remission
Probable minimal residual disease	Aggregates of lymphoid cells or lymphoid nodules in LP/ MM and/or SM	Absent	Empty LP and/or fibrosis	Complete remission
Responding residual disease	Dense, diffuse, or nodular extending around glands in the LP	Focal LEL or absent	Focal empty LP and/or fibrosis	Partial remission
No change	Dense, diffuse, or nodular	Present, may be absent	No changes	Stable disease or progressive disease

Abbreviations: GELA, Groupe d'Etude des Lymphomes de l'Adulte; LEL, lymphoepithelial lesions; LP, lamina propria; MALT, mucosa-associated lymphoid tissue; MM, muscularis propria; SM, submucosa.
Data from Copie-Bergman C, Gaulard P, Lavergne-Slove A, et al. Proposal for a new histological grading system for post-treatment evaluation of gastric MALT lymphoma. Gut 2003;52:1656; and Ruskoné-Fourmestraux A, Fischbach W, Aleman BM, et al. EGILS consensus report. Gastric extranodal marginal zone B-cell lymphoma of MALT. Gut 2011;60:747–58.

We performed a large-scale multicenter study of 420 Japanese patients with gastric MALT lymphoma to investigate the long-term outcome of the disease after *H pylori* eradication.[6] As a result, complete remission was achieved by *H pylori* eradication in 77% of patients. During the follow-up periods up to 14.6 years (mean, 6.5 years; median, 6.04 years), treatment failure was observed in 9% of patients (37 patients; 10 relapse, 27 progressive disease). The long-term prognosis was excellent; probability of freedom from treatment failure, overall survival, and event-free survival after 10 years was 90%, 95%, and 86%, respectively. **Table 4** summarizes 31 previously published studies that included more than 20 patients initially treated by *H pylori* eradication.[6,35–37] In those studies, complete remission was achieved in 1470 of 2031 patients (72%), progressive disease was observed in 17 of 1599 patients (1.1%), relapse was recorded in 63 of 1470 complete remission patients (4.3%), and treatment failure (progressive disease or relapse) was found in 121 of all 2031 patients (6.0%). These data are similar to those in our multicenter study,[6] except for progressive disease rate (1.1% vs 6.4%).

It is of interest that antibiotic therapy with the same regimen as *H pylori* eradication is also effective in some cases with *H pylori*–negative gastric MALT lymphoma.[10,11,38–40] A systematic review of the published cases revealed that 17 of 110 *H pylori*–negative cases (15%) achieved complete remission only by antibiotic therapy.[39] In responders, mechanisms for successful antibiotic treatment in such *H pylori*–negative cases are unclear. Removal of undetectable bacteria or potential

Table 4
Review of literature on efficacy of *Helicobacter pylori* eradication for gastric MALT lymphoma

Author (Year)	No. of Patients	CR Cases (%)	Median FW (Years)	PD (%)	Relapse (%)	Treatment Failure[a] (%)
Hancock (2009)	199	92 (46)	ND	ND	ND	25 (13)
Wündisch (2006)	193	146 (76)	2.3	0	5 (3.1)	5 (2.6)
Wündisch (2005)	120	96 (80)	6.3	0	3 (3.1)	3 (2.5)
Stathis (2009)	102	66 (65)	6.3	ND	ND	16 (16)
Kim (2007)	99	84 (85)	3.4	0	5 (5.9)	5 (5.1)
Nakamura (2005)	96	62 (65)	3.2	7 (7.3)	4 (6.4)	11 (11)
Hong (2006)	90	85 (94)	3.8	0	8 (9.4)	8 (8.9)
Fischbach (2004)	88	73 (83)	3.8	2 (2.3)	4 (5.5)	6 (6.8)
Nakamura (2008)	87	57 (66)	3.5	1 (1.1)	1 (1.8)	2 (2.3)
Savio (2000)	76	71 (93)	2.3	0	6 (8.5)	6 (7.9)
Terai (2008)	74	66 (89)	3.9	0	3 (4.5)	3 (4.1)
Sumida (2009)	66	47 (71)	3.3	0	0	0
Weston (1999)	58	40 (69)	1.8	0	0	0
Ono (2010)	58	48 (83)	6.3	2 (3.4)	1 (2.1)	3 (5.2)
Choi (2013)[35]	56	40 (71)	2.8	0	3 (7.5)	3 (5.4)
Andriani (2009)	53	42 (79)	5.4	0	9 (21)	9 (17)
Yapes (2012)[36]	50	33 (66)	2.4	ND	ND	0
Ryu (2014)[37]	48	36 (75)	ND	ND	ND	0
Akamatsu (2006)	47	30 (64)	3.1	1 (2.1)	1 (3.4)	2 (4.3)
Pinotti (1997)	44	30 (68)	1.8	0	2 (6.7)	2 (4.6)
Urakami (2000)	44	42 (95)	1.7	0	0	0
Ruskoné-Fourmestraux (2001)	44	19 (43)	2.9	1 (2.3)	2 (11)	3 (6.8)
Steinbach (1999)	34	14 (41)	3.4	2 (5.9)	0	2 (5.9)
Takenaka (2004)	33	26 (79)	ND	ND	ND	0
Chen (2005)	32	24 (75)	5.8	0	3 (13)	3 (9.4)
Lee (2004)	28	24 (86)	2.0	0	1 (4.2)	1 (3.6)
Montalban (2005)	24	22 (92)	4.6	0	1 (4.5)	1 (4.2)
de Jong (2001)	23	13 (57)	3.1	1 (4.3)	0	1 (4.4)
Raderer (2001)	22	15 (68)	2.1	0	1 (6.7)	1 (4.6)
Dong (2008)	22	13 (59)	1.5	0	0	0
Yamashita (2000)	21	14 (67)	0.8	0	0	0
Total of above	2031	1470 (72)	3.3	17 (1.1[b])	63 (4.3[c])	121 (6.0)
Nakamura (2012)[6]	420	323 (77)	6.04	27 (6.4)	10 (3.1)	37 (8.8)

Abbreviations: CR, complete remission; FW, follow-up; ND, not described; PD, progressive disease.
[a] PD or relapse.
[b] 17/1599 patients.
[c] 63/1470 CR patients.
Data from Nakamura S, Sugiyama T, Matsumoto T, et al. Long-term clinical outcome of gastric MALT lymphoma after eradication of *Helicobacter pylori*: a multicentre cohort follow-up study of 420 patients in Japan. Gut 2012;61:507–13.

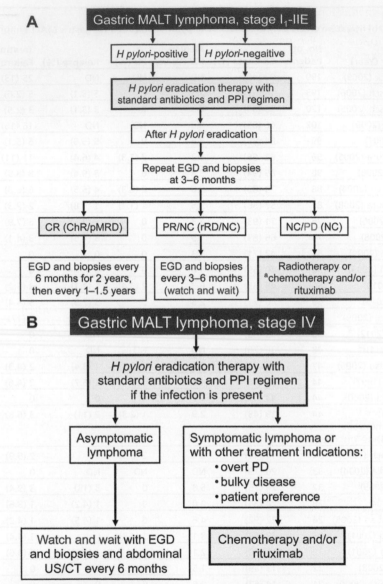

Fig. 2. Treatment algorithms for patients with gastric MALT lymphoma, which are modified versions shown in the European Society of Medical Oncology guideline.[23] Stage is defined by the Lugano system described in **Table 2**. (A) For patients with stage I_1-IIE disease. [a] When radiotherapy is not feasible or not indicated. (B) For patients with stage IV disease. ChR, complete histological response; CR, complete remission; EGD, esophagogastroduodenoscopy; NC, no change; PD, progressive disease; PPI, proton pump inhibitor; pMRD, probable minimal residual disease; PR, partial remission; rRD, responding residual disease; US, ultrasound. (*Adapted from* Zucca E, Copie-Bergman C, Ricardi U, et al; ESMO Guidelines Working Group. Gastric marginal zone lymphoma of MALT type: ESMO Clinical Practice Guidelines for diagnosis, treatment and follow-up. Ann Oncol 2013;24:vi146; with permission.)

immunomodulatory effect of antibiotics, such as clarithromycin, might have contributed some unknown antitumor effect.[10,40] Strategies for the management of patients with *H pylori*–negative gastric MALT lymphoma are controversial. Although EGILS consensus report recommends antibiotic therapy initially,[22] other guidelines recommend immediate oncologic treatments, such as radiotherapy.[23,41]

Therapeutic efficacy of *H pylori* eradication has also been reported in cases with gastric diffuse large B-cell lymphoma.[34,42,43] In those studies, 27% to 60% of *H pylori*–positive patients with diffuse large B-cell lymphoma in stage I/II$_1$ achieved complete remission after *H pylori* eradication. Not only cases with MALT lymphoma component, but also cases without any evidence of MALT lymphoma responded to eradication therapy.[42,43] Therefore, we believe that *H pylori* eradication should be performed in *H pylori*–positive patients with early stage gastric diffuse large B-cell lymphoma.

Strategies for Patients not Responding to Helicobacter pylori Eradication

The strategy for patients with gastric MALT lymphoma who do not respond to *H pylori* eradication is still controversial. Although patients with progressive disease or clinically evident relapse should undergo oncologic treatment, for patients with persistent histologic lymphoma without progressive disease (responding residual disease or no change), "watch and wait" strategy can be recommended up to 24 months after *H pylori* eradication.[22] The decision to continue a "watch and wait" follow-up or to start oncologic treatment should be individually tailored.[22]

As for the second-line oncologic treatment, radiotherapy, immunotherapy, and/or chemotherapy are recommended. Although radiotherapy and chemotherapy have a curative potential in localized (stage I/II$_1$) gastric MALT lymphoma, radiotherapy (30–40 Gy in 15–20 fractions) is generally preferred and is highly effective (response rate, 93%–100%).[6,22,23,41] Chemotherapy and/or immunotherapy with rituximab are also effective, and these systemic treatments are suitable for cases with histologic transformation to diffuse large B-cell lymphoma, disseminated disease, or advanced stage.[22,23] Although rituximab plus cyclophosphamide, doxorubicin, vincristine, prednisolone chemotherapy is relatively toxic for indolent MALT lymphoma, rituximab plus cyclophosphamide, vincristine, and prednisolone regimen seems well-tolerated and effective treatment.[44] Oral alkylating agents (ie, chlorambucil or cyclophosphamide) as a sole treatment are also well tolerated and effective, and achieved complete remission in 75% of patients, but the relapse rate is high (28%).[45] Recently, combination of rituximab and chlorambucil,[46] fludarabine,[47] or bendamustine[48] provided excellent responses in patients with MALT lymphoma of variable organs, including gastric cases. **Fig. 2** summarizes the treatment algorithms for patients with gastric MALT lymphoma in our institute, which are modified versions shown in the European Society of Medical Oncology guideline.[23]

SUMMARY/DISCUSSION

Based on a large amount of clinical evidence, the validity of *H pylori* eradication as the first-line treatment of gastric MALT lymphoma has been confirmed. Treatment strategies for patients not responding to *H pylori* eradication including "watch and wait" strategy, radiotherapy, chemotherapy, rituximab immunotherapy, and combination of these, should be tailored in consideration of the disease extent in each patient. Despite recent advances in the understanding of the pathogenesis of gastric MALT lymphoma, many questions still remain to be solved. Further basic and clinical research is necessary to clarify the molecular mechanisms in the development of the disease.

REFERENCES

1. Isaacson PG, Chott A, Nakamura S, et al. Extranodal marginal zone lymphoma of mucosa-associated lymphoid tissue (MALT lymphoma). In: Swerdlow SH, Campo E, Harris NL, et al, editors. WHO classification of tumours of haemato-poietic and lymphoid tissues. 4th edition. Lyon (France): IARC; 2008. p. 214–7.
2. Nakamura S, Matsumoto T, Iida M, et al. Primary gastrointestinal lymphoma in Japan: a clinicopathologic analysis of 455 patients with special reference to its time trends. Cancer 2003;97:2462–73.
3. Nakamura S, Matsumoto T. Gastrointestinal lymphoma: recent advances in diagnosis and treatment. Digestion 2013;87:182–8.
4. Nakamura S, Matsumoto T. *Helicobacter pylori* and gastric mucosa-associated lymphoid tissue lymphoma: recent progress in pathogenesis and management. World J Gastroenterol 2013;19:8181–7.
5. Zullo A, Hassan C, Cristofari F, et al. Effects of *Helicobacter pylori* eradication on early stage gastric mucosa-associated lymphoid tissue lymphoma. Clin Gastroenterol Hepatol 2010;8:105–10.
6. Nakamura S, Sugiyama T, Matsumoto T, et al. Long-term clinical outcome of gastric MALT lymphoma after eradication of *Helicobacter pylori*: a multicentre cohort follow-up study of 420 patients in Japan. Gut 2012;61:507–13.
7. Wotherspoon AC, Ortiz-Hidalgo C, Falzon MR, et al. *Helicobacter pylori*-associated gastritis and primary B-cell gastric lymphoma. Lancet 1991;338:1175–6.
8. Parsonnet J, Hansen S, Rodriguez L, et al. *Helicobacter pylori* infection and gastric lymphoma. N Engl J Med 1994;330:1267–71.
9. Nakamura S, Yao T, Aoyagi K, et al. *Helicobacter pylori* and primary gastric lymphoma: a histopathologic and immunohistochemical analysis of 237 patients. Cancer 1997;79:3–11.
10. Nakamura S, Matsumoto T, Ye H, et al. *Helicobacter pylori*-negative gastric mucosa-associated lymphoid tissue lymphoma: a clinicopathologic and molecular study with reference to antibiotic treatment. Cancer 2006;107:2770–8.
11. Asano N, Iijima K, Terai S, et al. Eradication therapy is effective for *Helicobacter pylori*-negative gastric mucosa-associated lymphoid tissue lymphoma. Tohoku J Exp Med 2012;228:223–7.
12. Du MQ. MALT lymphoma: many roads lead to nuclear factor-κb activation. Histopathology 2011;58:26–38.
13. Hussell T, Isaacson PG, Crabtree JE, et al. *Helicobacter pylori*-specific tumour-infiltrating T cells provide contact dependent help for the growth of malignant B cells in low-grade gastric lymphoma of mucosa-associated lymphoid tissue. J Pathol 1996;178:122–7.
14. D'Elios MM, Amedei A, Manghetti M, et al. Impaired T-cell regulation of B-cell growth in *Helicobacter pylori*-related gastric low-grade MALT lymphoma. Gastroenterology 1999;117:1105–12.
15. Craig VJ, Cogliatti SB, Arnold I, et al. B-cell receptor signaling and CD40 ligand-independent T cell help cooperate in *Helicobacter*-induced MALT lymphomagenesis. Leukemia 2010;24:1186–96.
16. Munari F, Lonardi S, Cassatella MA, et al. Tumor-associated macrophages as major source of APRIL in gastric MALT lymphoma. Blood 2011;117:6612–6.
17. Nakamura S, Ye H, Bacon CM, et al. Clinical impact of genetic aberrations in gastric MALT lymphoma: a comprehensive analysis using interphase fluorescence *in situ* hybridisation. Gut 2007;56:1358–63.

18. Liu H, Ye H, Ruskone-Fourmestraux A, et al. T(11;18) is a marker for all stage gastric MALT lymphomas that will not respond to *H. pylori* eradication. Gastroenterology 2002;122:1286–94.

19. Chuang SS, Lee C, Hamoudi RA, et al. High frequency of t(11;18) in gastric mucosa-associated lymphoid tissue lymphomas in Taiwan, including one patient with high-grade transformation. Br J Haematol 2003;120:97–100.

20. Chanudet E, Ye H, Ferry J, et al. A20 deletion is associated with copy number gain at the TNFA/B/C locus and occurs preferentially in translocation-negative MALT lymphoma of the ocular adnexa and salivary glands. J Pathol 2009;217:420–30.

21. Honma K, Tsuzuki S, Nakagawa M, et al. *TNFAIP3/A20* functions as a novel tumor suppressor gene in several subtypes of non-Hodgkin lymphomas. Blood 2009; 114:2467–75.

22. Ruskoné-Fourmestraux A, Fischbach W, Aleman BM, et al. EGILS consensus report. Gastric extranodal marginal zone B-cell lymphoma of MALT. Gut 2011; 60:747–58.

23. Zucca E, Copie-Bergman C, Ricardi U, et al. Gastric marginal zone lymphoma of MALT type: ESMO Clinical Practice Guidelines for diagnosis, treatment and follow-up. Ann Oncol 2013;24:vi144–8.

24. Wotherspoon AC, Doglioni C, Diss TC, et al. Regression of primary low-grade B-cell gastric lymphoma of mucosa-associated lymphoid tissue type after eradication of *Helicobacter pylori*. Lancet 1993;342:575–7.

25. Montalbán C, Castrillo JM, Abraira V, et al. Gastric B-cell mucosa-associated lymphoid tissue (MALT) lymphoma: clinicopathological study and evaluation of the prognostic factors in 143 patients. Ann Oncol 1995;6:355–62.

26. Taal BG, Boot H, van Heerde P, et al. Primary non-Hodgkin lymphoma of the stomach: endoscopic pattern and prognosis in low versus high grade malignancy in relation to the MALT concept. Gut 1996;39:556–61.

27. Fischbach W, Dragosics B, Kolve-Goebeler ME, et al. Primary gastric B-cell lymphoma: results of a prospective multicenter study. Gastroenterology 2000;119: 1191–2202.

28. Nakamura S, Akazawa K, Yao T, et al. Primary gastric lymphoma: a clinicopathologic study of 233 cases with special reference to evaluation with the MIB-1 index. Cancer 1995;76:1313–24.

29. Zullo A, Hassan C, Andriani A, et al. Primary low-grade and high-grade gastric MALT-lymphoma presentation. J Clin Gastroenterol 2010;44:340–4.

30. Rohatiner A, d'Amore F, Coiffier B, et al. Report on a workshop convened to discuss the pathological and staging classifications of gastrointestinal tract lymphoma. Ann Oncol 1994;5:397–400.

31. Ruskoné-Fourmestraux A, Dragosics B, Morgner A, et al. Paris staging system for primary gastrointestinal lymphomas. Gut 2003;52:912–3.

32. Matsumoto T, Nakamura S, Esaki M, et al. Double-balloon endoscopy depicts diminutive small bowel lesions in gastrointestinal lymphoma. Dig Dis Sci 2010;55:158–65.

33. Copie-Bergman C, Gaulard P, Lavergne-Slove A, et al. Proposal for a new histological grading system for post-treatment evaluation of gastric MALT lymphoma. Gut 2003;52:1656.

34. Nakamura S, Matsumoto T, Suekane H, et al. Predictive value of endoscopic ultrasonography for regression of gastric low grade and high grade MALT lymphomas after eradication of *Helicobacter pylori*. Gut 2001;48:454–60.

35. Choi YJ, Kim N, Paik JH, et al. Characteristics of Helicobacter pylori-positive and Helicobacter pylori-negative gastric mucosa-associated lymphoid tissue lymphoma and their influence on clinical outcome. Helicobacter 2013;18:197–205.

36. Yepes S, Torres MM, Saavedra C, et al. Gastric mucosa-associated lymphoid tissue lymphomas and Helicobacter pylori infection: a Colombian perspective. World J Gastroenterol 2012;18:685–91.
37. Ryu KD, Kim GH, Park SO, et al. Treatment outcome for gastric mucosa-associated lymphoid tissue lymphoma according to Helicobacter pylori infection status: a single-center experience. Gut Liver 2014;8:408–14.
38. Raderer M, Streubel B, Wöhrer S, et al. Successful antibiotic treatment of *Helicobacter pylori* negative gastric mucosa associated lymphoid tissue lymphomas. Gut 2006;55:616–8.
39. Zullo A, Hassan C, Ridola L, et al. Eradication therapy in *Helicobacter pylori*-negative, gastric low-grade mucosa-associated lymphoid tissue lymphoma patients: a systematic review. J Clin Gastroenterol 2013;47:824–7.
40. Raderer M, Wöhrer S, Kiesewetter B, et al. Antibiotic treatment as sole management of *Helicobacter pylori*-negative gastric MALT lymphoma: a single center experience with prolonged follow-up. Ann Hematol 2015;94(6):969–73.
41. NCCN Clinical Practice Guidelines in Oncology (NCCN Guidelines). Non-Hodgkin's lymphomas, Version 1. 2015. Available at: http://www.nccn.org/professionals/physician_gls/pdf/nhl.pdf. Accessed February 11, 2015.
42. Kuo SH, Yeh KH, Wu MS, et al. *Helicobacter pylori* eradication therapy is effective in the treatment of early-stage *H pylori*-positive gastric diffuse large B-cell lymphomas. Blood 2012;119:4838–44.
43. Tari A, Asaoku H, Kashiwado K, et al. Predictive value of endoscopy and endoscopic ultrasonography for regression of gastric diffuse large B-cell lymphomas after *Helicobacter pylori* eradication. Dig Endosc 2009;21:219–27.
44. Aguiar-Bujanda D, Llorca-Martínez I, Rivero-Vera JC, et al. Treatment of gastric marginal zone B-cell lymphoma of the mucosa-associated lymphoid tissue with rituximab, cyclophosphamide, vincristine and prednisone. Hematol Oncol 2014; 32:139–44.
45. Lévy M, Copie-Bergman C, Gameiro C, et al. Prognostic value of translocation t(11;18) in tumoral response of low-grade gastric lymphoma of mucosa-associated lymphoid tissue type to oral chemotherapy. J Clin Oncol 2005;23: 5061–6.
46. Zucca E, Conconi A, Laszlo D, et al. Addition of rituximab to chlorambucil produces superior event-free survival in the treatment of patients with extranodal marginal-zone B-cell lymphoma: 5-year analysis of the IELSG-19 Randomized Study. J Clin Oncol 2013;31:565–72.
47. Salar A, Domingo-Domenech E, Estany C, et al. Combination therapy with rituximab and intravenous or oral fludarabine in the first-line, systemic treatment of patients with extranodal marginal zone B-cell lymphoma of the mucosa-associated lymphoid tissue type. Cancer 2009;115:5210–7.
48. Kiesewetter B, Mayerhoefer ME, Lukas J, et al. Rituximab plus bendamustine is active in pretreated patients with extragastric marginal zone B cell lymphoma of the mucosa-associated lymphoid tissue (MALT lymphoma). Ann Hematol 2014;93:249–53.

Rationale for a *Helicobacter pylori* Test and Treatment Strategy in Gastroesophageal Reflux Disease

Nimish Vakil, MD, AGAF[a,b,*]

KEYWORDS

- *H pylori* • GERD • Proton pump inhibitors • Intestinal metaplasia • Gastric atrophy

KEY POINTS

- Proton pump inhibitors worsen corpus gastritis in patients infected with *Helicobacter pylori* and increase the rate of progression to intestinal metaplasia, both of which are precursor lesions for cancer.
- In animal models of gastric cancer, progression to gastric cancer can be demonstrated in infected animals that are treated with proton pump inhibitors.
- Eradicating *H pylori* prevents the progression to intestinal metaplasia and atrophy and should be offered to infected patients who are about to commence long-term proton pump inhibitor therapy, especially in countries and populations in which the incidence of gastric cancer is high.

INTRODUCTION

Helicobacter pylori infection causes a chronic gastritis that progresses to atrophy and intestinal metaplasia in a proportion of cases. Gastric atrophy and intestinal metaplasia are precursor lesions for gastric cancer. Eradication of *H pylori* infection can reverse atrophy, but intestinal metaplasia has not been reversible in most human studies. There is a great deal of interest in understanding the mechanisms for progression from chronic gastritis to atrophy and intestinal metaplasia. Identifying risk factors for the progression of atrophy is important in clinical practice because it offers a way to prevent gastric cancer. One risk factor that has been identified is the administration of proton pump inhibitors (PPIs) to patients infected with *H pylori* infection. In this article,

Disclosure: Consultant: Astra Zeneca, Ironwood, Bayer.
[a] University of Wisconsin School of Medicine and Public Health, 750 Highland Avenue, Madison, WI 53726, USA; [b] Aurora Summit Medical Center, 36500 Aurora Drive, Summit, WI 53066, USA
* Aurora Summit Medical Center, 36500 Aurora Drive, Summit, WI 53066.
E-mail address: nvakil@wisc.edu

Gastroenterol Clin N Am 44 (2015) 661–666
http://dx.doi.org/10.1016/j.gtc.2015.05.007
0889-8553/15/$ – see front matter © 2015 Elsevier Inc. All rights reserved.

the data on the risk of administering PPIs to patients with *H pylori* infection and the rationale for eradicating *H pylori* before initiating long-term PPI therapy are reviewed.

THE EFFECT OF PROTON PUMP INHIBITOR TREATMENT ON CHRONIC *HELICOBACTER PYLORI*-RELATED GASTRITIS

In 1996, Kuipers and colleagues[1] studied 2 cohorts of patients, one from Sweden treated with fundoplication for reflux disease and the other from the Netherlands who were treated with omeprazole 20 mg or 40 mg for gastroesophageal reflux disease (GERD). Both cohorts were followed for an average of 5 years. Patients in the fundoplication group did not receive acid inhibitory therapy over the course of the study. Histology was performed at baseline in the fundoplication group and histology and serology for *H pylori* were performed in the PPI therapy group. In the fundoplication group, there were 31 patients infected with *H pylori* at baseline, and none developed atrophic gastritis over the follow-up period. In the cohort of 59 *H pylori*–infected patients treated with omeprazole, corpus gastritis increased significantly from 59% to 81%. Atrophic gastritis increased from 0% at baseline to 4%, representing an annual increase of 0.8% in the prevalence of atrophy. Intestinal metaplasia did not develop in any of the patients. In patients who were not infected with *H pylori*, there was no progression to atrophy in either of the cohorts.

In another study, in 230 patients with GERD treated long term with omeprazole, 4.7% of the patients with moderate to severe gastritis who were infected with *H pylori* developed gastric atrophy. In contrast, only 0.7% of *H pylori*–negative subjects who had moderate to severe gastritis at baseline developed gastric atrophy.[2]

THE EFFECT OF *HELICOBACTER PYLORI* ERADICATION ON CHRONIC GASTRITIS AND ATROPHY RELATED TO *HELICOBACTER PYLORI* INFECTION

A randomized controlled trial evaluated the effect of *H pylori* eradication in patients with GERD who had been treated with PPIs for 12 months or longer. Two hundred thirty-one patients infected with *H pylori* were randomized to omeprazole or omeprazole triple therapy.[3] There was significant corpus gastritis at baseline in 50% of cases, and it remained unchanged at 1 and 2 years. In contrast, in the triple therapy group, moderate to severe gastritis was present at baseline in 55% of patients and decreased significantly to 4% and 5% at 1 and 2 years, respectively. Atrophy of the glands in the corpus was present in 24% of patients in the omeprazole group and remained unchanged at 1 and 2 years. In the triple therapy group, corpus glandular atrophy declined significantly with eradication from 27% at baseline to 19% and 14% at 1 and 2 years, respectively. When patients with moderate and severe atrophy were considered separately, the results were striking. Moderate to severe atrophy declined from 15% to 3% at 1 year and 5% at 2 years. These studies show an improvement in an intermediate marker on the progression to gastric cancer but do not prove that cancer can be prevented by eradication therapy. Long-term studies in humans to prove the hypothesis that cancer can be prevented have many challenges, including the prolonged duration of follow-up required and the ethics of not offering eradication therapy to controls. Animal models offer a potential solution to these challenges.

GASTRITIS AND ADENOCARCINOMA IN MONGOLIAN GERBILS

Mongolian gerbils infected with *H pylori* are a model for gastric cancer. The lesions created by *H pylori* are similar to the lesions produced in human gastric mucosa. In an experimental study, young Mongolian gerbils were infected with *H pylori* 1 month after birth. After 6 months, one-half of the gerbils were given omeprazole and followed for 6 months, whereas the other group received no medication.[4] A control group of *H pylori*–negative gerbils were treated similarly. There were no cases of adenocarcinoma in the *H pylori*–negative gerbils. In the infected gerbils, adenocarcinomas developed in significantly more infected gerbils (60%) treated with omeprazole than those who were infected but did not receive omeprazole (7%). Corpus atrophy scores were significantly higher in the infected gerbils treated with omeprazole compared with the untreated but infected gerbils and compared with *H pylori*–negative gerbils.

A CONTROLLED TRIAL OF PROTON PUMP INHIBITOR THERAPY IN INFECTED SUBJECTS WITH GASTROESOPHAGEAL REFLUX DISEASE

In a study from Taiwan, 325 patients with reflux esophagitis were studied.[5] All patients were treated with continuous esomeprazole therapy until their symptoms resolved; they were then placed on on-demand therapy. There was a control group of *H pylori*–negative patients (n = 115) and a study group of infected patients, half of whom were given eradication therapy (n = 105) before the esomeprazole therapy. The other half remained infected through the period of the study. Endoscopy was performed at entry and at 1 year and 2 years to assess the prevalence of atrophy and intestinal metaplasia and to assess progression over the course of the study. The *H pylori*–negative patients had no worsening of gastric atrophy or intestinal metaplasia. In the *H pylori*–eradication group, intestinal metaplasia and atrophy regressed during the follow-up period. In the untreated *H pylori*–infected patients, the prevalence of atrophy and intestinal metaplasia increased over the period of the study. These data are consistent with the results reported in Mongolian gerbils and demonstrate progression of gastritis and intestinal metaplasia in infected patients treated with PPIs.

THE CASE AGAINST *HELICOBACTER PYLORI* ERADICATION THERAPY IN GASTROESOPHAGEAL REFLUX DISEASE

Two studies are often cited as evidence that PPI therapy does not worsen atrophy or intestinal metaplasia. Both were randomized controlled trials that compared PPI therapy to fundoplication therapy for chronic reflux esophagitis. In the first of these studies, 155 patients were randomized to antireflux surgery and 155 to treatment with omeprazole.[6] There were 40 *H pylori*–infected patients in the omeprazole group and 53 in the surgery group. At 3 years of follow-up, nonsignificant increases in atrophy were noted, but there was no difference between the groups, and intestinal metaplasia rarely developed. The authors concluded that omeprazole therapy did not worsen atrophy of the corpus or increase the development of intestinal metaplasia. At 7 years, there were only a small number of patients left for evaluation: 13 in the omeprazole group and 12 in the antireflux surgery group.[7] There was a significant worsening of mucosal inflammation and a numerical but nonsignificant increase in the prevalence of atrophy. The small number of infected patients that were evaluated is a major limitation of both studies. When the 3-year data are recalculated focusing on the infected subjects alone (**Fig. 1**), progression of no or mild atrophy to moderate or severe atrophy was seen in 17.9% of patients. The magnitude of this effect is very similar to the results reported in the original study of Kuipers and colleagues[1] and supports the original premise that infected patients have progression of atrophy when they are treated with PPIs.

The second study was a randomized controlled trial of laparoscopic fundoplication to PPI therapy.[8] There were 158 patients in the surgery group and 180 in the PPI therapy group. Only a small number of patients were infected (10.8% in the surgery

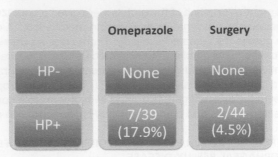

Fig. 1. Progression of no or mild atrophy to moderate or severe atrophy in a study of fundoplication versus PPI therapy. (*Data from* Yang HB, Sheu BS, Wang ST, et al. H. pylori eradication prevents the progression of gastric intestinal metaplasia in reflux esophagitis patients using long-term esomeprazole. Am J Gastroenterol 2009;104(7):1642–9.)

group and 16% in the PPI group). When the patients were evaluated overall, mucosal inflammation remained stable on esomeprazole but decreased slightly over time after fundoplication. Neither intestinal metaplasia nor atrophy developed in either group. When the data are recalculated focusing on the patients infected with *H pylori*, a different picture emerges. Although the numbers of patients are small, **Table 1** shows the data from this study and once again demonstrates progression of atrophy and intestinal metaplasia when only the infected patients are considered.

The case offered against progression of atrophy and intestinal metaplasia is weak and is based on small numbers of patients. When the group of *H pylori*–infected patients is considered in these studies, a progression of atrophy and intestinal metaplasia is demonstrated and is consistent with the studies described earlier in this article.

COST-EFFECTIVENESS ANALYSIS

A limitation of the available data is the absence of information on the cost-effectiveness of a strategy to eradicate *H pylori* in all infected patients who are about to commence long-term PPI therapy for GERD. Ultimately, the goal of such a strategy is to prevent the progression of atrophy and intestinal metaplasia to cancer. Because there are no

Table 1
Atrophy and metaplasia at 5 years in *H pylori*–infected subjects in another study of fundoplication versus proton pump therapy

	Baseline	1 y	3 y	5 y
Corpus atrophy				
PPI (n = 39)	3 (7.7%)	5 (13%)	3 (7.7%)	4 (10%)
Surgery (n = 53)	4 (2.5%)	2 (1.4%)	0	0
Intestinal metaplasia				
PPI (n = 39)	0	3 (7.7%)	0	3 (7.7%)
Surgery (n = 53)	1 (1.8%)	0	0	0

Data from Lundell L, Havu N, Miettinen P, et al. Changes of gastric mucosal architecture during long-term omeprazole therapy: results of a randomized clinical trial. Aliment Pharmacol Ther 2006;23(5):639–47.

data on the prevention of cancer by eradication of *H pylori* in the setting of chronic PPI use, only a nominal cost-effectiveness analysis can be performed. This technique helps to determine if the strategy of eradicating *H pylori* before commencing PPI therapy has the potential to be cost-effective. In 2012, there were 1,270,000 prescriptions for PPIs in the United States. Assuming a cost for *H pylori* testing of US $25 and a prevalence of *H pylori* of 15%, it can be calculated that there are 190,500 patients with *H pylori* infection who would be at risk of being exposed to PPI therapy. Assuming a treatment cost of $150, the total cost of treating these patients would be $28,575,000. The total cost of testing and treatment in this population would be $60,325,000. The lifetime risk for cancer in the United States is 0.9%. Therefore, it would be expected that there are 11,430 cancers in this population. If one were able to prevent all the cancers in this population, the cost of testing and treatment would be $5277 per cancer prevented. There are 2 key assumptions in this analysis, which may be challenged. The first is the lifetime risk of gastric cancer. This risk is a population-based risk and is not based on the select population being considered here. It is very likely that the risk is much greater in the population being considered in this article. The other assumption is that all the cancers can be prevented by eradication of *H pylori*. Clear data on the proportion of cancers that can be prevented are still lacking, but this analysis does suggest that a test and eradicate strategy have the potential to be cost-effective.

SUMMARY

PPIs worsen corpus gastritis in patients infected with *H pylori* and increase the rate of progression to intestinal metaplasia, both of which are precursor lesions for cancer. In animal models of gastric cancer, progression to gastric cancer can be demonstrated in infected animals that are treated with PPIs. Eradicating *H pylori* prevents the progression to intestinal metaplasia and atrophy and should be offered to infected patients who are about to commence long-term PPI therapy; this is especially true for countries and populations in whom the incidence of gastric cancer is high.

REFERENCES

1. Kuipers EJ, Lundell L, Klinkenberg-Knol EC, et al. Atrophic gastritis and Helicobacter pylori infection in patients with reflux esophagitis treated with omeprazole or fundoplication. N Engl J Med 1996;334(16):1018–22.
2. Klinkenberg-Knol EC, Nelis F, Dent J, et al, Long-Term Study Group. Long-term omeprazole treatment in resistant gastroesophageal reflux disease: efficacy, safety, and influence on gastric mucosa. Gastroenterology 2000;118(4):661–9.
3. Kuipers EJ, Nelis GF, Klinkenberg-Knol EC, et al. Cure of Helicobacter pylori infection in patients with reflux oesophagitis treated with long term omeprazole reverses gastritis without exacerbation of reflux disease: results of a randomised controlled trial. Gut 2004;53(1):12–20.
4. Hagiwara T, Mukaisho K, Nakayama T, et al. Long-term proton pump inhibitor administration worsens atrophic corpus gastritis and promotes adenocarcinoma development in Mongolian gerbils infected with Helicobacter pylori. Gut 2011; 60(5):624–30.
5. Yang HB, Sheu BS, Wang ST, et al. H. pylori eradication prevents the progression of gastric intestinal metaplasia in reflux esophagitis patients using long-term esomeprazole. Am J Gastroenterol 2009;104(7):1642–9.
6. Lundell L, Miettinen P, Myrvold HE, et al. Lack of effect of acid suppression therapy on gastric atrophy. Nordic GERD Study Group. Gastroenterology 1999;117(2): 319–26.

7. Lundell L, Havu N, Miettinen P, et al, Nordic GERD Study Group. Changes of gastric mucosal architecture during long-term omeprazole therapy: results of a randomized clinical trial. Aliment Pharmacol Ther 2006;23(5):639–47.

8. Fiocca R, Mastracci L, Attwood SE, et al, LOTUS Trial Collaborators. Gastric exocrine and endocrine cell morphology under prolonged acid inhibition therapy: results of a 5-year follow-up in the LOTUS trial. Aliment Pharmacol Ther 2012; 36(10):959–71.

Screening to Identify and Eradicate *Helicobacter pylori* Infection in Teenagers in Japan

Taiji Akamatsu, MD, PhD[a,b,*], Takuma Okamura, MD, PhD[b],
Yugo Iwaya, MD, PhD[b], Tomoaki Suga, MD, PhD[b]

KEYWORDS

- *Helicobacter pylori* • Gastric cancer • Prevention • Health screening • Teenager
- School children • Cost-effectiveness • Medical economy

KEY POINTS

- The rate of prevalence of *Helibobacter pylori* infection in Japanese teenagers is 4% to 5% at present.
- A very high participation rate of screening examination for *H pylori* infection using urine-based rapid test kit was achieved in high school health screening.
- The most common endoscopic findings for students with *H pylori* infection are nodular gastritis and closed-type atrophic gastritis.
- If this procedure was introduced nationwide, the cost of the prevention of a gastric cancer would be 481,144 yen ($4184 dollars) per person.
- This low rate of prevalence of *H pylori* infection makes it possible to perform this nationwide plan from a viewpoint of medical economy.

Author contributions: Each of the authors has been involved equally and has read and approved the final article. Each meets the criteria for authorship established by the International Committee of Medical Journal Editors and verifies the validity of the results reported. Supportive foundations: Dr T. Akamatsu and coauthors are not supported by any grants. Potential conflict: Dr T. Akamatsu and coauthors have nothing to declare.
 a Endoscopy Center, Suzaka Prefectural Hospital, Nagano Prefectural Hospital Organization, 1332 Suzaka, Suzaka, Nagano 382-0091, Japan; b Gastroenterology, Department of Internal Medicine, Shinshu University School of Medicine, 3-1-1 Asahi, Matsumoto, Nagano 390-8621, Japan
* Corresponding author. Endoscopy Center, Suzaka Prefectural Hospital, Nagano Prefectural Hospital Organization, 1332 Suzaka, Suzaka, Nagano 382-0091, Japan.
E-mail address: akamatsu-taiji@pref-nagano-hosp.jp

Gastroenterol Clin N Am 44 (2015) 667–676
http://dx.doi.org/10.1016/j.gtc.2015.05.008
0889-8553/15/$ – see front matter © 2015 Elsevier Inc. All rights reserved.

gastro.theclinics.com

INTRODUCTION

Helicobacter pylori infection is etiologically related to several gastric diseases, such as gastritis, gastroduodenal ulcer, gastric cancer, and mucosa-associated lymphoid tissue (MALT) lymphoma. Gastric cancer is one of the common malignant neoplasms in East Asia including Japan, and many people die of gastric cancer each year. Recently, it has been confirmed that *H pylori* infection is a significant risk factor for gastric cancer epidemiologically,[1,2] experimentally,[3,4] and clinically.[5] This has been proved by experiments using animals[6] and also by randomized clinical studies[7,8] showing that eradication of *H pylori* reduces the occurrence of gastric cancer. Furthermore, Nozaki and colleagues[9] reported that early stage eradication of *H pylori* was more effective in reducing the late occurrence of gastric cancer compared with late-stage eradication in animal experimentation. From these data, eradication of *H pylori* is thought to be beneficial for the prevention of human gastric cancer, and it is more effective to treat *H pylori* infection in young people compared with old people. Furthermore, *H pylori*–related diseases, especially complicated gastroduodenal ulcer, which can cause death and emergency operations because of perforation or bleeding, can be prevented by cure of *H pylori*. Most Japanese experts of *H pylori* infection agree that *H pylori* should be treated in young people, but the method of mass screening for *H pylori* infection and the most suitable age for receiving the treatment remain controversial.

This article presents our attempts at examination and treatment of *H pylori* infection in high school health screening between 2007 and 2013. The purpose of this study was to collect data regarding the screening for *H pylori* infection in health screenings in school, and to identify the actual effects of *H pylori* infection in Japanese teenagers.

AN EXAMINATION AND TREATMENT OF *HELICOBACTER PYLORI* IN HIGH SCHOOL STUDENTS

We have proposed that a screening for *H pylori* infection should be introduced into health screenings in school, and have performed this procedure in one Japanese high school since 2007.[10] The study was approved by the Ethics Committee of Shinshu University School of Medicine.

First Screening Examination for Helicobacter pylori Infection

All students of the second year in high school were annually examined about the status of *H pylori* infection using a urine-based rapid test kit (RUPIRAN; Otsuka Pharmaceutical Co, Tokyo, Japan). Students were between ages 16 and 17. Between 2007 and 2013, a total of 3251 of 3263 students (99.6%) received a first screening examination. One hundred and thirty-six of 3251 students (4.2%) were positive for *H pylori*; the remaining 3115 were negative (**Table 1**). A summary of the results is shown in **Fig. 1**.

Further Examination for Helicobacter pylori Infection

Seventy-four of 136 students who were determined to be *H pylori*–positive visited Shinshu University Hospital. Another 11 consulted other medical institution; the remaining 51 did not accept the invitation to visit a medical institution.

Seventy-two of the 74 students who visited Shinshu University Hospital underwent esophagogastroduodenoscopy (EGD) with sedation using 0.1 mg/kg of midazolam after providing written informed consent; two declined to undergo EGD.

H pylori status was assessed by histology (six sites) and culture (two sites) of biopsy specimens obtained from the antrum and corpus of the stomach. The biopsy samples were stained with hematoxylin and eosin, and immunostained for *H pylori* with rabbit

Table 1
Participation rate and positive rate of high school students in the screening examination of *Helicobacter pylori* infection

Year	Number of Participating Students	Number of Positive Students
2007	409/414 (98.8%)	14/409 (3.4%)
2008	370/373 (99.2%)	28/370 (7.6%)
2009	445/445 (100%)	22/445 (4.9%)
2010	478/480 (99.6%)	23/478 (4.8%)
2011	400/401 (99.8%)	12/400 (3.0%)
2012	539/539 (100%)	17/539 (3.2%)
2013	610/611 (99.8%)	20/610 (3.3%)
Total	3251/3263 (99.6%) (M, 1489; F, 1762)	136/3251 (4.2%) (M, 63; F, 73)

Abbreviations: F, female; M, male.

anti–*H pylori* polyclonal antibody (DAKO, Carpinteria, CA) if necessary. *H pylori* infection was deemed to be present if either or both tests were positive, and absent if both tests were negative. Furthermore, the results of a urea breath test (UBT) and a test for serum anti–*H pylori* antibody using an E-plate (Eiken Chemical, Tochigi, Japan) were examined if necessary to confirm the infection. Sixty of 72 students (83.3%) who underwent EGD were infected by *H pylori* and 12 (16.7%) were not infected. However, 3 of the 12 students without *H pylori* infection tested positive for serum anti–*H pylori* antibody.

Endoscopic Findings

The most common endoscopic appearance was nodular gastritis recognized in 50 of 60 students (83.3%) with *H pylori* infection (**Table 2**). Endoscopic findings of atrophic

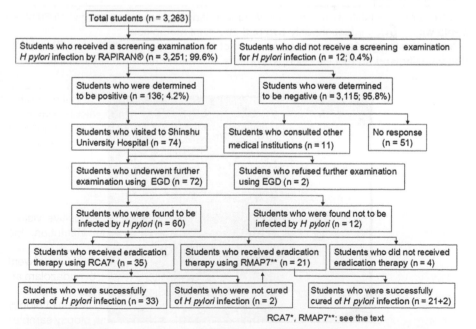

RCA7*, RMAP7**: see the text

Fig. 1. Summary of the results. EGD, esophagogastroduodenoscopy.

Table 2
Endoscopic findings in high school students

	Infected with *Helicobacter pylori* (N = 60)	Not Infected with *Helicobacter pylori* (N = 12)
Nodular gastritis	50 (83.3%)	0
Atrophic gastritis	36 (60.0%) (C-I, 9; C-II, 23; C-III, 4)	3 (25.0%)[a] (C-II, 1; O-II, 1; O-III, 1)
Duodenal erosion	4 (6.7%)	0
Duodenal ulcer scar	4 (6.7%)	0

Abbreviations: C, closed type; O, open type.
[a] Three cases show positive for serum anti–*H pylori* antibody.

gastritis were found in 36 of these students (60.0%). The endoscopic degree of atrophic gastritis according to Kimura-Takemoto classification[11] was the closed type (C-1:9, C-2:23, C-3:4) in all 36 cases. None had the open type atrophic gastritis. A scar from duodenal ulcer (**Fig. 2**) was present in 4 of the 60 students (6.7%) with *H pylori* infection; duodenal erosion (**Fig. 3**) was observed in another four (6.7%).

Normal endoscopic findings were present in 9 of the 12 students without *H pylori* infection. However, endoscopic findings of open-type severe atrophic gastritis (ie, extensive atrophy) were identified in two of the remaining three who were also positive for serum anti–*H pylori* antibody despite no active *H pylori* infection. Type A gastritis was ruled out because these students showed negative results for anti–parietal cell antibody and did not have hypergastrinemia. These three students were thought to have had *H pylori* infection in the past and to have rapidly developed atrophic changes caused by *H pylori* infection.

Histologic Findings

Inflammatory cell infiltration and focal atrophic changes were recognized in all 60 students with *H pylori* infection; only two had intestinal metaplasia.

Normal histologic findings were found in 9 of the 12 students without *H pylori* infection who showed normal endoscopic findings. However, inflammatory cell infiltration

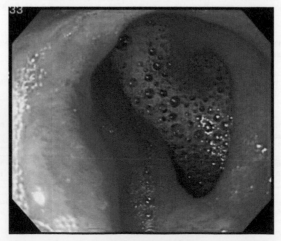

Fig. 2. Endoscopic picture of a scar from duodenal ulcer.

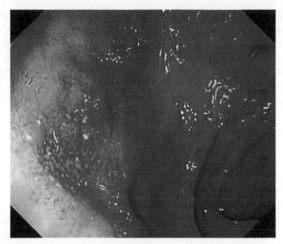

Fig. 3. Endoscopic picture of duodenal erosions.

and focal to moderate atrophic change was recognized in the remaining three who had endoscopic findings of atrophic change without currently active *H pylori* infections.

Susceptibility of Helicobacter pylori to Clarithromycin, Metronidazole, and Amoxicillin

The susceptibility of *H pylori* to clarithromycin (CAM), metronidazole (MNZ), and amoxicillin (AMC) was assessed by a modified agar plate dilution method (**Table 3**). The minimal inhibitory concentration of a given agent was defined here as the lowest concentration of the agent that was able to inhibit visual growth under the culture concentrations. Strains were considered to be resistant to CAM, MNZ, and AMC when the minimal inhibitory concentrations were equal to or above 1, 16, and 1 μg/mL, respectively.

CAM resistance was present in 24 of the 60 students (40%) with *H pylori* infection. MNZ resistance was present in 24 (40%); 15 students (25%) had dual CAM-MNZ resistance. No AMC resistance was present in any students.

Outcome of Helicobacter pylori Eradication Therapy

After informed consent, eradication therapy was performed. Students with *H pylori* that was not resistant to CAM received rabeprazole (2 × 10 mg/day), CAM (2 × 400 mg/day), and AMC (2 × 750 mg/day) for 7 days (RCA7). If *H pylori* had resistance to CAM, using rabeprazole (2 × 10 mg/day), MNZ (3 × 250 mg/day), AMC (2 × 750 mg/day), and pronase (3 × 18,000 U) for 7 days (RMAP7) was performed

Table 3 Susceptibility of *Helicobacter pylori* to antibiotics (N = 60)	
CAM-resistant	24 (40.0%)
MNZ-resistant	24 (40.0%)
AMPC-resistant	0 (0%)

Resistance: CAM, MIC ≥1 μg/mL; MNZ, MIC ≥16 μg/mL; AMPC, MIC ≥1 μg/mL.
Abbreviations: AMPC, amoxicillin; MIC, minimal inhibitory concentration.

whether or not *H pylori* had resistance to MNZ. The resolution of *H pylori* was assessed more than 8 weeks after treatment by a UBT (Otsuka Pharmaceuticals).

Fifty-six of the 60 students with *H pylori* infection and their parents agreed to receive eradication therapy. The 35 that had no resistance to CAM were administered with RCA7, and 33 of them (94.3%) were cured. The two students who failed therapy received the second treatment using RMAP7 and were cured. All 21 students (100%) with *H pylori* with CAM resistance were treated using RMAP7 and successfully cured by the first treatment.

Adverse Effects

No remarkable complications related to EGD, including taking biopsy specimens, were recognized in any of the 72 students who received EGD in Shinshu University Hospital. However, skin rash was observed in 4 of 56 students (7.1%) who received eradication therapy for *H pylori*. Two other students (3.6%) complained of slight diarrhea. All students but one with adverse effects related to eradication therapy were thought to be mild; however, one required hospitalization because of severe skin rash. Lymphocyte transformation for amoxicillin was recognized by mixed lymphocyte culture test in the student with severe skin rash.

Costs

The cost of the first screening using RUPIRAN was 700 yen for each student. The cost of further examination and treatment including endoscopy and eradication therapy for *H pylori* was 40,300 yen (**Table 4**). If this attempt was introduced into the nationwide health screening at Japanese high schools, the total cost would be 2,895,046,000 yen every year (**Table 5**).

DISCUSSION

Uemura and colleagues[5] reported that 2.9% of subjects with *H pylori* infection had been recognized to have gastric cancer in a mean period of 7.8 years. From these data, we calculated that the incidence rate of gastric cancer in people with *H pylori* was 0.37% per year. Furthermore, we assume that gastric cancer will appear between the ages of 40 and 80 (a period of 40 years), and that 14.8% (0.37% × 40 years) of people with *H pylori* infection will contact gastric cancer in their lifetime. From these data, it is

Table 4
Cost of the examination and treatment of *Helicobacter pylori* infection for each person

First screening	
Cost of detection of the antibody to *H pylori*	700 yen ($6.09[a])
Further examination and treatment of *H pylori* infection	
Cost of endoscopy and taking biopsy samples	14,500 yen ($126.09[a])
Cost of histologic examination	10,300 yen ($89.57[a])
Cost of culture and sensitivity	4100 yen ($35.65[a])
Charge for medicines	6000 yen[b] ($52.17[a])
Cost of urea breath test	5400 yen ($46.96[a])
Total	40,300 yen[c] ($350.04[a])

[a] US dollar is calculated at the rate of 115 yen to the US dollar.
[b] An average of clarithromycin-based regimen and metronidazole-based regime.
[c] These costs were calculated according to the present medical fee decided by the Ministry of Health, Labor and Welfare in Japan.

Table 5
Cost of the screening, further examination, and treatment of *Helicobacter pylori* infection in the nationwide health screening of high school students

Population of a 1-year generation in the present Japanese teenager	1,210,000 persons[a]
Cost of the screening examination for *H pylori* infection	700 yen ($6.09[b]) × 1,210,000 = 847000,000 yen ($7,365,217[b]) (A)
Positive rate in the screening examination for *H pylori* infection	4.2%[c]
The number of students who required further examination for *H pylori* infection	1,210,000 persons × 0.042 = 50,820 persons
Cost of further examination and treatment of *H pylori* infection	40,300 yen ($350.04[b]) × 50,820 = 2,048,046,000 yen ($17,809,096[b]) (B)
Total cost	A + B = 2,895,046,000 yen ($25,174,313[b]) (C)

[a] The present data of the Statistics Bureau in the Ministry of Public Management, Home Affairs, Posts, and Telecommunications.
[b] US dollar calculated at the rate of 115 yen to the US dollar.
[c] Our data are this study.

calculated that 7521 persons in a 1-year cohort of students will develop gastric cancer (**Table 6**). If the cure of *H pylori* infection in teenagers reduced 80% of the incidence of gastric cancer, a percentage estimated based on the results of an experiment using an animal model,[9] this would prevent the occurrence of gastric cancer in 6017 persons. The cost of the prevention of a gastric cancer was calculated to be 481,144 yen for each person (see **Table 6**). Treatment of patients with gastric cancer, especially those with advanced disease, is very costly. Furthermore, the cure of *H pylori* infection might also prevent many other *H pylori*–related diseases. Therefore, the screening examination and treatment of *H pylori* in young people is likely to be an effective method of reducing national medical expenses in Japan. If we conducted our study using UBT instead of endoscopy and treated *H pylori* using an MNZ-based regimen, the cost of this project would have been approximately halved (**Table 7**). We propose this second

Table 6
Expected cost-effectiveness of the prevention of gastric cancer by curing *Helicobacter pylori* infection in teenagers

The rate of persons with *H pylori* infection who will contract gastric cancer in their lifetime	14.8%[a]
The number of persons with *H pylori* infection who will contract gastric cancer in their lifetime	50,820 persons × 0.148 = 7521 persons
The rate of persons who will be prevented from contracting gastric cancer by curing *H pylori* infection in teenagers	80%[a]
The number of persons who will be prevented from contracting gastric cancer by cure of *H pylori* infection in teenagers	7521 persons × 0.8 = 6017 persons
Cost of prevention of gastric cancer for each person	C ÷ 6.017 = 481,144 yen ($4184[b])

C: 2,895,046,000 yen (see **Table 5**).
[a] See the text.
[b] US dollar is calculated at the rate of 115 yen to the US dollar.

Table 7
Simulation of cost-effective calculation on the assumption that the urea breath test would be used for further examination of *Helicobacter pylori* infection and that the eradication therapy would be performed using a metronidazole-based regimen as the first-line therapy

Further examination and treatment of H pylori infection for each person	
Cost of urea breath test (further examination and assessment after eradication therapy)	5400 yen ($46.96[a]) $\times$ 2 = 10,800 yen ($93.91[a])
A charge for medicines	438.6 yen ($3.81[a]) $\times$ 7 = 3070 yen ($26.70[a])
	along with the entry 13,870 yen ($120.60[a])
Cost of further examination and treatment of H pylori infection in the nationwide health screening of high school students	
13,870 yen ($120.60[a]) $\times$ 1,210,000 $\times$ 0.042 = 704,873,400 yen ($6,129,334[a]) (D)	
Total cost of adding screening examination of H pylori infection per year	
700 yen ($6.09[a]) $\times$ 1,210,000 + D = 1,551,873,400 yen ($13,494,551[a]) (E)	
Cost of prevention of gastric cancer for each person	
E $\div$ 6017[b] = 257,915 yen ($2243[a])	

[a] US dollar is calculated at the rate of 115 yen to the US dollar.
[b] See **Table 6**.

plan as a more realistic method for the examination and treatment of *H pylori* infection in nationwide high school health screening.

Other Effectiveness Except Preventing of Gastric Cancers

The cure of *H pylori* infection would prevent not only gastric cancers but also many other *H pylori*–related diseases, such as gastritis, gastroduodenal ulcer, and MALT lymphoma. Peptic ulcer especially has tormented people with recurrent abdominal pain, bleeding, and perforation for a long time without relation to aging. The examination and treatment for *H pylori* in young people will reduce these pains and complications in their lifetimes.

H pylori infection in Japanese young people has steadily decreased.[12] The main route of *H pylori* infection at present is thought to occur by person-to-person contact in childhood. Konno and colleagues[13] used the typing of *H pylori* by molecular biologic techniques to show that *H pylori* infection occurs through family contact, especially between mother and child. Therefore, *H pylori* infection should be cured before marriage or pregnancy to prevent transmission. The addition of examination and treatment of *H pylori* infection as part of the regular high school health screening would not only prevent *H pylori*–related diseases for those who received eradication therapy but also reduce the transmission of *H pylori* infection to their offspring.

Problems of Treatment of Helicobacter pylori Infection in High School Students

Almost all the students in our study received the screening examination for *H pylori* infection, and the participation rate was very high (99.6%). However, some declined to participate and despite repeated recommendations by a school doctor remain untreated. This emphasized the need for more efforts to educate students and their parents about *H pylori* infection, with the goal of increasing the rate of visits to medical institutions for further examination.

Fujisawa and colleagues[14] reported that the accuracy of RUPIRAN was 95.2% based on the biopsy test results, and was equivalent or superior to that of serum-based antibody test. However, 12 of 72 students (16.7%) who underwent further examination using the biopsy-based test were not found to be infected by *H pylori*. Furthermore, 9 of the 12 students without *H pylori* infection showed negative by serum anti–*H pylori* antibody, and their endoscopic findings were normal. However, the remaining three students were thought to show past infection with *H pylori*. From these findings, we believe that the ideal method of screening examination has not yet been identified and further research is needed.

CAM resistance was present in 40% of our students with *H pylori* infection, as was MNZ resistance, and 25% had dual resistance. We used susceptibility-guided therapy and all 54 of 56 were cured by the first treatment of *H. pylori* infection. Although CAM susceptibility can be determined by use of molecular techniques examining stool specimens,[15,16] MNZ resistance cannot. This study showed a rate of MNZ resistance that is higher than experienced by studies in adults in Japan. Identification of the best empiric therapy that can reliably cure the infection without the need for EGD remains a target for subsequent studies.

Other Studies of a Screen-and-Treat Approach for Helicobacter pylori Infection in Japanese Adolescents

Recently, some local governments have scheduled *H pylori* screening for junior high school students in Japan. In Maniwa City of Okayama Prefecture, free *H pylori* screening for junior high school students was performed from 2013 using the urine-based antibody. Other municipal governments, such as Wakkanai City, Fukushima Town, and Bihoro Town of Hokkaido Prefecture, are starting to take a similar approach to Maniwa City.[17] There are many controversies concerning who should receive screening and treatment of *H pylori*. Persons with *H pylori* infection should be treated before irreversible damage occurs, which typically implies at a younger age. However, reinfection of *H pylori* is considered more common in very young children. We believe that introduction of an examination and treatment of *H pylori* infection in high school or junior high school health screening is most suitable and efficient because a very high participant rate is expected. Importantly, many seem to believe that childhood *H pylori* infections are benign. Here we show that scars from duodenal ulcers and duodenal erosions were found in more than 10% and some children had already developed more extensive atrophic changes. Noninvasive methods to assess gastric damage in children are needed.

SUMMARY

We agree with mass screening and individual screening of gastric cancer in middle- and old-aged adults (for second prevention) but suggest that the addition of programs to identify and cure of *H pylori* infection in young people (for primary prevention) is needed to eliminate gastric cancer in Japan. The low rate of prevalence of *H pylori* infection in present Japanese teenagers makes it possible and cost-effective to perform examinations and carry out treatment of this infection in nationwide health screenings of high school or junior high school students. Furthermore, the occurrence of *H pylori*–related diseases, such as gastritis, gastroduodenal ulcer, and gastric MALT lymphoma, will be reduced simultaneously.

REFERENCES

1. Nomura A, Stemmermann GN, Chyou PH, et al. *Helicobacter pylori* infection and gastric carcinoma among Japanese Americans in Hawaii. N Engl J Med 1991; 325:1132–6.

2. Kikuchi S, Wada O, Nakajima T, et al. Serum anti-*Helicobacter pylori* antibody and gastric carcinoma among young adults. Research Group on Prevention of Gastric Carcinoma among Young Adults. Cancer 1995;75:2789–93.
3. Sugiyama A, Maruta F, Ikeno T, et al. *Helicobacter pylori* infection enhances N-methyl-N-nitrosourea-induced stomach carcinogenesis in the *Mongolian gerbil*. Cancer Res 1998;58:2067–9.
4. Honda S, Fujioka T, Tokieda M, et al. Development of *Helicobacter pylori*-induced gastric carcinoma in Mongolian gerbil. Cancer Res 1998;58:4255–9.
5. Uemura N, Okamoto S, Yamamoto S, et al. *Helicobacter pylori* infection and the development of gastric cancer. N Engl J Med 2001;345:784–9.
6. Shimizu N, Ikehara Y, Inada K, et al. Eradication diminishes enhancing effects of *Helicobacter pylori* infection on glandular stomach carcinogenesis in *Mongolian gerbils*. Cancer Res 2000;60:1512–4.
7. Wong BC, Lam SK, Wong WM, et al. *Helicobacter pylori* eradication to prevent gastric cancer in a high-risk region of China: a randomized controlled trial. JAMA 2004;29:187–94.
8. Fukase K, Kato M, Kikuchi S, et al. Effect of eradication of *Helicobacter pylori* on incidence of metachronous gastric carcinoma after endoscopic resection of early gastric cancer: an open-label, randomized controlled trial. Lancet 2008;372: 392–7.
9. Nozaki K, Shimizu N, Ikehara Y, et al. Effect of early eradication on *Helicobacter pylori*-related gastric carcinogenesis in *Mongolian gerbils*. Cancer Sci 2003;94: 235–9.
10. Akamatsu T, Ichikawa S, Okudaira S, et al. Introduction of an examination and treatment for *Helicobacter pylori* infection in high school health screening. J Gastroenterol 2011;46:1353–60.
11. Kimura K, Takemoto T. An endoscopic recognition of the atrophic border and its significance in chronic gastritis. Endoscopy 1969;1:87–97.
12. Fujisawa T, Kumagai T, Akamatsu T, et al. Changes in seroepidemiological pattern of *Helicobacter pylori* and hepatitis A virus over the last 20 years in Japan. Am J Gastroenterol 1999;94:2094–9.
13. Konno M, Yokota S, Suga T, et al. Predominance of mother-to-child transmission of *Helicobacter pylori* infection detected by random amplified polymorphic DNA fingerprinting analysis in Japanese families. Pediatr Infect Dis 2008;27:999–1003.
14. Fujisawa T, Kaneko T, Kumagai T, et al. Evaluation of urinary rapid test for *Helicobacter pylori* in general practice. J Clin Lab Anal 2001;15:154–9.
15. Fontana C, Favaro M, Pietroiusti A, et al. Detection of clarithromycin-resistant *Helicobacter pylori* in stool samples. J Clin Microbiol 2003;41:3636–40.
16. Rimbara E, Noguchi N, Yamaguchi T, et al. Development of a highly sensitive method for detection of clarithromycin-resistant *Helicobacter pylori* from human feces. Curr Microbiol 2005;51:1–5.
17. Asaka M, Mabe K. Strategies for eliminating death from gastric cancer in Japan. Proc Jpn Acad Ser B Phys Biol Sci 2014;90:251–8.

Current Status and Prospects for a *Helicobacter pylori* Vaccine

Thomas G. Blanchard, PhD*, Steven J. Czinn, MD

KEYWORDS

- *Helicobacter pylori* • Vaccine • Cancer • Clinical trials • Inflammation

KEY POINTS

- Vaccination against *Helicobacter pylori* remains an important goal in countries with high *H pylori* incidence and where gastric cancer remains common.
- Large and small animal models have been useful for demonstrating the feasibility of protecting the host against *H pylori* through vaccination.
- Regulatory T cells are a dominant aspect of the host response to *H pylori* infection, whereas vaccine-induced protective immunity requires a proinflammatory T_H1 or T_H17 response.
- Phase 3 clinical trials to test prophylactic and therapeutic vaccination against *H pylori* have been unsuccessful.
- Improvement of a vaccine against *H pylori* has been stalled because of the lack of safe but potent adjuvants or carriers to induce mucosal immunity.

THE NEED FOR AN *HELICOBACTER PYLORI* VACCINE: LATE DIAGNOSIS OF *HELICOBACTER PYLORI*-ASSOCIATED GASTRIC CANCER

The gram-negative bacterium *H pylori* remains prevalent, infecting the stomachs of more than half the world's population. More than 80% of infected individuals experience no untoward effects from being infected, and some studies indicate that infection may actually be beneficial for resistance to childhood asthma or esophageal diseases.[1–3] *H pylori* is, however, a major cause of significant pathologic conditions, such as gastritis, gastric and duodenal ulcers, and gastric cancer.[4–8] For most of these individuals, a diagnosis of *H pylori* infection followed by an appropriate course of antimicrobial therapy would be sufficient treatment, as eradication rates can exceed

Department of Pediatrics, University of Maryland School of Medicine, 655 West Baltimore Street, Baltimore, MD 21201, USA
* Corresponding author. University of Maryland School of Medicine, 655 West Baltimore Street, Bressler Research Building, 13-043, Baltimore, MD 21201.
E-mail address: tblanchard@peds.umaryland.edu

Gastroenterol Clin N Am 44 (2015) 677–689
http://dx.doi.org/10.1016/j.gtc.2015.05.013
0889-8553/15/$ – see front matter © 2015 Elsevier Inc. All rights reserved.

90%.[5] Nevertheless, many would benefit from an *H pylori* vaccine. Treatment, however, requires several antibiotics in combination with a proton pump inhibitor (PPI) taken several times a day for at least 7 days. In addition, the most common antibiotics for *H pylori* eradication, clarithromycin and metronidazole, are becoming less effective in some countries because of the increasing prevalence of antibiotic-resistant strains,[9] and eradication of *H pylori* infection does not provide continued protection against reinfection. Some countries have reported rates of reinfection as high as 15% to 30% per year.[9–11]

A more compelling justification for development of an *H pylori* vaccine is the relationship between *H pylori* and gastric cancer. Individuals who develop gastric cancer typically remain asymptomatic until cancer is well established. Therefore, by the time they have been diagnosed with *H pylori* infection the prognosis is poor. Approximately 1% of *H pylori*-infected individuals develop gastric adenocarcinoma and less than 1% develop mucosa-associated lymphoid tissue lymphoma.[12] Identifying these individuals is impossible, but the costs of identifying all infected people within a country and providing antimicrobial therapy to all infected individuals would be prohibitive, particularly in many of the African and south Asian countries where *H pylori* and its associated diseases are most prevalent. A vaccine administered in early life therefore would provide the most cost-effective means of preventing gastric cancer in a nation where the incidence is high.

HIGH INCIDENCE OF GASTRIC CANCER IN DEVELOPING NATIONS

Gastric cancer disproportionately affects developing nations. The prevalence of *H pylori* infection ranges from 10% to 60% in Western countries but can approach 100% in developing countries.[13] This prevalence is consistent with data demonstrating that infection rates increase significantly within the US population for individuals living below the poverty level and even higher for those living in overcrowded homes or individuals without an education.[14] The high incidence of *H pylori* in many nations translates to a high incidence of gastric cancer. The incidence of gastric cancer in the United States is 7.5 per 100,000 people, whereas many South and Central American countries have rates of more than 10 per 100,000 and many Asian countries have rates more than 20 per 100,000, including China at 22.7, Japan at 29.9, and The Republic of Korea at 41.8.[15,16] The lifetime risk of developing gastric cancer in these countries (approximately 10% in some districts of Japan and Korea) illustrates the dire need of developing preventive therapies.[17,18] A model developed in 2001 predicted the benefits to the United States of a vaccine administered in childhood if available by 2010.[19] It predicted a decrease in prevalence to only 0.7% by the year 2100 with a concomitant decrease in gastric cancer incidence of only 0.4 per 100,000. Extrapolating this model to countries with a higher cancer incidence predicted a decrease in Japan to 1 per 100,000 and for countries with a higher incidence a reduction to 5.8 per 100,000. Therefore, despite the low incidence of *H pylori* in the West, most of the world would benefit greatly from vaccination against *H pylori*.

CHALLENGES IN INDUCING PROTECTIVE *HELICOBACTER PYLORI* IMMUNITY AT THE GASTRIC MUCOSA

All vaccines must meet at least 4 requirements to optimize efficacy; an appropriate antigen, an optimum dose and frequency of administration, an optimum route of vaccination, and strong immunogenicity typically achieved by inclusion of an adjuvant or carrier. However, in the case of inducing immunity in the gastrointestinal tract, there is an additional impediment. Most traditional immunizations are designed to increase the immunogenicity of something already treated as foreign by the host, whereas a vaccine designed to stimulate immunity in the gastrointestinal tract must overcome the inherent natural local immune mechanisms to suppress immunity to luminal antigens, food, and microbes. The propensity of the host to limit immunity at mucosal surfaces may explain the paucity of vaccines for venereal diseases and gastrointestinal pathogens. It was against this background that much of the experimental *H pylori* vaccine research in animals was performed, primarily in mice but including some larger animals as well.[20] Results from all these animal studies are too numerous to recount in detail, but several findings should be highlighted for their influence on the design of vaccines against *H pylori* in clinical trials.

RESULTS FROM THE MOUSE MODEL THAT CONTRIBUTED TO VACCINE DEVELOPMENT

First, protective immunity against *H pylori* in mice can be achieved through almost any route of delivery. Early dogma held that oral or mucosal vaccination would be required to induce immunity in the stomach because *H pylori* resides in the lumen and is noninvasive. The first challenge studies, therefore, using the *Helicobacter felis* mouse model in the years before development of mouse-adapted *H pylori* strains, delivered live *H felis* to the peritoneal cavity or *H felis* lysate and cholera toxin (CT) adjuvant by oral gavage before challenge.[21,22] Immunized mice achieved significant reductions in bacterial load compared with nonvaccinated control mice. Subsequent studies by many laboratories confirmed these results and used this model to study the protective host immune response. In the process it was also determined that protection could be induced through vaccination targeting other mucosal tissues including orogastric, intranasal, and rectal.[21–27] Protective immunity in these models is generally defined as a significant reduction in bacterial load, although sterilizing immunity has been reported in some mice in gerbil studies using intranasal, oral, and rectal immunizations.[28–31] Intranasal immunization has been demonstrated to be at least as good as orogastric immunization with the added benefit of requiring less antigen and with less risk of detrimental effects due to bacterial exotoxin adjuvants such as CT or *Escherichia coli* heat labile toxin (LT); yet this technology has not been incorporated into human clinical trials (see later discussion).[28,30] Perhaps most surprising has been the observation that protective immunity equivalent to orogastric delivery can be induced through the use of systemic routes, including subcutaneous and intraperitoneal.[32–34] These results are in contrast to the failure of systemic immunization to protect against other mucosal pathogens but have been the impetus for at least 1 phase 3 clinical trial using parenteral immunization described later.[35]

Second, protection in mice can be achieved using numerous distinct *H pylori* protein antigens. It is likely that protection is mediated by a cellular inflammatory response promoted by T_H1 and T_H17 cells (**Fig. 1**). In addition, several laboratories have demonstrated that vaccine-induced protective immunity can be achieved in the absence of antibodies.[36–38] A partial list of antigens demonstrated to afford protection against *H pylori* in mice includes the urease subunits,[24] CagA,[23] VacA,[23] catalase,[39] flagellin,[40] heat shock proteins,[41] *H pylori* adhesion A,[42] and neutrophil activating protein (NAP).[43] Killed whole-cell bacteria may also suffice, as whole-cell lysates have been used extensively in mice as described in the original *Helicobacter* vaccine reports.[21,22] Such whole-cell preparations have been incorporated into the clinical trial described later.[44] The large number of antigens may prove beneficial if it is determined that a multivalent vaccine provides better efficacy in clinical trials. Ferrero and colleagues[41] demonstrated that improved efficacy could be achieved in mice by combining heat shock protein A (HspA) with a urease subunit vaccine to achieve protection in 100%

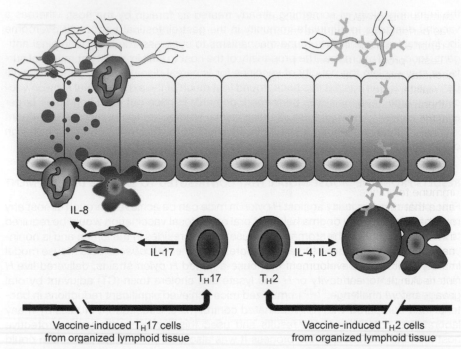

Fig. 1. Protection against *H pylori* mediated by distinct T-helper-cell responses. Immunizations delivered therapeutically or prophylactically with adjuvant systems that activate T$_H$17 or T$_H$1 immune responses promote robust inflammation and granulocyte recruitment and activity that can reduce the bacterial load or eradicate infection. Immunizations that activate T$_H$2 cells and humoral-based immune responses may prevent infection through antibody-mediated clearance of low-load bacterial challenge.

of mice compared with 80% of mice when immunized with either urease or HspA alone. This concept has been supported by a study using a canine model. As stated earlier, complete protection has been difficult to achieve in animal models. However, a multivalent vaccine consisting of VacA, CagA, and NAP was shown to be completely protective when given therapeutically in beagle dogs as determined by immunohisto-chemical detection of *H pylori* in histologic sections.[45]

A third principal derived from numerous animal studies, which has already been incorporated into clinical trials, is the use of therapeutic immunization to treat a preexisting *Helicobacter* infection. The initial experiment was performed in mice using the *H felis* infection model and demonstrated that protection was not limited to the timing of immunization but rather to the activation of an immune response that is not activated by chronic *Helicobacter* infection.[46,47] This experiment was subsequently performed using *H pylori* in mice.[38] In addition, as noted earlier, a trivalent subunit vaccine was used to eradicate *H pylori* from beagle dogs through systemic immunization.[45] Therapeutic immunization was also tested in the ferret model for treatment of *Helicobacter mustelae* infection.[48] *H mustelae* is an indigenous infection of the ferret stomach and induces gastric disease with high similarity to *H pylori* infection of humans. It was speculated that unlike the *H felis* and *H pylori* animal models mentioned earlier, the nature of the *H mustelae* ferret model would more closely approximate the host pathogen relationship of human *H pylori* infection and give a better impression of vaccine efficacy. In this light, although sterilizing immunity was achieved for some animals, this protection was observed in only 30% of immunized ferrets. This study was performed with purified recombinant *H pylori* urease plus CT, similar to 1 of the 2 reported therapeutic immunization clinical trials described later.[49]

Lastly, prophylactic immunization against *H pylori* is effective when administered to neonatal mice.[32] This experiment has important implications if a vaccine is to be administered to humans at an early age. Although there may be utility in administering a therapeutic vaccine to the adult population in countries where *H pylori*-associated gastric cancer remains prevalent, a more effective strategy for long-term reductions in *H pylori* infections and associated pathology may be to immunize children because most infections occur in early childhood. As mentioned earlier, there is a consensus that eradication of *H pylori* requires a T_H1- or T_H17-mediated inflammatory response. Immunization of neonatal mice has historically been associated with the induction of immune tolerance.[50] Early exposure in life to infectious agents can also lead to tolerance that can result in the inability of adults to clear the infection.[51] In this light, the number and activity of regulatory T cells is increased in the stomachs of children infected with *H pylori* relative to infected adults.[52,53] Therefore, the ability to protect neonatally immunized mice from challenge with *H pylori* at levels comparable to vaccinated adult mice is encouraging.[32] These mice responded with strong interferon γ, interleukin (IL)-4, and IL-5 responses when immunized subcutaneously or intraperitoneally and with either Freund incomplete or complete adjuvant.

CLINICAL TRIALS

To date there have been 4 major published clinical studies to test the efficacy of an *H pylori* vaccine (**Table 1**) in addition to several studies to determine safety and immunogenicity.[35,44,49,54] Each of these trials was distinguishable from the others based on the antigens used, the adjuvant or delivery system used, the route of delivery, or

Table 1						
Clinical trials for vaccine efficacy against *H pylori*						
Year	Route	Antigens	Adjuvant	Timing	Challenge	Result
1999[49]	Oral	Urease	LT	Therapeutic	Natural	Significant reduction in bacterial load in some vaccine groups
2001[44]	Oral	Whole cell	LT$_{mutant}$	Therapeutic	Natural	No clearance
2008[54]	Oral	Urease or Hp0231	*Salmonella enterica* serovar Typhi Ty21a	Prophylactic	Experimental	Some clearance in both vaccine and control groups
2012[35]	Intramuscular	CagA VacA Nap	Alum	Prophylactic	Experimental	Clearance equivalent between vaccine and controls groups
2014[82,84]	Oral	Urease	Undisclosed	Prophylactic	Natural	Efficacy, 72%

the timing of immunization compared with initiation of infection. Although all are considered unsuccessful based on the lack of protective immunity induced, some insight may be gained from an evaluation of the detailed results. The first of these studies used recombinant urease B in combination with E coli LT to treat volunteers already demonstrated to be naturally infected with H pylori.[49] A range of doses was tested (180, 60, and 20 mg) by the oral route, but none of the vaccine formulations induced protective immunity. However, immunization induced a significant increase in urease-specific circulating IgA-producing B cells compared with placebo. The group of volunteers receiving the lowest dose of urease antigen had a significant reduction in bacterial load. These data demonstrate that it is possible to positively affect the host immune response to H pylori through oral immunization. It is particularly meaningful because the volunteers had long-standing H pylori infections and therefore a well-established downregulated immune response to H pylori that could be overcome, if not to the degree necessary to achieve bacterial eradication. Another aspect of this study is that more than 60% of volunteers receiving the LT adjuvant experienced diarrhea after only a single dose, resulting in the discontinuation of the protocol that used the higher 10-μg dose of LT before completion of the study. Many individuals receiving the 5-μg dose, however, also experienced diarrhea. A subsequent study on safety and immunogenicity with human volunteers determined that a dose of 2.5 μg of LT was necessary to achieve immune induction but that 50% of the subjects still experienced diarrhea.[55] A separate study by the same group tested H pylori urease and LT combinations delivered by enema in an attempt to circumvent toxicity.[56] Volunteers received 3 immunizations during the course of 4 weeks, with no adverse events reported even in the group receiving 25 μg of LT. Unfortunately, although an immunologic response to LT was achieved as measured by LT-specific B cells in the blood that were induced, no immunologic response to H pylori urease was achieved, even in individuals receiving 60 mg of urease.

Efforts to eliminate the toxicity of the LT adjuvant have also used genetically modified LT derivatives containing amino acid substitutions that limit its enzymatic activity such as LT_{R192G},[57,58] which have been tested in murine models of H pylori infection using CagA, VacA, and urease protein antigens.[23,57] This adjuvant was used in a clinical vaccine trial in combination with formalin-inactivated whole-cell H pylori (HWC).[44] A dose of 25 μg LT_{R192G} in combination with up to 2.5 × 10^{10} HWC was administered orally to H pylori-uninfected and infected volunteers. The levels of H pylori-specific salivary and fecal antibodies increased in those volunteers infected with H pylori and who received the highest dose of vaccine. Peripheral blood lymphocyte memory immune responses, however, were only observed in uninfected volunteers. These data indicate that a nontoxic derivative of LT can induce immunogenicity against H pylori. The therapeutic efficacy of vaccination in infected volunteers was determined using the noninvasive ^{13}C urea breath test to determine the presence or absence of H pylori, but no eradication was observed when evaluated up to 7.5 months after vaccination. Diarrhea was reported in 18% of vaccinated individuals receiving adjuvant LT_{R192G}, a toxicity that might be ameliorated with reduced doses of the mutant LT. Research on nontoxic derivatives of LT continues, and a double amino acid mutant of LT has been evaluated as an adjuvant in a vaccine against H pylori challenge in mice.[58] It was demonstrated to be as immunogenic and efficacious as the single mutant LT_{R192G}. The above-mentioned studies highlight the difficulties associated with developing safe and efficacious adjuvants for mucosal immunization in humans and demonstrate a need for continued development of nontoxic mucosal adjuvants. Notwithstanding the results achieved in animal models, these results indicate that it may not be possible to achieve a dose of LT or LT derivative that retains adjuvanticity without toxicity. Another disappointing aspect of this study was the lack of efficacy achieved when using a complex, multivalent antigen such as HWC. Prior studies in mice had indicated that efficacy is improved when administering more than one *H pylori* antigen.[41] Because the bacterial load of vaccinated volunteers could not be determined using the ^{13}C urea breath test, it is impossible to determine whether the investigators did indeed achieve at least a reduction in bacterial load.

The third reported oral vaccine study was performed using attenuated recombinant *Salmonella* Ty21a as an immunogenic carrier vehicle to deliver either *H pylori* urease or the HP0231 antigen to the intestines.[54] Prior clinical work using recombinant *Salmonella* Ty21a expressing urease proteins demonstrated the safety of the vaccine, and, although antibody responses were not induced, a T-cell memory response was measured in many individuals.[59,60] For their challenge study, the investigators used *H pylori*-negative individuals. Participants received multiple doses of vaccine before being challenged with a human strain of *H pylori* that had been previously characterized for use in clinical studies.[61] The volunteers developed the host response that generally characterizes *H pylori* infection, including increased serum cytokine levels and histologic gastritis.[54] Challenge resulted in an increase in the number of urease-specific, circulating antibody-secreting cells that had not been observed before the challenge. Of 33 volunteers receiving the vaccine, 8 experienced a decrease in bacterial load, although a decrease was also observed in 5 of 25 subjects immunized with the Ty21a control vector. This experiment therefore, similar to those using the LT adjuvant described earlier, demonstrates that the host mucosal immune response against *H pylori* can be manipulated to favor eradication of *H pylori* and may indeed prove protective with expression of additional antigens or with the coexpression of factors designed to boost the immune response. Similar to the prior studies with the Ty21a vaccine, the constructs were well tolerated, demonstrating that intestinal delivery with an immunogenic carrier rather than using a mucosal adjuvant may prove more useful for continued development of an oral vaccine against *H pylori*.

The most recently reported clinical study investigated an alum-based trivalent vaccine including *H pylori* CagA, VacA, and NAP delivered by intramuscular immunization.[35] Previous studies in mice had demonstrated that vaccine-induced protective immunity against *H pylori* might be more reliant on inducing a strong immune response in draining lymph nodes rather than local delivery to the gut where immunosuppressive mechanisms are prevalent.[62] Indeed, subcutaneous or intraperitoneal delivery with alum-based candidate vaccines was demonstrated to be at least as effective as oral immunization using bacterial exotoxin adjuvants.[33,34] Following a phase 1 trial demonstrating strong antigen-specific antibody and T-cell memory responses in the absence of adverse effects,[63] the vaccine was tested on *H pylori*-negative volunteers for efficacy.[35] Volunteers received 3 monthly doses of vaccine (n = 19) or placebo (n = 15) followed by challenge 1 month after the final boost. The end point for protection was set at 12 weeks postchallenge. Volunteers were determined to be infected in 42% of vaccinated subjects versus 53% of subjects receiving placebo. Therefore, clearance of *H pylori* was observed in approximately 50% of all subjects. Based on the number of subjects in this study, the investigators were unable to demonstrate improved efficacy compared with control subjects.

RETROSPECTIVE ANALYSIS AND NEW CONSIDERATIONS IN *HELICOBACTER PYLORI* VACCINE DEVELOPMENT

The results of the clinical studies performed to date warrant a reevaluation of the understanding of *H pylori* immunity. At the very least it must be acknowledged that the mouse model, although extremely useful in helping to define differences in the nature of the immune responses to infection and immunization, may lack predictive ability when designing an efficacious vaccine. As discussed earlier, most studies defined protection as a significant reduction in bacterial load, with only occasional reports of sterilizing immunity.[28–31] The comparison with the domestic model of indigenous *H mustelae* infection in which 30% of animals could be protected by therapeutic immunization would seem to suggest that studies in animals with nonnative infections may not provide the stringency required to accurately gauge a vaccine strategy for use in humans. Additional evidence that the levels of protection observed in mice might not translate to humans comes from nonhuman primate studies in which rhesus macaques found to harbor native *H pylori* infections have been used. Results have been mixed but confirm that in a model of indigenous *H pylori* infection, vaccines similar to those tested on mice are much less efficacious.[64–67]

Clinical and animal model studies also highlight the difficulty in overcoming the immunoregulatory nature of *H pylori* infection. The host response to *H pylori* is actively suppressed by Treg cells and IL-10-producing Tr1 cells.[68–73] In vitro lymphocyte recall assays on infected and noninfected subjects demonstrate comparable responses to *H pylori* antigen.[74–79] Depletion of CD25^{hi} T cells (Treg cells), however, results in significant activity in the T cells isolated from *H pylori*-infected donors.[80] Subsequent experiments have documented the presence of Treg cells in the infected human stomach, and the authors and others have demonstrated in mouse models that blocking or deleting Treg cells results in significantly increased T_H cell activity and gastric inflammation, which significantly reduces or eliminates the bacterial load from the stomach.[68,71,72] The host gastrointestinal tract inherently suppresses immune responses to commensal bacteria, and it is likely that the host responds in a similar manner to *H pylori* because it is a noninvasive colonizer of the epithelium with no outright cytotoxic activity. Therefore, future strategies might incorporate mechanisms of limiting regulatory T-cell activity or preferentially activating proinflammatory T cells that can overcome regulatory T-cell activity. In that light, administration of IL-12 to *H felis*-infected mice was sufficient to achieve eradication of the bacteria in the absence of immunization.[81]

Finally, although the results have yet to be published, a large-scale phase 3 clinical trial was completed in China to test a prophylactic oral vaccine against natural acquisition of *H pylori*.[82] The vaccine was tested on children aged 6 to 15 years who were negative for *H pylori*. The oral vaccine contained the urease B protein subunit, but additional details remain unknown. It was administered in three 15-mg immunization doses, and the children were monitored to determine the rate of natural *H pylori* infection compared with a control group that received a placebo. Press reports indicate that this study involved several thousand subjects and that vaccine efficacy against infection was 72% at the initial postimmunization evaluation. If this information is accurate, such results may contribute significantly to the understanding of host protection against *H pylori*. The nature of the adjuvant used, if at all, could be informative as to the type of immunity induced. This study also highlights issues such as the likely dose of natural *H pylori* exposure compared with experimentally applied challenges. It is possible that difficulties in eradicating *H pylori* such as by therapeutic immunization or to protect against a bolus experimental challenge become less important if mucosal antibodies are capable of preventing colonization by the low dose exposure experienced naturally (see **Fig. 1**). Studies in mice indicate that antibodies are sufficient to prevent infection when present at challenge.[83] There may also be fundamental differences in the type or strength of the vaccine-induced immune response in children compared with adults that have gone unaddressed in the previously published clinical trials. Ultimately, achieving such efficacy in such a large-scale study should bring renewed energy and optimism at the prospects for vaccine against *H pylori*.

REFERENCES

1. Chen Y, Blaser MJ. *Helicobacter pylori* colonization is inversely associated with childhood asthma. J Infect Dis 2008;198:553–60.
2. Corley DA, Kubo A, Levin TR, et al. *Helicobacter pylori* infection and the risk of Barrett's oesophagus: a community-based study. Gut 2008;57:727–33.
3. Dellon ES, Peery AF, Shaheen NJ, et al. Inverse association of esophageal eosinophilia with *Helicobacter pylori* based on analysis of a US pathology database. Gastroenterology 2011;141:1586–92.
4. Eurogast Study Group. An international association between *Helicobacter pylori* infection and gastric cancer. Lancet 1993;341:1359–62.
5. NIH Consensus Conference. *Helicobacter pylori* in peptic ulcer disease. J Am Med Assoc 1994;272:65–9.
6. Parsonnet J, Friedman GD, Vandersteen DP, et al. *Helicobacter pylori* infection and the risk of gastric carcinoma. N Engl J Med 1991;325:1127–31.
7. Warren JR, Marshall BJ. Unidentified curved bacilli on gastric epithelium in active chronic gastritis. Lancet 1983;1:1273–5.
8. World Health Organization. Infection with *Helicobacter pylori*. Schistosomes, liver flukes and *Helicobacter pylori*, vol. 61. Lyon (France): International Agency for Research on Cancer; 1994. p. 177–241.
9. Frenck RW Jr, Clemens J. *Helicobacter* in the developing world. Microbes Infect 2003;5:705–13.
10. Gisbert JP. The recurrence of *Helicobacter pylori* infection: incidence and variables influencing it. A critical review. Am J Gastroenterol 2005;100:2083–99.
11. Parsonnet J. What is the *Helicobacter pylori* global reinfection rate? Can J Gastroenterol 2003;17(Suppl B):46B–8B.
12. Luther J, Kao JY. Considering global vaccination against *Helicobacter pylori*. South Med J 2010;103:185–6.
13. Graham DY, Malaty HM, Evans DG, et al. Epidemiology of *Helicobacter pylori* in an asymptomatic population in the United States. Effect of age, race, and socioeconomic status. Gastroenterology 1991;100:1495–501.
14. Kruszon-Moran D, McQuillan GM. Seroprevalence of six infectious diseases among adults in the United States by race/ethnicity: data from the third national health and nutrition examination survey, 1988–94. Adv Data 2005;9:1–9.
15. Ferlay J, Soerjomataram I, Dikshit R, et al. Cancer incidence and mortality worldwide: sources, methods and major patterns in GLOBOCAN 2012. Int J Cancer 2015;136:E359–86.
16. World Cancer Research Fund International. Stomach Cancer Statistics, 2013. Available at: http://www.wcrf.org/int/cancer-facts-figures/data-specific-cancers/stomach-cancer-statistics.
17. Cancer incidence in five continents. Volume VIII. IARC Sci Publ 2002;(155):1–781.
18. Yaghoobi M, Bijarchi R, Narod SA. Family history and the risk of gastric cancer. Br J Cancer 2010;102:237–42.
19. Rupnow MF, Shachter RD, Owens DK, et al. Quantifying the population impact of a prophylactic *Helicobacter pylori* vaccine. Vaccine 2001;20:879–85.
20. Blanchard T, Nedrud J. *Helicobacter pylori* vaccines. In: Sutton P, Hazel M, editors. *Helicobacter pylori* in the 21st century. Wallingford (United Kingdom): CABI; 2010. p. 167–89.

21. Chen M, Lee A, Hazell S, et al. Immunisation against gastric infection with *Helicobacter* species: first step in the prophylaxis of gastric cancer? Zentralbl Bakteriol 1993;280:155–65.

22. Czinn SJ, Cai A, Nedrud JG. Protection of germ-free mice from infection by *Helicobacter felis* after active oral or passive IgA immunization. Vaccine 1993;11: 637–42.

23. Ghiara P, Rossi M, Marchetti M, et al. Therapeutic intragastric vaccination against *Helicobacter pylori* in mice eradicates an otherwise chronic infection and confers protection against reinfection. Infect Immun 1997;65:4996–5002.

24. Lee CK, Weltzin R, Thomas WD Jr, et al. Oral immunization with recombinant *Helicobacter pylori* urease induces secretory IgA antibodies and protects mice from challenge with *Helicobacter felis*. J Infect Dis 1995;172:161–72.

25. Marchetti M, Arico B, Burroni D, et al. Development of a mouse model of *Helicobacter pylori* infection that mimics human disease. Science 1995;267:1655–8.

26. Michetti P, Corthesy-Theulaz I, Davin C, et al. Immunization of BALB/c mice against *Helicobacter felis* infection with *Helicobacter pylori* urease. Gastroenterology 1994;107:1002–11.

27. Weltzin R, Kleanthous H, Guirdkhoo F, et al. Novel intranasal immunization techniques for antibody induction and protection of mice against gastric *Helicobacter felis* infection. Vaccine 1997;15:370–6.

28. Garhart CA, Redline RW, Nedrud JG, et al. Clearance of *Helicobacter pylori* infection and resolution of postimmunization gastritis in a kinetic study of prophylactically immunized mice. Infect Immun 2002;70:3529–38.

29. Jeremy AH, Du Y, Dixon MF, et al. Protection against *Helicobacter pylori* infection in the Mongolian gerbil after prophylactic vaccination. Microbes Infect 2006;8: 340–6.

30. Jiang W, Baker HJ, Smith BF. Mucosal immunization with *Helicobacter*, CpG DNA, and cholera toxin is protective. Infect Immun 2003;71:40–6.

31. Kleanthous H, Tibbitts TJ, Gray HL, et al. Sterilizing immunity against experimental *Helicobacter pylori* infection is challenge-strain dependent. Vaccine 2001;19:4883–95.

32. Eisenberg JC, Czinn SJ, Garhart CA, et al. Protective efficacy of anti-*Helicobacter pylori* immunity following systemic immunization of neonatal mice. Infect Immun 2003;71:1820–7.

33. Gottwein JM, Blanchard TG, Targoni OS, et al. Protective anti-*Helicobacter* immunity is induced with aluminum hydroxide or complete Freund's adjuvant by systemic immunization. J Infect Dis 2001;184:308–14.

34. Guy B, Hessler C, Fourage S, et al. Systemic immunization with urease protects mice against *Helicobacter pylori* infection. Vaccine 1998;16:850–6.

35. Malfertheiner P, Selgrad M, Wex T, et al. Efficacy of an investigational recombinant antigen based vaccine against a CagA *H. pylori* infectious challenge in healthy volunteers. Gastroenterology 2012;142:S-184.

36. Blanchard TG, Czinn SJ, Redline RW, et al. Antibody-independent protective mucosal immunity to gastric *Helicobacter* infection in mice. Cell Immunol 1999; 191:74–80.

37. Ermak TH, Giannasca PJ, Nichols R, et al. Immunization of mice with urease vaccine affords protection against *Helicobacter pylori* infection in the absence of antibodies and is mediated by MHC class II-restricted responses. J Exp Med 1998; 188:2277–88.

38. Sutton P, Wilson J, Kosaka T, et al. Therapeutic immunization against *Helicobacter pylori* infection in the absence of antibodies. Immunol Cell Biol 2000;78:28–30.

39. Radcliff FJ, Hazell SL, Kolesnikow T, et al. Catalase, a novel antigen for *Helicobacter pylori* vaccination. Infect Immun 1997;65:4668–74.
40. Skene C, Young A, Every A, et al. *Helicobacter pylori* flagella: antigenic profile and protective immunity. FEMS Immunol Med Microbiol 2007;50:249–56.
41. Ferrero RL, Thiberge JM, Kansau I, et al. The GroES homolog of *Helicobacter pylori* confers protective immunity against mucosal infection in mice. Proc Natl Acad Sci U S A 1995;92:6499–503.
42. Sutton P, Doidge C, Pinczower G, et al. Effectiveness of vaccination with recombinant HpaA from *Helicobacter pylori* is influenced by host genetic background. FEMS Immunol Med Microbiol 2007;50:213–9.
43. Satin B, Del Giudice G, Della Bianca V, et al. The neutrophil-activating protein (HP-NAP) of *Helicobacter pylori* is a protective antigen and a major virulence factor. J Exp Med 2000;191:1467–76.
44. Kotloff KL, Sztein MB, Wasserman SS, et al. Safety and immunogenicity of oral inactivated whole-cell *Helicobacter pylori* vaccine with adjuvant among volunteers with or without subclinical infection. Infect Immun 2001;69:3581–90.
45. Rossi G, Ruggiero P, Peppoloni S, et al. Therapeutic vaccination against *Helicobacter pylori* in the beagle dog experimental model: safety, immunogenicity, and efficacy. Infect Immun 2004;72:3252–9.
46. Corthesy-Theulaz I, Porta N, Glauser M, et al. Oral immunization with *Helicobacter pylori* urease B subunit as a treatment against *Helicobacter* infection in mice. Gastroenterology 1995;109:115–21.
47. Doidge C, Crust I, Lee A, et al. Therapeutic immunisation against *Helicobacter* infection. Lancet 1994;343:914–5.
48. Cuenca R, Blanchard TG, Czinn SJ, et al. Therapeutic immunization against *Helicobacter mustelae* in naturally infected ferrets. Gastroenterology 1996;110:1770–5.
49. Michetti P, Kreiss C, Kotloff KL, et al. Oral immunization with urease and *Escherichia coli* heat-labile enterotoxin is safe and immunogenic in *Helicobacter pylori*-infected adults. Gastroenterology 1999;116:804–12.
50. Billingham RE, Brent L, Medawar PB. Actively acquired tolerance of foreign cells. Nature 1953;172:603–6.
51. Cihak J, Lehmann-Grube F. Immunological tolerance to lymphocytic choriomeningitis virus in neonatally infected virus carrier mice: evidence supporting a clonal inactivation mechanism. Immunology 1978;34:265–75.
52. Freire de Melo F, Rocha AM, Rocha GA, et al. A regulatory instead of an IL-17 T response predominates in *Helicobacter pylori*-associated gastritis in children. Microbes Infect 2012;14:341–7.
53. Harris PR, Wright SW, Serrano C, et al. *Helicobacter pylori* gastritis in children is associated with a regulatory T-cell response. Gastroenterology 2008;134:491–9.
54. Aebischer T, Bumann D, Epple HJ, et al. Correlation of T cell response and bacterial clearance in human volunteers challenged with *Helicobacter pylori* revealed by randomised controlled vaccination with Ty21a-based *Salmonella* vaccines. Gut 2008;57:1065–72.
55. Banerjee S, Medina-Fatimi A, Nichols R, et al. Safety and efficacy of low dose *Escherichia coli* enterotoxin adjuvant for urease based oral immunisation against *Helicobacter pylori* in healthy volunteers. Gut 2002;51:634–40.
56. Sougioultzis S, Lee CK, Alsahli M, et al. Safety and efficacy of E coli enterotoxin adjuvant for urease-based rectal immunization against *Helicobacter pylori*. Vaccine 2002;21:194–201.
57. Marchetti M, Rossi M, Giannelli V, et al. Protection against *Helicobacter pylori* infection in mice by intragastric vaccination with *H. pylori* antigens is achieved

using a non-toxic mutant of *E. coli* heat-labile enterotoxin (LT) as adjuvant. Vaccine 1998;16:33–7.

58. Summerton NA, Welch RW, Bondoc L, et al. Toward the development of a stable, freeze-dried formulation of *Helicobacter pylori* killed whole cell vaccine adjuvanted with a novel mutant of *Escherichia coli* heat-labile toxin. Vaccine 2010; 28:1404–11.

59. Bumann D, Metzger WG, Mansouri E, et al. Safety and immunogenicity of live recombinant *Salmonella enterica* serovar Typhi Ty21a expressing urease A and B from *Helicobacter pylori* in human volunteers. Vaccine 2001;20:845–52.

60. Metzger WG, Mansouri E, Kronawitter M, et al. Impact of vector-priming on the immunogenicity of a live recombinant *Salmonella enterica* serovar typhi Ty21a vaccine expressing urease A and B from *Helicobacter pylori* in human volunteers. Vaccine 2004;22:2273–7.

61. Graham DY, Opekun AR, Osato MS, et al. Challenge model for *Helicobacter pylori* infection in human volunteers. Gut 2004;53:1235–43.

62. Blanchard TG, Eisenberg JC, Matsumoto Y. Clearance of *Helicobacter pylori* infection through immunization: the site of T cell activation contributes to vaccine efficacy. Vaccine 2004;22:888–97.

63. Malfertheiner P, Schultze V, Rosenkranz B, et al. Safety and immunogenicity of an intramuscular *Helicobacter pylori* vaccine in noninfected volunteers: a phase I study. Gastroenterology 2008;135:787–95.

64. Dubois A, Lee CK, Fiala N, et al. Immunization against natural *Helicobacter pylori* infection in nonhuman primates. Infect Immun 1998;66:4340–6.

65. Lee CK, Soike K, Hill J, et al. Immunization with recombinant *Helicobacter pylori* urease decreases colonization levels following experimental infection of rhesus monkeys. Vaccine 1999;17:1493–505.

66. Lee CK, Soike K, Giannasca P, et al. Immunization of rhesus monkeys with a mucosal prime, parenteral boost strategy protects against infection with *Helicobacter pylori*. Vaccine 1999;17:3072–82.

67. Solnick JV, Canfield DR, Hansen LM, et al. Immunization with recombinant *Helicobacter pylori* urease in specific-pathogen-free rhesus monkeys (*Macaca mulatta*). Infect Immun 2000;68:2560–5.

68. Anderson KM, Czinn SJ, Redline RW, et al. Induction of CTLA-4-mediated anergy contributes to persistent colonization in the murine model of gastric *Helicobacter pylori* infection. J Immunol 2006;176:5306–13.

69. Eaton KA, Mefford M, Thevenot T. The role of T cell subsets and cytokines in the pathogenesis of *Helicobacter pylori* gastritis in mice. J Immunol 2001;166: 7456–61.

70. Matsumoto Y, Blanchard TG, Drakes ML, et al. Eradication of *Helicobacter pylori* and resolution of gastritis in the gastric mucosa of IL-10-deficient mice. Helicobacter 2005;10:407–15.

71. Rad R, Brenner L, Bauer S, et al. CD25+/Foxp3+ T cells regulate gastric inflammation and *Helicobacter pylori* colonization in vivo. Gastroenterology 2006;131:525–37.

72. Raghavan S, Suri-Payer E, Holmgren J. Antigen-specific in vitro suppression of murine *Helicobacter pylori*-reactive immunopathological T cells by CD4CD25 regulatory T cells. Scand J Immunol 2004;60:82–8.

73. Sayi A, Kohler E, Toller IM, et al. TLR-2-activated B cells suppress *Helicobacter*-induced preneoplastic gastric immunopathology by inducing T regulatory-1 cells. J Immunol 2011;186:878–90.

74. Fan XJ, Chua A, Shahi CN, et al. Gastric T lymphocyte responses to *Helicobacter pylori* in patients with H pylori colonisation. Gut 1994;35:1379–84.

75. Karttunen R. Blood lymphocyte proliferation, cytokine secretion and appearance of T cells with activation surface markers in cultures with *Helicobacter pylori*. Comparison of the responses of subjects with and without antibodies to *H. pylori*. Clin Exp Immunol 1991;83:396–400.
76. Karttunen R, Andersson G, Poikonen K, et al. *Helicobacter pylori* induces lymphocyte activation in peripheral blood cultures. Clin Exp Immunol 1990;82: 485–8.
77. Karttunen R, Karttunen T, Ekre HP, et al. Interferon gamma and interleukin 4 secreting cells in the gastric antrum in *Helicobacter pylori* positive and negative gastritis. Gut 1995;36:341–5.
78. Lindholm C, Quiding-Jarbrink M, Lonroth H, et al. Local cytokine response in *Helicobacter pylori*-infected subjects. Infect Immun 1998;66:5964–71.
79. Sharma SA, Miller GG, Perez-Perez GI, et al. Humoral and cellular immune recognition of *Helicobacter pylori* proteins are not concordant. Clin Exp Immunol 1994; 97:126–32.
80. Lundgren A, Suri-Payer E, Enarsson K, et al. *Helicobacter pylori*-specific CD4+ CD25high regulatory T cells suppress memory T-cell responses to *H. pylori* in infected individuals. Infect Immun 2003;71:1755–62.
81. Ding H, Nedrud JG, Blanchard TG, et al. Th1-mediated immunity against *Helicobacter pylori* can compensate for lack of Th17 cells and can protect mice in the absence of immunization. PLoS One 2013;8:e69384.
82. ClinicalTrials.gov. A phase III clinical trial with oral recombinant *Helicobacter pylori* vaccine in Chinese children, 2014. Bethesda, Maryland: National Institutes of Health; 2015.
83. Blanchard TG, Czinn SJ, Maurer R, et al. Urease-specific monoclonal antibodies prevent *Helicobacter felis* infection in mice. Infect Immun 1995;63:1394–9.
84. IHS, editor. China develops world's first *H. Pylori* vaccine, given green light by SFDA. April 23, 2009, Englewood, Colorado. Available at: https://www.ihs.com/country-industry-forecasting.html?ID=106595607.

Index

Note: Page numbers of article titles are in **boldface** type.

A

Adherence, to bismuth quadruple therapy, 543–546
Adjuvant therapy, probiotics as, 567–569
Age factors, in gastric cancer, 611–612, 616
AID protein, in gastric cancer, 630–631
Allele-specific primer polymerase chain reaction, for antibiotic resistance, 584, 588
Amoxicillin
    in bismuth quadruple therapy, 552
    in hybrid therapy, 526–527
    in triple therapy, 525–526, 528–529
    resistance to, 521, 590–591
    susceptibility to, 671
Antibiotics, resistance to. *See* Resistance, to antibiotics.
APOBEC family, in gastric cancer, 630–631
APRIL (A proliferation-inducing ligand), in MALT lymphoma, 650
Atrophic gastritis, 601–603, 611–613, 661–666

B

Bifidobacterium formulations, 530, 568–570
Biopsy, 508–510, 614
Bismuth quadruple therapy, **537–563**
    acceptability of, 546–548
    adherence to, 543–546
    amoxicillin in, 552–553
    bismuth forms in, 538
    clinical trials of, 552, 554
    components of, 540
    doxycycline in, 547, 549
    duration of, 543–546
    efficacy of, 524–528
    failure of, 547, 550–552
    for eradication, 540–542
    history of, 538
    in sequential therapy, 552
    meal considerations in, 554–555
    metronidazole resistance and, 542
    outcome of, 547, 550–552
    packaging of, 545–546
    pathogenic considerations in, 538–540
    proton pump inhibitor dosage in, 556
    recommendations for, 556–557

Gastroenterol Clin N Am 44 (2015) 691–698
http://dx.doi.org/10.1016/S0889-8553(15)00087-4
0889-8553/15/$ – see front matter © 2015 Elsevier Inc. All rights reserved.

Printed and bound by CPI Group (UK) Ltd, Croydon, CR0 4YY

03/10/2024

01040488-0019